Paths to Asian Medical Knowledge

COMPARATIVE STUDIES OF
HEALTH SYSTEMS AND MEDICAL CARE

For a complete list of titles in this series, please contact the
Sales Department
University of California Press
2120 Berkeley Way
Berkeley, CA 94720

Paths to Asian Medical Knowledge

EDITED BY

Charles Leslie and Allan Young

UNIVERSITY OF CALIFORNIA PRESS

Berkeley   Los Angeles   Oxford

University of California Press
Berkeley and Los Angeles, California

University of California Press
Oxford, England

Library of Congress Cataloging-in-Publication Data
Paths to Asian medical knowledge / Charles Leslie and Allan Young,
editors.
 p. cm.—(Comparative studies of health systems and medical
care)
 Many chapters presented as papers at the 84th Meeting of the
American Anthropological Association in Washington, D.C., Dec. 1985.
 Includes bibliographical references and index.
 ISBN 0-520-07317-7 (cloth : alk. paper); 0-520-07318-5 (pbk)
 1. Medicine, Oriental—East Asia—Congresses. 2. Medicine,
Ayurvedic—Congresses. I. Leslie, Charles M., 1923– .
II. Young, Allan, 1938– . III. American Anthropological
Association, Meeting (84th : 1985 : Washington, D.C.) (84th :
Washington, D.C.) IV. Series.
 [DNLM: 1. Medicine, Oriental Traditional—Asia—congresses. WB
50 JA1 P29 1985]
 R581.P38   1992
 610'.95—dc20
 DNLM/DLC
 for Library of Congress   91-796
                                                              CIP

Printed in the United States of America

1 2 3 4 5 6 7 8 9

For Lita Osmundsen,
who helped to create medical anthropology
through her foresight
in establishing and
sponsoring conferences long before this
field was a recognized specialty, and who
saw, in particular, the theoretical importance of
research on Asian medicine.

CONTENTS

vii

PART II · ĀYURVEDA, COSMOPOLITAN MEDICINE, AND OTHER TRADITIONS IN SOUTH ASIA

PART III · ISLAMIC HUMORAL TRADITIONS

ACKNOWLEDGMENTS

The chapters in this book, with the exception of the contributions by Charles Leslie and Margaret Trawick, were first presented as papers at the 1985 meeting of the American Anthropological Association in Washington, D.C., for a conference on "Permanence and Change in Asian Medical Systems." Separate informal symposia were held at the Woodrow Wilson Center of the Smithsonian Institution.

We thank the Tanaguchi Foundation for permission to reprint a slightly different version of Charles Leslie's essay from the *History of Diagnostics: Proceedings of the 9th International Symposium on the Comparative History of Medicine, East and West*, edited by Yosio Kawakita, and published by the Tanaguchi Foundation, Osaka, Japan, 1987.

Pergamon Press granted permission to print a revised version of Margaret Trawick's essay, which was first published in *Social Science and Medicine*, volume 17, number 14, 1983.

The American Anthropological Association granted permission to print the conference papers by Margaret Lock and Mark Nichter. Earlier versions of their essays appeared as "New Japanese Mythologies: Faltering Discipline and the Ailing Housewife" in *American Ethnologist*, volume 15, number 1, 1988, and as "Kaysanur Forest Disease: An Ethnography of a Disease of Development" in *Medical Anthropology Quarterly*, New Series, volume 1, number 4, 1987.

We thank the Wenner-Gren Foundation for Anthropological Research for sponsoring the conference, the American Anthropological Association for including it in the program for its 84th Annual Meeting, and the Department of Anthropology of the National Museum of Natural History for cosponsoring conference symposia at the Smithsonian Institution.

Lee Mullett assisted our entire enterprise from the initial application for a grant through arrangements for the symposia and the preparation of manuscripts. We are grateful to her.

Introduction

Charles Leslie
Allan Young

Western interest in Asian medicine has a long history, extending back to classical times. Until relatively recently, however, this interest has been predominantly practical, reflecting a venerable Western tradition of seeing all forms of non-Western medicine as a potentially exploitable source of efficacious substances and procedures that might be added to the Western medical armamentarium. Even Western scholars who were students of Asian society, and who were ordinarily interested in understanding people's behavior in the context of their cultural meanings, tended to look at Asian medical beliefs and practices from an essentially pragmatic point of view, seeing them as technologies for managing illnesses and to be understood mainly in terms of efficacy. Indologists and sinologists, Western scholars who might be expected to have a more global perspective on Asian medicine, showed little interest in this subject, and were content to let Asian medicine languish in the shadow of Asian religion, art, and philosophy, the *locus classicus* of Western interest in Asian conceptions of the self, the body, and the world.

A similar situation recently prevailed in other areas of academia. Among anthropologists, for example, relatively few scholars were familiar enough with Asian languages to have studied Asian medicine, and those few who had the knowledge tended to concentrate on the traditional interests of their discipline—kinship, caste, and ritual. But now things are different. We take for granted that Asian medical systems are worth studying in their own right, no matter how unsatisfactory their beliefs or how useless their practices appear to biomedical ways of thinking. Yet three decades ago most Westerners would have found this proposition simultaneously dubious and indulgent.

One should not press this point too far. Not all Asian medical traditions were ignored in the past, at least not to the same degree. Because of the

Greco-Roman origins of both Arabic and European medical traditions, Western historians have been less negligent of Islamic medicine. The medical traditions of India, China, and Japan, however, are another matter. A glance along a library shelf shows that, with some notable exceptions, Asian medicine has attracted the attention of indigenous scholars rather than Westerners. And where Westerners did turn their interest to Asian medicine, the scholarly convention was to concentrate on written texts abstracted from the stream of contemporary history and the context of everyday clinical practice.

Western pragmatism—in its tendency to view medical systems as technologies—does not necessarily prevent a Western observer from being curious about the ideas and theories that inform Asian therapies and procedures. If one starts off with the assumption that the ability to discover efficacious treatments is somehow connected to the discoverer's ideas about the etiology of disease, pathophysiology, and pharmacology, then pragmatic interests might lead one deeper into these ideas, and into the theories and epistemologies that support them. Therein lies the rub: it is precisely this assumption that Western observers of Asian medicine have tended to reject. Given the history of Western medicine that has shaped Western attitudes, these observers have had good reasons for this attitude. We all know this triumphalist history: it begins in the sixteenth century, with the rapid and progressive accumulation of knowledge of anatomy and physiology; then it moves on to the nineteenth century, in which one great discovery follows another—germ theory, antisepsis, and anaesthesia; and it arrives in our time to record the discovery of antibiotics and the development of diagnostic imaging technologies and microsurgery, to name a few. The history of Western medicine moves relentlessly from triumph to triumph, leaving far behind every other medical system.

Insofar as Western attitudes toward Asian medical beliefs are concerned, it is this history's subtext rather than its details that makes it interesting. Briefly, its message is that biomedicine's extraordinary progress is a consequence of its scientific epistemology, that distinctive set of rules by which biomedicine knows what it knows. In this account, the fact that Asian medicine had so little to give to the West in the way of superior cures is evidence of both the uniqueness of biomedicine and the irrelevance of the theories and explanations with which Asians have embroidered their few authentic discoveries. To Western pragmatists, the ideas of Asian medicine were entirely ignorable. It made more sense to believe that the few successes that Asian medicine could claim, such as the drug rauwolfia, a hypotensive that originated in Āyurvedic medicine and was later incorporated into the Western pharmacopoeia, were products of Asian empiricists—indigenous protoscientists who stumbled on their remedies through trial and error—rather than the work of savants reasoning from indigenous systems of medical knowledge.

The derogation of Asian medical theories and epistemologies was not an isolated event. Rather, it was an expression of a more general cultural phenomenon—that collection of attitudes, interpretations, and theories that we bundle together under the labels "modernization" and "westernization." Modernization, according to writers and researchers on this topic, is irresistible, both as an interpretation of culture and history and as a force for change, because it embodies an ontologically privileged understanding of the world and because it represents the victory of reason and pragmatism over culture and tradition. In retrospect, it is clear that many of the putatively culture-free ideas that these universalizing thinkers found in biomedicine— the idea that mind-body dualism is a self-evident fact of nature, for instance—reiterate notions that are particular to Western culture. What interests us here, though, is not so much the modernizers' particular mistakes but, rather, the source of their remarkable presumption. How could they claim to know the point where culturally configured knowledge leaves off and reality takes over, the point at which the knowledge claims of biomedicine separate from those of, say, Āyurveda?

The modernizers based their claims on what was then the dominant philosophy of science—logical empiricism. According to this philosophy, reality—in our case, the objects, events, and processes that constitute the domains of health, sickness, and healing—is something that exists prior to and independent of people's attempts to understand and control it, and what science (biomedicine) says about reality closely corresponds with reality. This correspondence between reality and the way science represents reality, a match guaranteed by science's epistemology, makes scientific representations not merely useful, but also true. Yet, non-Western epistemologies and systems of belief, Āyurvedic and Chinese medicine, for example, inevitably culturalize reality and deserve our attention only to the extent that they create obstacles to instructing people in the lessons of biomedicine. Within this frame of reference, the theories and ideas that surround Asian medicine are simultaneously untrue and impermanent because human nature is intrinsically pragmatic (freed from tradition, people are rational maximizers and satisficers). Since biomedicine is patently superior to traditional Asian medicine, resistance to it will decline over time and Asian medicine can be expected to gradually fade away.

Ironically, the theory of modernization, a conception of cultural change that seemed compelling to Western social science only a short time ago, has been undermined by historical processes it failed to grasp, and by social and political developments it failed to predict, while Asian medicine continues on.

Like the theory of modernization, the correspondence theory of scientific knowledge has also been left behind. Beginning in the 1960s with the publication of T. S. Kuhn's *The Structure of Scientific Revolutions*, philosophers and sociologists of science persuasively challenged two previously accepted claims of logical empiricism: that scientific knowledge is ontologically privileged (it corresponds to external reality) and that scientific knowledge is the product of scientists following distinctive rules (either rules that can verify its facts or, following Karl Popper, rules that can show that the facts are not yet falsified).

In place of the philosophy of logical empiricism, students of culture and society now largely follow what they consider to be a more edifying account of scientific knowledge. This is naturalism, and it says that in its origins, scientific knowledge is essentially no different from other kinds of knowledge. All knowledge is the product of a natural process, social and cognitive in character rather than logical and axiomatic, through which human beings and groups of human beings struggle to make sense of the world. By socializing and historicizing scientific knowledge, by calling attention to the role played by individual and social interests in overriding epistemological principles, for instance, naturalism uncoupled the link that heretofore joined biomedicine's ability to predict, control, and manipulate objects and events with biomedicine's particular knowledge-claims about these objects and events—the point being that the superior technologies of biomedicine do not logically entail privileged ontologies.

The ascendancy of naturalist and relativist epistemologies of science, like the decline of the concept of modernization, are symptoms of a transformation that is now taking place in Western intellectual sensibilities. As a consequence, this transformation has opened a space for cultural studies of Asian medical systems.

The opening up of this space was signaled by the Introduction to *Asian Medical Systems* (Leslie 1976), a collection of articles that originated, like the present volume, in a conference sponsored by the Wenner-Gren Foundation for Anthropological Research. The introduction made four points which, taken together, map a field for cultural studies of Asian medical systems.

The first point starts from a very general observation that the medical systems of contemporary Asia—Āyurveda, Unani, Chinese medicine—are intellectually coherent. Each system consists of beliefs and practices connected by an underlying logic and each is underpinned by a coherent network of assumptions about pathophysiology, therapeutics, and so forth. The systems are connected to one another conceptually and historically by ideas about bodily humors and their relation to sickness and healing. Prior to the rise to dominance of allopathic medicine in Europe, similar humoral ideas and practices, commonly traced to Galen, also dominated medicine in the West and linked it to the Asian systems. Homeopathic medicine, whose professional rivalry with allopathic medicine continued into the twentieth century in the United States, and which is now enjoying a renaissance in Western Europe and francophone Canada, represents such a link among Asian, European, and North American humoral traditions. The cultivation of T'ai Chi Chuan and Yoga exercises, along with Āyurvedic and Chinese medicine, by students and consumers of "alternative medicines" further perpetuates this connection.

The second point is that, like medical systems elsewhere, these Asian systems are each embedded in distinctive cultural premises and symbols. Thus, while it is reasonable to talk about *Asian* medical systems in the same way that we reason about *humoral* or *allopathic* systems, it is important to identify the cultural features that distinguish between the classic, literate medical system of a given Asian society and its local appearances, for example, the distinction between an urban pundit's and a village vaidya's versions of Āyurveda.

The third point is that Asian medical systems cannot be fully understood outside the stream of history. Because history is a process running through the present into the future, and because a people's or a culture's history is the product of both endogenous and exogenous forces, it is unsatisfactory to see Asian medicine as something frozen in time or insulated from the influences that have connected Asia with the rest of the world over the ages.

All societies are permeable to exogenous influences. Technical systems—whether they are military, industrial, or medical—seem to be particularly permeable. The permeability of Asian medicine—the fact that over the centuries, Asians have "discovered" and adopted European practices and notions, for instance—has been consistently misinterpreted by both Western modernizers and Western celebrants of Asian traditions. Among modernizers, the tendency has been to see the permeability of Asian systems as evidence of the irresistible encroachment of Western medicine, presaging either the disappearance of Asian medicine or its marginalization as "superstition." Among celebrants of Asian medicine, the tendency has been to identify permeability with the transformation of hitherto unchanging medical traditions. Given the continuing vitality of Asian pharmaceutical and other health care traditions, the modernizers' conclusion is, at best, very premature. The second view often sees permeability as contamination, and is a view shared by a number of Asian keepers of the literate, high tradition. It is difficult to dismiss, since this issue is largely philosophical or conceptual and not empirical. The argument is analogous to the familiar debate over the identity and continuity of particular languages, that is, the dispute between essentialists who see their language as a fixed system whose constituent elements must be defended against exogenous influences and corruptions, and advocates of the idea that every language is an evolving system, constantly borrowing from the outside while ceaselessly transforming itself on the inside.

The position adopted in the introduction to *Asian Medical Systems*, and the view now shared by a majority of scholars in this field, is that Asian medical systems are intrinsically dynamic, and, like the cultures and societies in which they are embedded, are continually evolving.

The final point was the introduction's most controversial, and returns us full circle to the challenge of reconciling our understanding of "science" with our interest in cultural studies of Asian medicine. The introduction suggested that henceforth writers should reject using terms such as "Western," "scientific," and "modern" as ways of identifying the dominant medical tradition of the industrial societies. In their place, it proposed "cosmopolitan medicine." The term "biomedicine" serves the same purpose and is now widely used by writers in this field, but perhaps "cosmopolitan medicine" can be retained as a synonym for biomedicine when an author wants the connotation that the ideology and institutional forms of biomedicine are part of the capitalist world-system. The introduction rejected the term "Western" because biomedicine is clearly international. To take an obvious example, public and private research institutions are the main source of new biomedical knowledge and technologies. Fifty years ago, almost all of these research institutions were located in either Europe or the Americas or in the colonial possessions of Western powers, operating under imperial auspices. Today, well-established medical research institutions operate in Japan and in other Asian countries. The term "scientific medicine" was rejected on two grounds: clinical work necessarily includes much by way of inference, intuition, and judgment that is clearly medical but cannot reasonably be labeled science; "science," like the term "Western," implies a greater degree of homogeneity than this medical system can justifiably claim. "Modern" was rejected for reasons we have already given. Among other faults, it implies a spurious inevitability.

Unfortunately, some readers of *Asian Medical Systems* concluded that the argument over the appropriateness of terms such as "modernization" and "scientific" was a celebration of Asian medicine as a curative system, a rediscovery of an Oriental efficacy lost, and an advocacy of "alternative medicines." Far from making a case for the specifically medical power of Asian medicine, however, the introduction was an appeal to scholars to study Asian medicine as a civilizational process, to approach it in the same way that one might approach other sets of historically and culturally constituted beliefs and practices.

Nearly two decades later, these points are no longer remarkable. What needed arguing in the 1970s is common sense for most medical anthropologists and students of Asian medicine today. The original problem, resistance to the idea that Asian medical systems are aspects of civilizational processes, had at least two sources. The first of these was a tendency to cite medical anthropology, as an academic specialty, within a discrete division of labor—

more specifically, a tendency to see anthropologists as collectors of local knowledge in the service of physicians and public health specialists who needed help recognizing cultural and social obstacles to the programs they wished to introduce into traditional and non-Western communities. This once-pervasive attitude (which today remains embedded in methodologies such as the "rapid ethnographic survey") is a narrowly empiricist view of medical anthropology. It is ahistorical, blind to its own apriority, and preoccupied with bits and pieces of belief rather than systems of knowledge.

Even those early researchers who were prepared to adopt a less empiricist view of their subject were at a distinct disadvantage. In Asian societies, they confronted long-established pluralistic and syncretic humoral traditions, along with the world system of biomedicine modified in numerous ways to accommodate local conditions. In trying to understand these complex medical systems and humoral traditions, medical anthropologists were blinkered by a paucity of comparative research. Up to this point, relatively little research had been conducted on the historical development of Asian medicine. The role played by humoral medicine in cultural revivalism, the creation of Asian medical institutions paralleling the schools and clinics of cosmopolitan medicine, the growth of an enormous pharmaceutical industry based on humoral preparations, the professionalization of humoral practitioners— each of these remarkable developments lay outside the gaze of medical anthropologists and sociologists.

Theoretically inclined ethnologists had long been interested in the symbolic aspects of ritual curing, but they did not think of themselves as medical anthropologists. Nor did they generally concern themselves with learning how instances of ritual curing fit into indigenous systems of diagnosis and treatment. Further, their most influential studies were written in the ethnographic present to describe "peoples without histories." And this ahistorical work was preoccupied with shamanism, witchcraft, and sorcery to the neglect of humoral concepts and treatments of ordinary illnesses. The 1971 conference on which *Asian Medical Systems* was based eschewed ritual curing and, instead, emphasized the history and ethnology of Islamic, Indian, and Chinese humoralism. Its theoretical interests were in the historical processes of conflict and accommodation between these traditions and the world system of cosmopolitan medicine.

The conference concluded by discussing ways to draw like-minded scholars into an invisible college that would promote new historically informed work. This resolution took form in 1979, when Professor A. L. Basham organized an international conference on traditional Asian medicine at the Australian National University and used the occasion to found the International Association for the Study of Traditional Asian Medicine (IASTAM). The Wenner-Gren Foundation awarded IASTAM a small start-up grant, and the three hundred scholars who attended the Canberra conference were enrolled.

Five years later, IASTAM sponsored a second major conference hosted by Airlangga University in Surabaya, Indonesia, and in 1990 IASTAM organized a third conference in Bombay, cosponsored by three Indian universities, and attended by over six hundred participants. Today, the Association publishes a newsletter and its chapters in Europe, North America, and India sponsor various scholarly activities in their respective regions.

Public interest in Asian medicine was stimulated in the early 1970s when the People's Republic of China, having opened its doors to foreign journalists, scholars, and tourists, promoted its "integrated system of Chinese and Western medicine" as an exemplar of Maoist enterprise. Widely published photographs showed alert patients undergoing major surgery while anesthetized solely by acupuncture, schoolchildren were shown gathering medicinal herbs, and stories were told and retold about the impressive achievements of barefoot doctors exploiting traditional medical resources. In the wake of these images and developments, numerous conferences on Chinese medicine were organized in Europe and North America. The most important of these for the ethnology of Chinese medicine was organized by Arthur Kleinman, Peter Kundstadter, Russell Alexander, and James Gale. (The proceedings are published in Kleinman et al. 1975, 1978.) Since social science research was not yet tolerated in the People's Republic of China, the papers reported research undertaken in Taiwan, Hong Kong, and overseas Chinese communities. The conference's focus was anthropological; for comparative purposes, it included a few papers on other Asian cultures.

Arthur Kleinman was the most influential medical anthropologist in North America during the 1980s. Besides editing a journal and a book series, he wrote four books, numerous articles, and conference papers, and helped to edit several large volumes of essays. His books on Chinese culture and medicine are *Patients and Healers in the Context of Culture* (1980), which centered on his ethnographic work in Taiwan, and *Social Origins of Distress and Disease* (1986), based on his research in a psychiatric unit in the People's Republic of China. Kleinman's enduring interest has been in the social construction of illness experiences, and in the ways that different popular, folk, and biomedical interpretations of illnesses are mediated in clinical settings. The main criticism directed at *Patients and Healers in the Context of Culture* was that his concepts and clinical observations neglected the large-scale political and economic forces that affect people's illness experiences, their access to therapy, and the epidemiology of the diseases that afflict them. *Social Origins of Distress and Disease* was an answer to this criticism in that Kleinman analyzed the Chinese disposition to somatize social and psychological distress, and the political and social reasons that the concept of neurasthenia, a somatizing conception of distress, has been maintained in China long after it became obsolete in Western psychiatry. His analysis attended to a historical context by showing how the persecution that occurred during the Cultural Revolution was a source of later disorders revealed in patient narratives and clinical histories. In this book, Kleinman was particularly concerned with what he called "the sociosomatic recticulum," the symbolic bridge between social and bodily distress. These ideas were further discussed in *The Illness Narratives* (Kleinman 1988), a book written in an intimate voice that drew largely on clinical experience in the United States.

Although Kleinman's books describe beliefs and practices associated with Chinese humoral medicine, they are not his main subject. Rather, they are treated as part of the cultural background needed for understanding clinical interactions in biomedical settings. Anthropological research has been severely restricted in the People's Republic of China and, so far, the best ethnographic work by Western scholars on the professional culture and the institutional practice of Chinese humoral medicine is based on research in Japan. Margaret Lock's book, *East Asian Medicine in Urban Japan* (1980), is a major study in this field. Lock centers her work on Kanpo (humoral) clinics and pharmacies in Kyoto. The book also includes descriptions of acupuncture, moxibustion, and massage, and briefly analyzes the practice of cosmopolitan medicine. Thus, her study takes full measure of the pluralistic context within which Kanpo is practiced in contemporary Japan. Lock has subsequently addressed the changing cultural role of biomedicine in Japan as part of an ambitious program of comparative research. (See Lock and Gordon 1988, Lock's essay in the present volume, and her contribution to Norbeck and Lock 1987.) The subject of medical pluralism in Japan is also treated by Emiko Ohnuki-Tierney in *Illness and Culture in Contemporary Japan* (1984), a book that provides detailed accounts of traditional conceptions of physiology and pollution, magical thinking in religious curing, and patterns of sociality connected with sickness. Ohnuki-Tierney's examination of Japanese medical culture is strongly influenced by the perspective of symbolic anthropology.

Despite the impressive contributions of Kleinman, Lock, Ohnuki-Tierney, and other social scientists during the past twenty years, philologists and historians can claim to have made greater progress in research on East Asian medicine than have anthropologists and sociologists. We will mention only four of these writers. The most reknown figure among Western historians of Chinese science is undeniably Joseph Needham. For an example of his work on Chinese medicine, see *Celestial Lancets: A History and Rationale of Acupuncture and Moxa* (1980), written together with Lu Gwei-djen. The German Sinologist, Manfred Porkert, has written an authoritative exposition of humoral theory in *The Theoretical Foundations of Chinese Medicine: Systems of Correspondence* (1974). Nathan Sivin, the leading specialist in the United States, translated part of a 1972 handbook published in Beijing. This is published in *Traditional Medicine in Contemporary China* (1987), together with a valuable two-hundred-page introduction that focuses on problems of understanding this system of knowledge and provides an analysis of the ways in which it is changing. Finally, Paul Unschuld, who contributes an essay to the present volume, has been enormously productive over the last two decades, having published, in German and in English, *Medical Ethics in Imperial China* (1979) and a three-volume work, *Medicine in China* (1985, 1986*a*, 1986*b*). The first volume, *A History of Ideas* (1985), emphasizes the development of medical pluralism from the earliest period to the present. The second volume is *A History of Pharmaceutics* (1986*a*). The concluding volume is a translation of *Nan-Ching: The Classic of Difficult Issues* (1986*b*) and includes commentaries by Chinese and Japanese scholars from the third through the twentieth century.

These authors have made the history of Chinese medicine (and, more particularly, Chinese medical texts) accessible to laypersons and scholars in other disciplines. Anthropologists interested in Asian medicine will find these texts essential reading. Readers who want to examine the Chinese texts directly should consult Unschuld's *Introductory Readings in Classical Chinese Medicine* (1988). This book contains sixty selections in Chinese, a list of all the characters in each selection, together with their meanings, a transliteration of each text in Western script, and an English translation.

Translation inevitably involves many issues of interpretation, and each of these scholars of Chinese medicine finds points of disagreement with the others. The proceedings of a conference that addressed these kinds of problems is published in *Approaches to Traditional Chinese Medical Literature* (Unschuld 1989), which includes three essays on problems of translating ancient and medieval Sanskrit, Arabic, and Latin texts.

Moving from East Asia to South Asia, G. Jan Meulenbeld was awarded the Basham Medal in 1990, during the Bombay meeting of IASTAM, for his English language translation and annotation of the *Mādhavanidāna*, a key Āyurvedic text (1974). Meulenbeld's *History of Sanskrit Medical Literature* (forthcoming) will be the first volume (or volumes, since it is a monumental work) in a new series to be published by the Royal Asiatic Society and the Wellcome Institute for the History of Medicine. The series is jointly edited by Lawrence Conrad, an Arabic specialist, Dominik Wujastyk, a Sanskritist, and Paul Unschuld. In addition, Meulenbeld has recently edited the proceedings of a conference that aimed at identifying priorities for historical and philological research on Āyurveda (Meulenbeld 1984). Also notable in this connection is the work of Kenneth Zysk, who has published two essential studies of the Hindu-Buddhist tradition in the period before the composition of classic medical texts. Zysk's work appears in *Religious Healing in the Veda* (1985), which includes translations and annotations of curing hymns from the Rigveda, and *Asceticism and Healing in Ancient India: Medicine in the Buddhist Monastery* (1991).

The most original historical analysis of Āyurveda to date is *The Jungle and the Aroma of Meats* (1987), by the French Indologist and anthropologist, Francis Zimmermann. In scope, a comparable work on humoral thinking in Chinese medicine is Manfred Porkert's *Theoretical Foundations* (1974). But Zimmermann's study is strongly grounded in an anthropological conception of science and culture and, in this respect, it is quite different from Porkert's. Influenced by the ideas of Louis Dumont, Claude Lévi-Strauss, and Gaston Bachelard, Zimmermann argues that the ecological contrasts between dry and wet regions of South Asia structured the Āyurvedic classification of therapeutic substances and the cosmic physiological processes that sustain life. Like Porkert, though, in this book he is primarily interested in describing a system of thought apart from particular historical circumstances that affected its development.

Students of Chinese and Sanskrit texts, writers like Nathan Sivin, Paul Unschuld, Kenneth Zysk, and Francis Zimmermann, have a sophisticated understanding of the social sciences, but anthropological and sociological perspectives are not conspicuous among students of Arabic texts. The only book we know of that deals in a sociologically informed way with the transition from learned humoral traditions to cosmopolitan medicine in a Muslim country is Nancy Elizabeth Gallagher's *Medicine and Power in Tunisia, 1780–1900* (1983). Gallagher argues that this transition was facilitated by the inability of the humoral traditionalists to deal with epidemics of plague, cholera, and typhus, in contrast with the abilities of nineteenth-century European physicians. We should also mention the work of LaVerne Kuhnke, who has written a sophisticated study of the introduction of cosmopolitan medicine into Egypt in the nineteenth century (Kuhnke 1990). Like Gallagher, Kuhnke emphasizes the political significance of nineteenth-century epidemics in the context of capitalist development and imperialism. However, Kuhnke focuses on conflicts within biomedicine—between advocates and critics of contagion theory, and between social and curative models of practice—and largely ignores indigenous medical traditions.

During this same period from 1970 to 1990, Asian scholars have also published significant works on the classic texts and their history. For example, Priya Vrata Sharma has published a new edition and English translation of the *Charaka Samhita*, the most important text in Āyurveda (1981, 1983). In 1990 IASTAM awarded Yamada Keiji of Kyoto University the Basham Medal for his research on ancient Chinese medicine. In Japan, an annual International Symposium on the Comparative History of Medicine, East and West, has been sponsored for many years by the Taniguchi Foundation, and its papers are published in English. However, fewer critically trained Asian scholars work in medical anthropology and sociology than in history and philology. The exception may be India. Here, the most notable writer is the psychoanalyst, Sudhir Kakar, author of *Shamans, Mystics and Doctors: A Psychological Inquiry into India and Its Healing Traditions* (1982). But the prevailing tendency among Indian ethnologists and sociologists has been to neglect research on Āyurveda, Unani, and other forms of indigenous medicine, in favor of biomedical institutions (Banerji 1986, 1988; Madan 1980).

Medical anthropology as a special field of research has been very largely a creation of North American scholars, and the majority of Asianists among them have worked in South and Southeast Asia. For various reasons— political, economic, linguistic, and professional—anthropologists have had easier access to these regions. Several symposia on Asian medicine have been published during the 1980s in *Social Science and Medicine* and *Culture, Medicine and Psychiatry*, and they reflect the range of topical and regional interests represented in this anthropological literature. (See Crandon 1987; Dutt 1980; Elling 1981; Good, Good, and Fischer 1988; Laderman and Van Esterik 1988; Manderson 1987; Pfleiderer 1988; Rifkin 1983; Weisberg and Long 1984.)

One of the most original works in medical anthropology in the last twenty years is *Jero Tapakan: Balinese Healer* (1986), by the ethnologist Linda Connor, and the anthropological filmmakers, Patsy and Timothy Asch. The book is accompanied by four films on the life and work of Jero Tapakan. The book has chapters on the process of making the films and on their ethnographic content, and one film shows the shaman watching herself and commenting on her performance as a spirit medium in another film. This unique combination of film and text gives the viewer/reader access to the working relations between the ethnologist and filmmakers and their subject, Jero Tapakan, but it maintains a spare style, in contrast to the self-indulgence that mars much of the current discourse on anthropological reflexivity.

Although numerous medical anthropologists have worked in Thailand, the most accomplished and ambitious book on the indigenous medical system to date is *Traditional Herbal Medicine in Northern Thailand* (1987) by Viggo Brun, a linguist, and Trond Schumacher, a physician-botanist. Brun and Schumacher are Scandinavian scholars and their book is a source of detailed information that sets a standard of excellence for ethnobotany. However, it is a book that readers are likely to consult topically, rather than read through from start to finish. In contrast, Carol Laderman, working in an adjacent region, has written two monographs in the best tradition of literary ethnology. Her *Wives and Midwives: Childbirth and Nutrition in Rural Malaysia* (1983) began as a doctoral dissertation at Columbia University, where there was a strong tradition of biocultural studies. In this book, Laderman employs ethnographic, ecological, and biomedical data (including dietary analyses) to criticize the assumption, common among biomedical planners, that village cultures are intrinsically obstacles to improving health care in developing countries. Her main point is a familiar one to anthropologists: villagers are flexible and pragmatic in acting on and interpreting their cultural ideologies, even though these systems of belief appear rigid and self-limiting to outsiders. Laderman's second book, *Taming the Wind of Desire: Psychology, Medicine, and Aesthetics in Malay Shamanistic Performance* (1991), includes a comprehensive ethnographic description of Malay curing rites. Other recent books describe comparable rituals in other Asian cultures, for example, Laurel Kendall has published on Korean shamanism (1985, 1988) and Bruce Kapferer on the ritual dramas of the famous Singalese devil dancers (1983). However, Laderman's monograph is distinctive in the scope of her ethnography. After analyzing the elaborate poetic performances of the Malay shaman in the context of village medicine and cosmology, she goes on to describe the historical relationship of these performances to medieval Islamic medicine and indigenous traditions of theater.

For Āyurveda, we have already mentioned Francis Zimmermann's historical work. Zimmermann is presently translating into English an ethnological study that he published in French (1989), *The Discourse on Remedies in the Land of Spices*, based on study with Astavaidyan Vayaskara N. S. Mooss, an Āyurvedic physician of the Malabar Coast. This new book reports the most thorough and elegant ethnographic research so far published on any system of humoral medicine.

Among American ethnologists, Mark Nichter's work in South India and Sri Lanka stands out. Nichter's book, *Anthropology and International Health: South Asian Case Studies* (1989), has the descriptive fullness and complexity that distinguish first-rate ethnography. *Labour Pains and Labour Power* (1989) by Patricia Jeffery, Roger Jeffery, and Andrew Lyon—a study of women and childbearing in neighboring villages, one Muslim and the other Hindu, in North India—is likewise a combination of first-rate ethnography and critical analysis.

We close this inventory by mentioning two other studies on South Asia, although they deal with governmental agencies rather than with indigenous health cultures. Roger Jeffery's *The Politics of Health in India* (1988) is a sociological analysis of the historical development of cosmopolitan medicine in India. Judith Justice's *Policies, Plans and People: Culture and Health Development in Nepal* (1986) analyzes the ways in which international agencies operate in developing countries. Her research breaks new ground for anthropologists, who usually study villagers and townspeople, by focusing on international bureaucrats and showing that major problems of development lie with the developers themselves.

This brief review of literature which has appeared since the publication of *Asian Medical Systems* indicates the great variety of current work. The Wenner-Gren conference on which the present volume is based brought together scholars whose research spans a wide range of topics and regional cultures, but these essays have been selected to focus on a particular set of interests: the sources and modalities of medical knowledge. A more diverse collection of essays drawn from the same conference and edited by Beatrix Pfleiderer has been published as "Permanence and Change in Asian Health Care Traditions" (Pfleiderer 1988).

The chapters in *Paths to Asian Medical Knowledge* are about the ongoing evolution of Āyurveda as a professionalized system of knowledge in a modern state (Leslie); the persistence of meanings of death and nurturance in Indian medicine (Trawick); the cultural assimilation of knowledge of epidemic disease in south India (Nichter); the place of experimentation and ideas about proofs in Āyurvedic clinical practice (Obeyesekere); the epistemology of the case study in Chinese medicine (Farquhar); the role of epistemology in relation to changing notions of legitimacy in Chinese medicine (Unschuld); continuities in folk concepts of physiology and etiology in Chinese geomancy (Seaman); the medicalization of the lifeworld in a rapidly changing Japan (Lock); and the role of Islamic humoralism in Malay medicine (Laderman). One chapter splits the arena of inquiry between Asian and Western societies: an account of the "discovery" and reinterpretation of Āyurveda by Westerners who have rejected Western therapeutics (Zimmermann). While other essays concern particular twentieth-century settings, one chapter (Kuriyama) examines eighteenth-century Japan's extraordinary encounter with Western medicine via Dutch anatomical engravings, and another chapter (Good and DelVecchio-Good) is an account of Islamic medicine as a symbol system encompassing the breadth of Asia.

The shared perspective throughout the book is epistemological. Authors ask: How do patients and practitioners know what they know? What are their various rules of evidence, what kinds and categories of information do they find persuasive, and under what circumstances? How do they know when a medical judgment is wrong or correct? What do "wrong" and "correct" mean to patients, to village practitioners, and to experts trained in the great tradition? What sorts of inductive logic and analogy are at work here? Under what circumstances are these people inclined to accept or ignore novel medical ideas and practices?

REFERENCES

Banerji, Debabar
    1982   *Poverty, Class and Health Culture in India.* New Delhi: Prachi Prakashan.
    1986   *Social Sciences and Health Service Development in India: Sociology of Formation of an Alternative Paradigm.* New Delhi: Lok Paksh.
Brun, Viggo, and Trond Schumacher
    1987   *Traditional Herbal Medicine in Northern Thailand.* Berkeley, Los Angeles, London: University of California Press.

Connor, Linda, Patsy Asch, and Timothy Asch
1986   *Jero Tapakan: Balinese Healer; An Ethnographic Film Monograph.* Cambridge: Cambridge University Press.

Crandon, Libbet, ed.
1987   Beyond the cure: anthropological inquiries in medical theories and epistemologies. *Social Science and Medicine* 24 (12): 997–1124.

Dols, Michael W.
1984   *Medieval Islamic Medicine: Ibn Ridwan's Treatise on the Prevention of Bodily Ills in Egypt.* Berkeley, Los Angeles, London: University of California Press.

Dutt, Ashok K., ed.
1980   Contemporary perspectives on the medical geography of South and Southeast Asia. *Social Science and Medicine* 14D (3): 271–347.

Elling, Ray, ed.
1981   Traditional and modern medical systems. *Social Science and Medicine* 15A (2): 87–192.

Gallagher, Nancy Elizabeth
1983   *Medicine and Power in Tunisia, 1780–1900.* Cambridge: Cambridge University Press.

Good, Mary-Jo DelVecchio, Byron J. Good, and Michael M. J. Fischer, eds.
1988   Emotion, illness and healing in Middle Eastern societies. *Culture, Medicine and Psychiatry* 12 (1): 1–135.

Jeffery, Patricia, Roger Jeffery, and Andrew Lyon
1989   *Labour Pains and Labour Power: Women and Childbearing in India.* London: Zed Books Ltd.

Jeffery, Roger
1988   *The Politics of Health in India.* Berkeley, Los Angeles, London: University of California Press.

Justice, Judith
1986   *Policies, Plans, and People: Culture and Health Development in Nepal.* Berkeley, Los Angeles, London: University of California Press.

Kakar, Sudhir
1981   *Shamans, Mystics and Doctors: A Psychological Inquiry into India and Its Healing Traditions.* New York: Alfred A. Knopf.

Kapferer, Bruce
1983   *A Celebration of Demons: Exorcism and the Aesthetics of Healing in Sri Lanka.* Bloomington: Indiana University Press.

Kendall, Laurel
1985   *Shamans, Housewives, and Other Restless Spirits: Women in Korean Ritual Life.* Honolulu: University of Hawaii Press.
1988   *The Life and Hard Times of a Korean Shaman.* Honolulu: University of Hawaii Press.

Kleinman, Arthur
1980   *Patients and Healers in the Context of Culture.* Berkeley, Los Angeles, London: University of California Press.
1986   *Social Origins of Distress and Disease: Depression, Neurasthenia and Pain in Modern China.* New Haven: Yale University Press.

1988   *The Illness Narratives: Suffering, Healing, and the Human Condition.* New York: Basic Books, Inc.

Kleinman, Arthur, Peter Kunstadter, E. Russell Alexander, and James L. Gale, eds.

1975   *Medicine in Chinese Cultures: Comparative Studies of Health Care in Chinese and Other Societies.* Washington: U.S. Department of Health, Education, and Welfare, National Institutes of Health.

1977   *Culture and Healing in Asian Societies: Anthropological, Psychiatric and Public Health Studies.* Cambridge, Mass.: Schenkman Publishing Company.

Knorr-Cetina, Karin D., and Michael Mulkay, eds.

1983   *Science Observed: Perspectives on the Social Study of Science.* Beverly Hills: Sage Publications.

Kuhn, Thomas S.

1962   *The Structure of Scientific Revolutions.* Chicago: University of Chicago Press.

Kuhnke, LaVerne

1990   *Lives at Risk: Public Health in Nineteenth-Century Egypt.* Berkeley, Los Angeles, Oxford: University of California Press.

Laderman, Carol

1983   *Wives and Midwives: Childbirth and Nutrition in Rural Malaysia.* Berkeley, Los Angeles, London: University of California Press.

1991   *Taming the Wind of Desire: Psychology, Medicine, and Aesthetics in Malay Shamanistic Performance.* Berkeley, Los Angeles, Oxford: University of California Press.

Laderman, Carol, and Penny Van Esterik, eds.

1988   Techniques of healing in Southeast Asia. *Social Science and Medicine* 27 (8): 747–877.

Leslie, Charles, ed.

1976   *Asian Medical Systems: A Comparative Study.* Berkeley, Los Angeles, London: University of California Press.

1980   Medical pluralism. *Social Science and Medicine* 14B (4): 191–296.

1983   New research on traditional medicine in South Asia. *Social Science and Medicine* 17 (14): 933–989.

Lock, Margaret

1980   *East Asian Medicine in Urban Japan: Varieties of Medical Experience.* Berkeley, Los Angeles, London: University of California Press.

Lock, Margaret, and Deborah Gordon, eds.

1988   *Biomedicine Examined.* Dordrecht, Holland: Kluwer Academic Publishers.

Lu Gwei-djen, and Joseph Needham

1980   *Celestial Lancets: A History and Rationale of Acupuncture and Moxa.* Cambridge: Cambridge University Press.

Madan, Triloki Nath

1980   *Doctors and Society: Three Asian Case Studies: India, Malaysia, Sri Lanka.* Ghaziabad, U.P. India: Vikas Publishing House.

Manderson, Lenore, ed.

1987   Hot-cold food and medical theories: cross-cultural perspectives. *Social Science and Medicine* 25 (4): 329–417.

Meulenbeld, G. Jan
1974 *The Madhavanidana and Its Chief Commentary: Chapters 1–10, Introduction, Translation, and Notes.* Leiden, Holland: E. J. Brill.
1984 *Proceedings of the International Workshop on Priorities in the Study of Indian Medicine.* Groningen, Holland: Institute of Indian Studies, University of Groningen.
Forth- *History of Sanskrit Medical Literature.* London: Royal Asiatic Society and
coming Wellcome Institute for the History of Medicine.
Needham, Joseph
1970 *Clerks and Craftsmen in China and the West: Lectures and Addresses on the History of Science and Technology.* Cambridge: Cambridge University Press.
Nichter, Mark
1989 *Anthropology and International Health: South Asian Case Studies.* Dordrecht, Holland: Kluwer Academic Publishers.
Norbeck, Edward, and Margaret Lock, eds.
1987 *Health, Illness, and Medical Care in Japan.* Honolulu: University of Hawaii Press.
Ohnuki-Tierney, Emiko
1984 *Illness and Culture in Contemporary Japan: An Anthropological View.* Cambridge: Cambridge University Press.
Pfleiderer, Beatrix, ed.
1988 Permanance and change in Asian health care traditions. *Social Science and Medicine* 27 (5): 411–567.
Porkert, Manfred
1974 *The Theoretical Foundations of Chinese Medicine: Systems of Correspondence.* Cambridge: Massachusetts Institute of Technology Press.
Rechung Rinpoche
1976 *Tibetan Medicine: Illustrated in Original Texts Presented and Translated by the Venerable Rechung Rinpoche Jampal Kunzang.* Berkeley, Los Angeles, London: University of California Press.
Rifkin, Susan B., ed.
1983 Primary health care in Southeast Asia. *Social Science and Medicine* 17 (19): 1409–1496.
Sharma, Priya Vrata
1981–83 *Carakasamhitā, Text with English Translation.* 2 volumes. Varanasi: Chaukhambha Orientalia.
Sivin, Nathan
1987 *Traditional Medicine in Contemporary China.* Ann Arbor: Center for Chinese Studies, University of Michigan.
Trawick, Margaret
1987 The Ayurvedic physician as scientist. *Social Science and Medicine* 24 (12): 1031–1050.
1991 An Ayurvedic theory of cancer. *Medical Anthropology.* In press.
Ullmann, Manfred
1978 *Islamic Medicine.* Islamic Surveys II. Edinburgh: Edinburgh University Press.

Unschuld, Paul U.
1979   *Medical Ethics in Imperial China: A Study in Historical Anthropology.* Berkeley, Los Angeles, London: University of California Press.
1985   *Medicine in China: A History of Ideas.* Berkeley, Los Angeles, London: University of California Press.
1986*a*   *Medicine in China: A History of Pharmaceutics.* Berkeley, Los Angeles, London: University of California Press.
1986*b*   *Nan-Ching: The Classic of Difficult Issues.* Berkeley, Los Angeles, London: University of California Press.
1988   *Introductory Readings in Classical Chinese Medicine: Sixty Texts with Vocabulary and Translation, a Guide to Research Aids and a General Glossary.* Dordrecht, Holland: Kluwer Academic Publishers.
1989   *Approaches to Traditional Chinese Medical Literature.* Dordrecht, Holland: Kluwer Academic Publishers.
Van Der Geest, Sjaak, and Susan Reynolds Whyte, eds.
1988   *The Context of Medicines in Developing Countries: Studies in Pharmaceutical Anthropology.* Dordrecht, Holland: Kluwer Academic Publishers.
Weisberg, Daniel H., and Susan Orpett Long, eds.
1984   Biomedicine in Asia: transformations and variations. *Culture, Medicine and Psychiatry* 8 (2): 117–205.
Zimmermann, Francis
1987   *The Jungle and the Aroma of Meats: An Ecological Theme in Hindu Medicine.* Berkeley, Los Angeles, London: University of California Press.
1989   *Le Discours des Remedes au Pays des Epices: Enquete sur la Medecine Hindoue.* Paris: Editions Payot. (English translation forthcoming, Berkeley, Los Angeles, Oxford: University of California Press.)
Zysk, Kenneth Gregory
1985   *Religious Healing in the Veda, with Translations and Annotations of Medical Hymns from the Rgveda and the Atharvaveda.* Philadelphia: American Philosophical Society.
1991   *Asceticism and Healing in Ancient India. Medicine in the Buddhist Monastery.* New York: Oxford University Press.

PART ONE

Chinese Medicine, Cosmopolitan Medicine, and Other Traditions in East Asia

The relationships between theory and practice and between historical continuity and change are key issues in these essays. The authors' choices of topics emphasize one or another line of interpretation. For example, Shigehisa Kuriyama and Paul Unschuld set out to analyze historical discontinuities in Chinese and Japanese medical thought, but Judith Farquhar describes the historical continuity of Chinese medicine in her explication of a modern case history.

The discontinuity that Kuriyama analyzes in chapter 1 was marked by the Japanese translation of a Dutch anatomy book. He describes the role of European medical illustrations in the conceptual transformation of Japanese medical thought. During a period in which traditional social institutions were failing, the new style of perspective drawing and chiaroscuro enabled Gempaku, the physician translator, to see anatomical features in dissection that he had not seen before, and led him to advocate a new way of looking at the world. Kuriyama comments, "By learning a new style of representing the world the Japanese in the eighteenth century learned a new style of perceiving the world."

Like the long-standing controversies about the relative significance of genetic inheritance and social conditioning in human behavior, scholars disagree about the nature and importance of historical continuity and change, or about the primacy of forms of thought or practice in human affairs. Paul Unschuld observes in chapter 2 that the social structure and ideology that historically provided the "legitimizing circumstances" of humoral thought no longer dominate Chinese society. He lists three strategies in this century to restore the legitimacy of Chinese medicine, and judges them all to be failures. This is in striking contrast to the premises of Judith Farquhar's interpretation of a modern case history in chapter 3. She analyzes the pub-

19

lication of a contemporary physician to reveal his virtuosity in drawing upon a "medical archive" that preserves "several thousand years of experience on the part of laboring people of China." Farquhar and Unschuld agree that the archive of Chinese medicine has been incorrectly interpreted by modern scholars as an intellectually coherent body of knowledge. In Farquhar's view, Chinese medical science does not reside in a systematically consistent set of humoral theories but in highly variable clinical practices. She claims that the historical documents of Chinese medicine accurately record the clinical experiences of physicians, and that knowledge in this tradition is fundamentally different from knowledge based on the "essentialist and reductionist biases" of Western tradition. On this point, Unschuld would seem to disagree, for he asserts that scholars have greatly exaggerated the epistemological differences between Chinese and Western traditions. He claims that they are both philosophically heterogenous, and more alike than different from each other. In his view, the important but neglected difference between them derives from Chinese religious pluralism in contrast to the monotheistic Judeo-Christian paradigm for truth seeking in Western scientific discourse.

Readers who are not already acquainted with Chinese medicine might well begin this book with Gary Seaman's essay in chapter 4. He describes the general forms of thought involved in medicine and in geomancy, the practice of divination to determine where buildings should be cited or graves dug. Here the division between theory and practice is not one made by the outside observer, but an indigenous distinction played out by learned "Professors" and illiterate "Dirt Masters," two kinds of specialists who publicly accept each other's expertise while "undercutting each other's reputations in private consultations."

In the final essay of this section, Margaret Lock, like Kuriyama, deals with biomedicine in Japan. Again, the central theme is the relationship between cultural theory and practice, which Lock describes as the discontinuity between the popular conception of modern, urban, post-World War II Japan presented by the mass media, and the reality of contemporary life. The contrast between mythic images and actual practices exposes the rhetoric that medicalizes social issues. Her central example is the "climacterium syndrome" that is now covered by health insurance in Japan, and is tied to stereotypes that denigrate middle-class housewives who are said particularly to suffer from it. But Lock's essay requires close reading, for her skepticism is thoroughgoing. Social science analyses of medicalization are riddled with assumptions that Lock rejects. Her essay is a complex analysis of social issues and the moralistic rhetoric that portrays them as health care problems.

ONE

Between Mind and Eye: Japanese Anatomy in the Eighteenth Century

Shigehisa Kuriyama

It has long been a commonplace of Japanese historiography that the publication of Sugita Gempaku's (1733–1817) *Kaitai Shinsho* (1774) was a major turning point in Japanese cultural history. As one of the earliest translations of a Western anatomical text, *Kaitai Shinsho* represented the beginning of two epoch-making developments. First, and most directly, Gempaku's work set in motion the modern transformation of Japanese medicine, revealing not only many anatomical structures hitherto unknown in traditional medicine, but also and more fundamentally introducing the very notion of an anatomical approach to the body—the idea of visual inspection in dissection as the primary and most essential way of understanding the nature of the human body. Second, and more generally, *Kaitai Shinsho* inspired the rise of Dutch studies (*Rangaku*) in Japan, thus giving birth to one of the most decisive influences shaping modern Japanese history, namely, the study of Western languages and science.[1]

Not surprisingly, *Kaitai Shinsho* has been the subject of frequent and meticulous study. The tale of how Sugita Gempaku, a physician, with no training in foreign languages, no foreign teachers, no dictionary, and no precedents to rely on, managed through heroic struggles to produce a remarkably sound translation of a Dutch medical text is a story that has fascinated generations. The lives of Sugita Gempaku and his collaborators, the challenges they encountered in this pioneering effort of translation, and the role of *Kaitai Shinsho* in the development of Western studies in Japan have all been repeatedly chronicled in painstaking detail.[2]

This paper will suggest some new perspectives on this old and familiar material and will raise some questions that have previously not been asked. More specifically, *Kaitai Shinsho* will be reconsidered in the context of the history of visual perception. My contention is that questions about the relationship between eye and mind and between looking and seeing constitute the conceptual challenge of *Kaitai Shinsho*, and that without addressing the relationships framed by these questions we cannot hope to apprehend the deeper implications of the cultural transformation that was taking place in late eighteenth-century Japan.

1

An expression that figures prominently in the writings of Sugita Gempaku, and which defines the leitmotif of his thought, is *memboku o aratameru*, "changing one's outlook." In its general intent, the meaning of the phrase is clear. It presupposes Gempaku's sense of the profound divide separating the new world, which he is initiating, from the past world of his predecessors; and it expresses his call for a fundamental rethinking of the nature and method of medical knowledge, a radical transformation of habits of mind. In his introduction to *Kaitai Shinsho* Gempaku urges "all those who read this book to change their outlook."[3] He promises a lucidity about the body totally unknown in the past, a new realm of clear and certain perceptions. But, he stipulates, "without a change in outlook, it is impossible to enter this realm."[4] In fact, as Gempaku modestly concludes, it was precisely because he himself was able to change his outlook that, despite his natural ineptitude, he was able to achieve insights he could be proud of.[5]

As Gempaku conceived it, the idea of "changing one's outlook," of *memboku o aratameru*, represented both a prerequisite for, and a consequence of, the transition from Oriental medicine to Dutch medicine, and summarized his conviction that the past and future constituted two entirely different worlds. But this idea naturally gives rise to a number of questions. First, in what ways were the worlds different? That is, what was the precise nature of this "changed outlook"? And how did Gempaku envisage the new realm of medical understanding and experience? Any serious attempt to understand Gempaku and *Kaitai Shinsho* must address these issues.

To begin, the word "outlook" may be somewhat ambiguous. Generally, "outlook" refers to a conceptual orientation, a set of attitudes. That is, the visual metaphor implicit in "out-look" is usually construed as just that, a metaphor. This common metaphorical interpretation of outlook as conceptual perspective does not, however, capture the full or even primary thrust of Gempaku's call for reform. Rather, "changing one's outlook" must be interpreted literally as well as metaphorically; Gempaku's phrase is as much an expression of a new way of seeing as a call for a new way of thinking. The transformation represented by *Kaitai Shinsho* was first and foremost perceptual; *memboku o aratameru* corresponded to a novel mode of visual experience.

Traditionally, the interpretation of Gempaku's changed outlook has focused on the new primacy of anatomy, and this interpretation is certainly correct—as far as it goes. In one of his late writings, Gempaku first reiterates how he realized the necessity of rejecting long-standing misconceptions and adopting a totally new outlook in medicine. He then goes on to explain: "After that, I understood that true medicine was to be found in the far West, in Holland. The foundation of medicine consists in the detailed investigation of the human body's natural structures, of the appearance of its interior and exterior; and it is when this investigation is accepted as the heart of medicine that medical science in our country will be securely founded."[6] What made Dutch medicine true medicine, in other words, and what set it irrevocably apart from the traditional medicine of China and Japan, was its stress on the observations of dissection. The essence of changing one's outlook was learning to conceive of the body anatomically.

This much is straightforward. What is less apparent, however, is exactly what it could mean to conceive of the body anatomically. Here we encounter a critical theoretical lacuna in the historiography of Japanese medicine. If scholars have unanimously recognized the centrality of the dissector's vision in Gempaku's call for medical reform, none to my knowledge has thought to inquire about what *kind* of looking this vision involves. Yet it is precisely this question of the particular mode of seeing that we must be most concerned with. To grasp the meaning of Gempaku's call for a changed outlook, common schematic notions of anatomy—of anatomy as simply cutting open the body and peering inside—are inadequate. We need to inquire further and pursue the specific character of anatomical observation.

In his introduction to *Kaitai Shinsho*, Gempaku stresses that the study of anatomy is in itself neither an unprecedented endeavor nor one unique to the West. Physicians throughout Chinese history had often discussed the internal organs and the skeleton, and some had even pursued dissections. But, he laments,

> because their minds were hardened by chronic misconceptions (*kyûsen ni kosuru*), even in the case of these physicians, even though they looked at the difference between accepted beliefs and the actual structure of the organs and the skeleton, they wavered haplessly in suspicions and doubts. It is just like the story about the man from Yen who had his native country before his eyes and yet could not recognize it. Even though they dissected they were not thereby suddenly able to see clearly; instead they remained in utter confusion.[7]

According to Gempaku, then, the failure of traditional medicine ultimately lay in a peculiar failure of vision. Earlier physicians *had* been interested in the internal organs, and dissections *had* been performed. Despite this interest, however, and despite cutting open the body and looking inside, they somehow had not seen the body as Gempaku saw it. It is here, in the differing perspicuity of vision, that past and present stood radically opposed, and that *Kaitai Shinsho* opened up a new world. Gempaku plants himself confidently in the present, awake and clairvoyant, instead of in the past, where human beings, their minds enslaved by the strange power of old beliefs, could not see what was before their eyes. "Because their eyes and ears were confused by turbid traditions (*oshû*)," Gempaku eloquently concludes, "they were ultimately unable to sweep away the foggy obscurity and see the clarity of blue skies."

It is difficult in these translations to bring out the full force of Gempaku's language. Expressions such as "hardened by chronic misconceptions" and "turbid traditions" only vaguely hint at the distinct connotations of taint, pollution, and disease implicit in the terms *kyûsen ni kosuru* and *oshû*. In the original Japanese, the misapprehensions of traditional medicine appear not simply as mistaken beliefs, but as pathological states of mind, diseases that somehow incapacitated basic powers of discernment and perception. At the same time, the contrast between foggy obscurity and the clarity of blue skies intimates something further; it suggests that Gempaku conceived of this process of "changing one's outlook" as nothing less than a form of spiritual transformation, of quasi-religious enlightenment.

This contrast between a defiled and clouded past, and a present of clear and lucid vision was intended, at least in part, to be taken quite literally. As Gempaku points out, the failure of traditional medicine stemmed neither from a lack of interest in the internal organs nor even from a failure to inspect them. Rather, physicians in the past had been unable to perceive what was before their very eyes because of certain long-standing delusions, owing to certain dispositions of the mind. They had looked but had not seen.

What were these confused precedents that Gempaku was setting himself off against? They were of two sorts. First, there were the early Chinese investigations into anatomy. References to dissection appear in China as early as the Han dynasty (206 B.C.–A.D. 221).[8] The sources of this period, however, provide only sketchy, general accounts of what was discerned from dissection at this time, and it is not until the Song dynasty (960–1279) that the first anatomical charts appear. These Song charts were based on the dissection in 1045 of the rebel Ou Xifan as well as on dissections performed at the beginning years of the twelfth century, and they eventually became the basis on which later physicians in China and Japan imagined the body's interior. Copies of the charts appeared thereafter not only in various Chinese medical texts, but by the fourteenth century had made their way into the works of the Japanese monk-physician Kajiwara Shozen.[9]

By the mid-eighteenth century, however, a number of Japanese physicians had begun to question the conception of human structure represented in this tradition of Song charts. The pioneering efforts of Yamawaki Tôyô (1705–1762), a leading member of the "Ancient Practice" school (*kohôha*) of physicians, spearheaded the movement that sought to purify medicine of metaphysical speculation and return it to the supposedly more empirical and certain foundations of ancient times. In much the same way that contemporary Confucian scholars of the "Ancient Learning" school (*kogakuha*) criticized postclassical interpretations of the Confucian canon as distortions of the sage's original teachings, Tôyô and other members of the "Ancient Practice" school rejected the systematic theorizing characteristic of medieval Chinese medicine, and subjected accepted doctrines to searching doubt.

Among other things, Tôyô was skeptical of the account of human structure current in his time. In 1754 he arranged for the first recorded dissection of a human cadaver in Japan, and on the basis of this experience he pointed out many discrepancies between accepted doctrine and what is actually found in the body. This dissection and the subsequent publication, with illustrations, of the anatomical treatise based on it—the *Zôshi* (1759)—inspired a minor flurry of dissections in Japan, and Gempaku himself acknowledged how Tôyô's discoveries had fired his imagination.[10]

In a certain sense, then, *Kaitai Shinsho* can be seen as the culmination of the surge of anatomical interest that began with Tôyô. Gempaku himself, however, as evidenced by his repeated calls for "changing one's outlook," saw more discontinuity rather than continuity. It was probably Tôyô and his imitators that Gempaku had uppermost in his mind when he made his remarks about the strange failures of vision. Tôyô, in Gempaku's view, despite the heroic and essentially sound character of his intentions, had, when he peered into the cadaver, "merely looked with vague incomprehension," unable to distinguish what was what. And this was also the case with the dissectors after him. Gempaku cites the example of the government physicians Okada Yôsen and Fujimoto Ryôsen who were said to have dissected seven or eight cadavers—a remarkably large number for the time. Yet they, too, in Gempaku's judgment, seemed to have been "unable to break old habits; in any case, they failed to accomplish anything useful."[11] All these efforts, no matter how praiseworthy in intent, still belonged to a past era of vague and clouded perceptions. They belonged to a different world.

What was it then about the way in which Gempaku looked at the body that fundamentally differed from his predecessors? How is it that earlier dissectors did not see what he saw? In what sense could Gempaku claim to see "the clarity of blue skies"? These questions define the puzzle of *Kaitai Shinsho*.

2

In terms of content, in terms of *what* they saw, the difference between Gempaku and his predecessors is not hard to pinpoint; it is a difference in visual guides. Anyone who has dissected human or animal cadavers knows that anatomical study is far from a straightforward ostensive procedure. It is messy and complex, and for the most part we are able to distinguish what we distinguish only because we are guided by teachers and texts. In other words, we see what we are taught to look for.

Perhaps the most familiar manifestation of this dependence on guides appears in the universally conservative tendency of anatomical traditions. We may recall for example how even so acute an observer as Leonardo da Vinci "saw" in his dissections pores connecting the two ventricles of the heart—imagined, that is, those pores that had been standard in anatomical teaching since the time of Galen, but which present-day anatomists can no longer see. Nor can we forget Vesalius's scathing critique of his predecessors—of generations of anatomy professors directing dissections without ever noticing the discrepancies between the Galenic texts they read aloud and the realities before their eyes.[12]

Gempaku's *Dawn of Western Science in Japan* (*Rangaku Kotohajime*) tells of similar failures of vision in traditional Japan. The context is familiar: in Japan as in pre-Vesalian Europe we find the actual dissection left in the hands of nonphysicians, with the outcast *eta* (who provided the executioners and butchers of traditional Japan) filling the role played by barber-surgeons in Europe; and as in Europe we encounter the same perfunctory attitude toward anatomical inspection, the use of dissection merely to confirm textual knowledge. Consider the account of the first dissection that Gempaku attended—the dissection of a female criminal in 1771:

> Toramatsu, an Eta and skillful dissector, was expected to perform the task, but he failed to appear on account of sudden illness. His ninety-year-old grandfather, a sturdy-looking man, took his place. He said that he had performed a number of dissections ever since his youth. In dissecting the human body, the custom till then was to leave everything up to such outcast people. They would cut open the body and point out such organs as the lungs, the liver, and the kidneys, and the observing doctors simply watched them and came away. All they could say then was: "We actually viewed the inside of a human body." With no sign attached to each organ, all they could do was listen to the dissector's words and nod.
>
> On this occasion, too, the old man went on explaining the various organs such as the heart, the liver, the gallbladder and the stomach. Further, he pointed to some other things and said: "I don't know what they are, but they have always been there in all the bodies which I have so far dissected." Checking them with the Dutch charts, we were able to identify them to be the main arteries and veins and suprarenal glands. The old man also said: "In my past experience of dissection, the doctors present never showed puzzlement or asked questions specifically about one thing or another."[13]

It is not difficult to appreciate how dissections of this sort could contribute little to medical innovation. By glancing at and assenting to what the dissector indicated, physicians merely confirmed what was already common knowledge. We recognize here the psychology of the tourist who visits sites solely for the satisfaction of saying that he has seen them. Gempaku identifies the intriguing feature of human perception that conditions this attitude when he writes, "With no sign attached to each organ, all they could do was listen to the dissector's words and nod." Without pictures, words, or gestures guiding and illuminating our vision we cannot attend to what is before our eyes. Or, to put it positively, such guides enable us to discern the body's articulated structure. In this peculiar indirectness of our senses, this dependence on mediating "signs" to make the world visible, we begin to explore the territory that separates mere looking from seeing.

This is in fact the first reason that Gempaku offers for the "vague incomprehension" of Tôyô's gaze; Tôyô could not clearly distinguish anatomical structures because he had nothing to tell him what was what.[14] By contrast, Gempaku had the guidance of the *Anatomische Tabellen* of Johann Adam Kulmus,[15] and using it he and his companions came to recognize the arteries, veins, and suprarenal glands—to name them, picture them, and thus stabilize their existence. The real contrast, however, is perhaps not so much between "vague incomprehension" and clear perception as between different visions of anatomy. After all, Tôyô did distinguish many important structural features of the body. But the illustrations and descriptions of his *Zôshi* did not resemble the anatomy of European physicians. The body he saw was not the body that Gempaku saw. Tôyô's anatomical vision was guided by his fundamental suspicion, as a member of the Ancient Practice school, that the medical tradition in his time distorted the insights of the most ancient Chinese physicians. By pointing out the absence of those structures postulated by contemporary teachings, he wished to demonstrate the need for medical reform, and he directed reform toward what he imagined to be the pristine vision of the golden past.

Tôyô regarded his chief anatomical find to be his famous "theory of nine organs" (*kyûzô setsu*). This theory was based on his "discovery" that the small intestine, which had long formed part of Chinese medical theory, could not be found when the body is dissected. Tôyô claimed that the small intestine was a myth, a fictional entity postulated by medieval physicians to fit their metaphysical schemes. Thus, there were actually nine organs, rather than the ten of accepted doctrine.[16] But the organs Tôyô observed were, as he himself noted, precisely the organs listed in the *Zhouli* and in the "Pangeng" section of the *Book of Documents*. That is, the dissection confirmed what he took to be among the oldest Chinese works. Tôyô was guided in dissection by texts he took to be free from the distortions of later Chinese medicine.

Viewed in this way, matters seem simple; the divergence separating Gempaku from his predecessors reduces to a difference in the texts that guided their seeing. They saw different things because they looked for different things. Tôyô looked for and found the organs described in the oldest Chinese references; Gempaku looked for and found the structures depicted in the texts of Western anatomy. But beyond the idea that observations are theory-laden, the real novelty of Gempaku's visual world consisted not just in *what* he saw, but more fundamentally in *how* he saw, in a new perceptual style. The key to this altered style of seeing must be sought in another development in late eighteenth-century Japanese culture, namely, the changing understanding of artistic representation.

3

The illumination provided by Western anatomical labels and illustrations allowed Gempaku to apprehend a whole array of structures that had been previously looked at in Japan but not seen. Nerves, blood vessels, and glands were all suddenly made visible by the selective detail found in Kulmus's *Anatomische Tabellen.* Now it might be objected that this reverses the order of things, since words and pictures shaped what Gempaku saw, whereas common sense teaches that seeing and other sense experiences constitute the ground in which our words and pictures are rooted. After all, not only does the act of looking at something precede the act of drawing it, but the very term "representation" seems to imply that words and pictures are but secondary schematic substitutes for original perceptions.

Yet how perspicuous are our perceptions? Consider the witness trying to describe to a police artist the criminal he has seen. Almost invariably requests for detail uncover uncertainties: Did the assailant have long or short earlobes? Were his eyelids single or double-fold? As the witness struggles to answer such questions, the mental image that he had assumed to be lucid and complete turns out to be remarkably fragmentary. Based on initial recollections of the witness, the artist makes a preliminary sketch and asks, "Did he look something like this?" "I think he looked older than that," the witness might comment, "and his eyes were more sly, and his lips seemed more fleshy." Through exchanges of this sort an increasingly nuanced and detailed portrait is crafted. In this process the witness also clarifies his vision. The image that seemed to disappear under scrutiny gradually reemerges. By looking at and criticizing successive drawings, the witness discovers more exactly what he saw. Pictures here serve in part as mnemonic aids to an imperfect memory; but the matter also goes deeper. Anyone who has ever tried to sketch a model is familiar with a similar dialectic whereby picturing and seeing go hand in hand: while looking at our model helps us to draw, the drawing in turn helps us to refine our visual grasp of the model. The "seeing" of the model emerges through a dialectical interaction of looking and representing.

This discussion only hints at the complexities joining perception and representation.[17] But it indicates the particular sense of the indirectness of the senses: pictures sharpen, articulate, and illuminate our perception of the world, and vice versa, or, to put it differently, perception, *tout court*, has its object neither in the world nor in pictures, but in their dynamic interplay in the mind.

Moving back and forth between pictures and the world, between the body depicted and the actual cadaver, was precisely Gempaku's experience of the eye-opening dissection of 1771. By a coincidence, both Gempaku and Maeno Ryôtaku, the physician Gempaku invited to accompany him, possessed copies of Kulmus's *Tabellen*, and both brought their copies to the dissection. Gempaku's description is revealing: "Comparing the things we saw with the pictures in the Dutch books Ryôtaku and I had with us, we were amazed at their perfect agreement."[18] We are invited here to imagine a situation in which seeing the body and seeing the pictures of the body were inseparable. The revelation of the striking fidelity of the Western anatomical illustrations went hand in hand with the revelation of the body's articulated structure. One was not possible without the other. Kulmus's anatomical illustrations not only guided what Gempaku saw but also how he saw. By learning a new style of representing the world the Japanese in the eighteenth century learned a new style of perceiving the world; they acquired a new visual style.

The argument is a logical one based on the commonplace observation that style and content are inseparable. If Western anatomical charts allowed Gempaku to see in the body *what* his predecessors had never seen, then it stands to reason that they also allowed him to see in *a way* that set him apart. This argument also does not lack historical evidence. Of special interest here is Gempaku's reaction to Lorenz Heister's *Surgery*, the first Western medical text he saw:

> Needless to say, I could not read the book, not a word or a line. But the illustrations of the book looked markedly different from those in Japanese or Chinese books. *Just viewing their exquisite precision I felt as though being enlightened* (emphasis added). So I borrowed the book for some time as I wanted to copy the pictures at least.[19]

These remarks must be taken with Gempaku's comment that when he and his companions first examined Kulmus's anatomical charts, "They looked so different from the pictures in the Chinese anatomical books that many of us felt rather dubious of their truth."[20] In other words, what so excited Gempaku about Western anatomical drawings was not any sense of their self-evident veracity, or simply the curiosity aroused by their content. It was their striking difference in style, their "exquisite precision." Underlying Gempaku's refrain of *memboku o aratameru*, of changing one's outlook, then, was the intense visual experience of an entirely new mode of representation. The quasi-religious revelation of "clear blue skies" was an expression of this eye-opening experience.

4

If Western anatomical charts made Gempaku's experience of enlightenment possible, they did not by themselves make it necessary.[21] Pictures may provide fresh ways of looking at the world, but only if one has a way of looking at pictures. The importance of Western illustrations in shaping the way Gempaku and his contemporaries saw the world raises the question of how these illustrations were themselves perceived. What did Japanese in the late eighteenth century see in Western pictures? How are we to understand Gempaku's immediate and enthusiastic response to a foreign mode of representation?

Gempaku provides no direct insight into these issues. Though we have noted the eagerness with which he took in the Western style of representation, he never explicitly theorized about why he was so receptive, or recorded what it was exactly that he found so appealing in Western pictures. We must therefore approach the question obliquely—but only slightly obliquely, for Gempaku was not alone in his enthusiasm for Western illustrations. The years when he and his collaborators were struggling with their translation of Kulmus's anatomy also correspond precisely to the period in which Japanese artists were beginning to study and imitate Western techniques of representation. Historically, this temporal coincidence is significant because the contemporary investigations of Western representational technique helped make *Kaitai Shinsho* what it was. Adorned by skillful copies of Western anatomical charts, *Kaitai Shinsho* simply looked strikingly different from *Tôyô's Zôshi* or any other previous work in Oriental medical history.

However, the pioneers of Western-style art in Japan were self-conscious about the aims and uses of representation in a way that nonartists like Gempaku were not. Two contemporaries of Gempaku, whose attitudes typify those of the Western-style artists in this period, are Satake Shozan (1748–1785), whose *Gahô Kôryô* is now recognized as the first theoretical treatise on illusionism in Japan, and Shiba Kôkan (1738–1818), the foremost exponent of Western art in his time, and the first Japanese to master the technique of copperplate prints. Both were pupils of Odano Naotake (1749–1780), the artist who executed the masterful copies of Western anatomical illustrations for *Kaitai Shinsho*.[22] Their reflections on art are early and direct sources for understanding the Japanese response to illusionism. The writings of Shozan and Kôkan make plain that they discerned two great virtues in the Western style, two principles that made it incomparably superior to the traditional Chinese and Japanese approach to painting. One was the illusionistic princi-

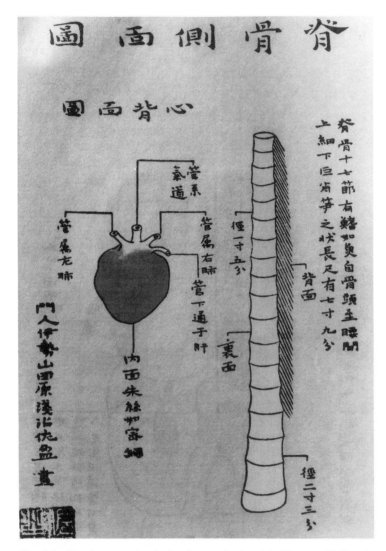

Fig. 1.1. The heart and spinal column, depicted in Yamawaki Toyo's *Zoshi*.

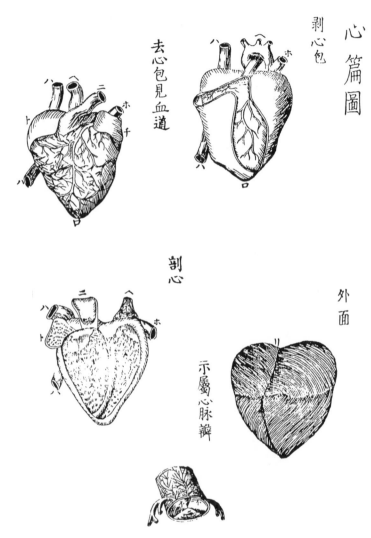

心篇圖

剥心包

去心包見血道

剖心

外面

示屬心脉瓣

Fig. 1.2. Views of the heart in Sugita Gempaku's *Kaitai Shinsho*.

ple of "resemblance," the notion that pictures should look like what they depict, and the other was the principle of *yô*, or utility.

Of these principles it is especially the latter that we must come to terms with. Usefulness, for both Shozan and Kôkan, defined the ultimate goal of representation: the realism of a picture, its resemblance to the object represented, was valued because it was the essential means to actualizing the utilitarian end. Thus, when in *Gahô Kôryô* we read, "In judging the usefulness of a picture one should value resemblance," we must realize (and a consideration of the treatise as a whole makes this unmistakable) that Shozan was not setting up "usefulness" as one possible criterion of judgment as opposed to another, such as beauty. Usefulness was the only real criterion of judgment, the one standard that truly mattered. To judge the utility of a picture was to judge the picture. Since enthusiasm for the Western style of representation focused on the style's "utility," our problem is what utility meant as well as what its connection was to resemblance.

In 1773, Hiraga Gennai—Gempaku's friend, brilliant polymath, and, among other things, an expert on mining—was hired by the domain (*han*) of Akita to help develop the domain's copper resources. This represented part of Akita's effort to stave off the economic disaster brought on by a recent series of floods and fires. As it turned out, mining in Akita never developed to the extent that domain leaders had hoped. But Gennai's visit did have an effect of perhaps even greater historical moment. During his stay he introduced local artists to Western representational techniques. This was the origin of the so-called Akita school of Dutch art. The most brilliant of Gennai's disciples was Odano Naotake, the illustrator of *Kaitai Shinsho*, and the teacher of Satake Shozan and Shiba Kôkan.

These details bring out an essential point; namely, that the study of Western methods of representation originated in the context of an impoverished domain's search for fiscal solvency. Shozan, the author of the first theoretical defense of illusionism, was also and more important the lord of the beleaguered Akita domain. The point is more revealing than one might at first suspect, for the problems in Akita were in fact merely one local manifestation of a more general crisis in mid-Tokugawa society. Throughout the course of the eighteenth century the transition from an agrarian to a commercial economy had steadily eroded the feudal foundations of Tokugawa rule, and produced increasing strains and contradictions in the old social order. The Tanuma era (1760–1786),[23] the era in which Sugita Gempaku, Satake Shozan, and Shiba Kôkan first encountered the Western style of depicting the world, was also the era in which these strains and contradictions were beginning to appear in especially grotesque and frightening forms. The Tanuma era was as notorious for the extravagant banquets and outrageous orgies of the urban elite as for the famines and epidemics that devastated the countryside, a period when despite the deepening debt that threatened the very sur-

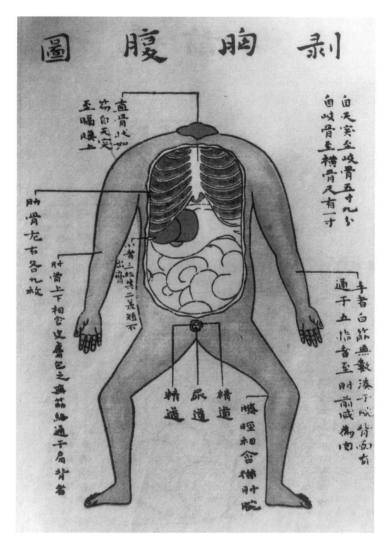

Fig. 1.3. Anatomical perspective in *Zoshi*.

門
脈
篇
圖

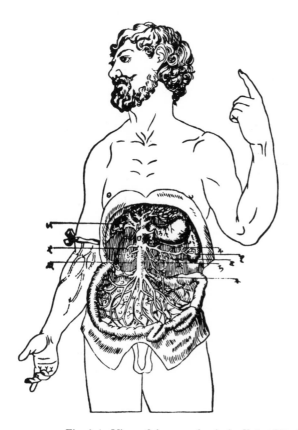

Fig. 1.4. View of the portal vein in *Kaitai Shinsho*.

vival of the samurai class, and despite official prohibitions to the contrary, samurai went in droves to the pleasure quarters and whiled away the hours. The period saw the birth of the geisha, and the quest for sensual gratification became a refined art; but it also witnessed widespread infanticide among the peasantry.[24]

Against this background, we must interpret the insistence of Shozan and Kôkan that art must have "practical utility" (*jitsuyô*), and that it must be "an instrument of national utility" (*kokuyô no gu*). The call for usefulness was sloganeering that expressed an acute sense of a world gone seriously wrong; it was a call for positive action and reform in a nation perceived to be slipping rapidly toward ruin. Thus for Shozan and Kôkan utility meant first and above all "national utility" (*kokuyô*); it referred to whatever might serve the state in its time of crisis. Construed in this broad sense, the preeminence of usefulness in art is not difficult to comprehend. In the minds of reformers—and all proponents of Westernism were by definition reformers—usefulness was the supreme value in representation because it was the supreme value in all things.

Still, we may wonder about how pictures could be useful. It is the specific usefulness of illusionistic pictures that we want to know about. Now, in one sense, there is no great mystery. For Shozan and Kôkan pictures were an unsurpassed tool of communication whose utility to the state lay in their power as instruments of enlightenment, in their ability to convey "what words cannot express." Unlike words, they could be understood by "even children and fools."[25] The necessary connection between resemblance and usefulness thus becomes clear. With its capacity to create pictures that resembled the reality they depicted, the Western style of representation created unprecedented possibilities for educating the people and disseminating information. As Shiba Kôkan explained:

> The marvel of pictures lies in their ability to allow one to directly see what one has not seen. If, therefore, a picture does not faithfully copy an object as it really is, it loses this marvelous usefulness (*myôyô*).
> [For example,] Mt. Fuji is a mountain found in no other land. If one wants to see it, one must see it in pictures. If, however, one just concentrates on the expressiveness and technique of the brushwork and the picture does not look like Mt. Fuji, then the marvelous usefulness of pictures is lost.[26]

In a similar but humorous vein, Shozan wrote, "If a picture of a lion looks like a dog, people will laugh at it."[27]

Another and perhaps even more fundamental aspect of the demand for usefulness was its negative critique. In large measure the notion of the useful defined itself in opposition to the traditional style. To appreciate the full appeal of Western illusionism for Shozan and Kôkan we must examine their deep dissatisfaction with the artistic culture of their time.

One source of disaffection concerned the contemporary uses of pictures. *Gahô Kôryô* sets forth the contrast between the practical, informational uses of art made possible by illusionism and the frivolous pastimes then prevalent. His contemporaries, Shozan complains, have landscapes painted on sliding doors so that they might enjoy them in the relaxed leisure of the home; or they hang up paintings just to entertain friends who come to visit; or again people paint as a form of Zen meditation, or even more commonly (and in Shozan's view, worst of all) simply as a diversion, like playing chess or the zither. All of these uses Shozan castigates as making pictures into "playthings which are useless to the state."[28] Practicality was defined here by opposition to the aestheticism of a privileged elite; and we can see in Shozan's austere utilitarianism a reaction against an era consumed by the pursuit of pleasure and the cultivation of sensibility, a culture oblivious to the practical problems that so urgently required attention.[29]

Yet it was not just a problem of the ways in which people used pictures. The question of social application was inseparable from the question of style. As Kôkan explained, the marvelous usefulness of pictures is realized only by pictures that resemble the thing they depict, but in Chinese-style depictions, Mt. Fuji did not look like Mt. Fuji. The failure to look like Mt. Fuji was not an accident. It arose from a highly sophisticated conception of representation that was not concerned with depicting the world but sought instead to evoke the artist's experience. The focus of the Chinese aesthetic was, as Kôkan reminds us, "the expressiveness and technique of the brushwork," the manifestation of the painter's sensibility as he blended his mind into nature and saw it, as it were, from within. This is why in traditional landscapes, depictions of Mt. Fuji might often be indistinguishable from depictions of other mountains. The individuating outer "form" was essentially irrelevant, for what mattered was the inner "spirit," the invisible inner vitality of things as intuited by the sensitive artist and expressed in the nuanced suggestions of his brushwork. From the perspective of reformers, this elitist aestheticism and its worship of sensibility was decadent self-indulgence. At best, the adulation of the suggestive brushstroke was useless, and contributed nothing to resolving the crisis of their time. At worst, a mind-set so preoccupied with the nuances of subjective experience could not clearly see objective and problematic reality and was itself a basic cause of this crisis.

"There is a theory that paintings should present that spirit rather than the form," Shozan wrote in *Gahô Kôryô*, "but such an approach abandons the practical usefulness of painting."[30] Gempaku, Shozan, and Kôkan all saw in Western illusionism an alternative to the decadent subjective orientation of the Tanuma era.[31] Thus, for Kôkan, the essence of the Western style was epitomized by the camera obscura, and in his enthusiasm for this foreign device he urged people to look at his pictures through it.[32] Instead of a world perceived through the haze of the painter's personal intuition, instead of the "spiritual" vision of the artist immersed in and harmonizing with nature, the camera obscura presented a world of independent objects, observed from without, mirrored with geometrical fidelity.[33] It was especially against the gaze of the traditional aesthete that the early defenders of Westernism in Japan championed Dutch art, which, as Kôkan put it, "Just depicts things as they really are" (*tada sono mono o shin ni utsusu*).[34]

Against the self-indulgent "spiritual" tradition of Chinese-style painting, with which they were so dissatisfied, Shozan and Kôkan championed an art of "forms," an art that depicted the world seen lucidly from without. This was the deepest meaning of usefulness—the clear separation of the human seer from the objects that are seen. For reformers in late eighteenth-century Japan the most compelling attraction of the Western style of representation was the recognition of the world as an independent and objective reality that had to be reckoned with.

5

In the first section of this essay I pointed out the strong language in which Sugita Gempaku set forth his call for reform, how his references to the "chronic misconceptions" and "turbid traditions" of the past hinted at moral failures, and how his conception of *memboku o aratameru* seemed to carry nuances of spiritual transformation. The preceding discussion of illusionism in the Tanuma era has further underlined the importance of coming to terms with the moral element in the changing outlook of the late eighteenth century. In this concluding section I will examine the way in which Gempaku's experience of a new visual lucidity was tied in with Confucian conceptions of self-cultivation.

What was the problem with the past? Recall that Gempaku compared the confusion of early dissectors to the confusion of the man from Yen. This is an allusion to a brief story found in the Chinese classic, the *Liezi*:

> There was a man who was born in Yen but grew up in Chu, and in old age returned to his native country. While he was passing through the state of Jin his companions played a joke on him. They pointed out a city and told him: "This is the capital of Yen."
>
> He composed himself and looked solemn.
>
> Inside the city they pointed out a shrine: "This is the shrine of your quarter."
>
> He breathed a deep sigh.
>
> They pointed out a hut: "This is your father's cottage."
>
> His tears welled up.
>
> They pointed out a mound: "This is your father's tomb."
>
> He could not help weeping aloud. His compansions roared with laughter. "We were teasing you. You are still only in Jin."

The man was very embarrassed. When he reached Yen, and really saw the capital of Yen and the shrine of his quarter, really saw his father's cottage and tomb, he did not feel it so deeply.[35]

The tale is a variation of a favorite Daoist theme: the subjectivity of perception. The source of individual unhappiness and social divisiveness, from the Daoist perspective, is that our perceptions are conditioned by artificial expectations and projections. We always see things *as* something; that is, we impose an arbitrary value structure on them. The painful confusion of the man from Yen reflects not only the embarrassment of having been gulled, but also the situation of an individual who suddenly confronts the artificiality of his deepest sentiments.

Aside from its piquant Daoist message, the story illustrates a basic assumption common to both the Daoist and Confucian traditions in China, namely that perception is a form of response. Seeing, hearing, smelling, tasting, and touching may or may not have the sentimental overtones of the reactions of the man from Yen, but they all involve, by their very nature, the active participation of the perceiver. The passive reception of images is foreign to the traditional Chinese scheme of experience. One sees in much the same way as one gets angry.

To appreciate how this understanding of perception helps us to interpret Gempaku's criticism of past medicine, I must add that in the Confucian conception of good and evil, particularly as interpreted by the influential Song Confucians, each is a matter of appropriateness of response. Anger, sorrow, and the various other feelings each has its proper place and measure; but only the sage is able to respond with the appropriate feeling in the appropriate degree to each of the countless situations that arises in daily life. It is, of course, not a matter of conscious calculation. Rather, by maintaining a careful watchfulness, the sage achieves a mental balance that allows him to react naturally with a just response. Neglect and carelessness can easily upset this balance and hence skew the ways in which we interact with the world; and thus most of us fall short of the goodness of the sage.

In *Keiei Yawa* (*Conversations with a Nocturnal Shadow*) Gempaku discusses a wide variety of issues in the form of a dialogue with an alter ego, Shadow. At one point the Shadow asks about human possibilities. He notes that great Confucians such as Arai Hakuseki and Ogyû Sorai had achieved the things they achieved because of naturally superior dispositions combined with great effort. But how, asks the Shadow, can the ordinary man hope for sagehood? Gempaku denies any radical divide separating sages and ordinary humans, and appeals to the vision of self-cultivation suggested by a passage in the Confucian classic, *The Great Learning* (*Daxue*). He only alludes to it, citing the phrase, "we look but do not see, listen but do not hear," for most of his readers would have known the text by heart:

What is meant by saying that the cultivation of the personal life depends on the rectification of the mind is that when one is affected by wrath to any extent, his mind will not be correct. When he is affected by fear to any extent, his mind will not be correct. When he is affected by fondness to any extent, his mind will not be correct. When the mind is not present, we look but do not see, listen but do not hear, and eat but do not know the taste of food. This is what is meant by saying that the cultivation of the personal life depends on the rectification of the mind.[36]

That perception and attention are intimately related is both a commonplace of academic psychology and a fact of daily experience. But in the Confucian perspective inattention represents the fundamental moral flaw. For the eye to see what is before it, and for the ear to hear the sounds around it are the natural responses of being human. But any sort of disturbance of the mind—preoccupations, worries, infatuations—will disturb the mind's natural balance, and hence its capacity to perceive. In extreme cases, Gempaku explains, people will not hear the roaring thunder, or see a sword held menacingly in front of them.[37] Such inattention is for Gempaku the root of spiritual failure. The foundation of self-cultivation is actually simple and accessible to all. If one is alert and attentive, then nothing will separate one from the great sages. "The essential thing," Gempaku concludes, "is attentiveness."[38]

We can now understand the moral taint associated with the oversights of past anatomists. A failure to see reveals a skewed state of mind. Conversely, the bright clarity of Gempaku's new outlook expressed not only his enthusiasm for the new world of illusionistic representation, but a corresponding sense of moral purification. It was the encounter with Western artistic techniques that taught Gempaku a visual style illuminating the world in sharp, vivid detail; but the meaning of this visual illumination was defined by traditional ideas of spirituality. This fusion of two traditions is perhaps the ultimate meaning of "changing one's outlook."

The essential novelty of Gempaku's visual world was a novelty of representation. The traditional historiography that situates Gempaku's anatomical contributions in the history of Japanese empiricism is certainly justified. But the history of empiricism itself needs to be reconsidered from the perspective of the history of visual perception. We need to examine more closely what it means to observe. I suggest that it is in the visual possibilities revealed by new representational techniques that we must seek the sources of Gempaku's vivid sense of a world suddenly seen clearly and afresh.

NOTES

1. Because of the privileged access enjoyed by Dutch traders to the port of Nagasaki, Japanese study of the West (*Yôgaku*) began with Dutch language and works in Dutch (*Rangaku*). The text that Gempaku translated, however, was actually a Dutch translation of a German anatomy.

2. Much of the essential factual detail surrounding the work is covered in Ogawa Teizô's *Kaitai Shinsho* (Tokyo: Chûôkôronsha, 1968). Basic background information in English can be found in Sugimoto Masayoshi and David L. Swain, eds., *Science and Culture in Traditional Japan* (Cambridge, Mass.: MIT Press, 1978), 316–336. But perhaps the best introduction to this remarkable story is Gempaku's own account, *Rangaku Kotohajime*, translated by Matsumoto Ryôzô and Kiyooka Eiichi as the *Dawn of Western Science in Japan* (Tokyo: Hokuseidô Press, 1969).

One of the most insightful analyses into Gempaku and his times appears in Haga Tôru's introduction to vol. 22 of the *Nihon no Meicho* series (Tokyo: Chûôkôronsha, 1971). Also worthy of special mention are Satô Shôsuke's remarks concerning the influence of Ogyû Sorai on Gempaku's thought in *Yôgakushi Kenkyû Josetsu* (Tokyo: Iwanami shoten, 1964), 59–70.

3. Saigusa Hiroto, ed., *Nihon Kagaku Koten Zensho* (Tokyo: Asahi Shinbunsha, 1978), 3: 240.

4. Ibid.

5. Ibid., 241.

6. *Sugita Gempaku Shû. Asada Sôhaku Shû.* Dai nihon shisô zenshû, vol. 12 (Tokyo, 1934), 208.

7. Saigusa, 240.

8. See the "Jingshui" chapter in the *Lingshu*, and the biography of Wang Mang in the *Hanshu*. On Chinese dissection at this time see Mikami Yoshio, "Omô jidai no jintai kaibô to sono tôji no jijô," *Nihon Ishigaku Zasshi* (January 1945): 1–29.

9. Miyasita Saburô, "A link in the westward transmission of Chinese anatomy in the later middle ages," in *Science and Technology in East Asia*, ed. Nathan Sivin (New York: Science History Publications, 1977), 201.

10. See Matsumoto and Kiyooka, *Dawn of Western Science*, 26–27; *Sugita Gempaku Shû. Asada Sôhaku Shû*, 207.

11. *Sugita Gempaku Shû. Asada Sôhaku Shû*, 217.

12. In the preface to the *Fabrica*, Vesalius explains that the barber-surgeons who actually do the dissections "are so ignorant of languages that they are unable to describe their dissections to the spectators and muddle what ought to be displayed according to the instructions of the physician who, since he has never applied his hand to the dissection of the body, haughtily governs the ship from a manual." Charles O'Malley, *Andreas Vesalius of Brussels. 1514–1564* (Berkeley, Los Angeles: University of California Press, 1964), 319–320.

13. Matsumoto and Kiyooka, *Dawn of Western Science*, 29–30. I have modified the translation slightly.

14. *Sugita Gempaku Shû. Asada Sôhaku Shû*, 217.

15. This is the title of the original German text. However, the version that Gempaku had access to was the Dutch translation. See note 1.

16. Actually many texts of his time listed twelve organs, but the nature and anatomical status of two of the organs had been debated even in classical times.

17. For the reader interested in pursuing this issue in greater depth I would like to make special reference to the following sources: first the classic study by E. H. Gombrich, *Art and Illusion: A Study in the Psychology of Pictorial Representation* (New York: Pantheon Books, 1960); Richard Wollheim, *On Art and the Mind* (Cambridge, Mass.: Harvard University Press, 1974), 3–30 and 261–289; and the provocative series of

articles in *Social Research* 51 (Winter 1984), which is devoted to the topic of "Representation" (I am indebted to Dr. Ariel Mack for this last reference). For a more general consideration of the relationship between vision and cognition see, Ludwik Fleck, "To look, to see, to know," in *Cognition and Fact: Materials on Ludwik Fleck*, ed. Robert S. Cohen and Thomas Schnelle (Dordrecht: D. Reidel, 1986), 129–151; and Rudolf Arnheim, *Visual Thinking* (Berkeley, Los Angeles: University of California Press, 1969).

18. Matsumoto and Kiyooka, *Dawn of Western Science*, 29–30.

19. Ibid., 18–19.

20. Ibid., 29.

21. In fact, more than a decade and a half before *Kaitai Shinsho*, Yamawaki Tôyô had already seen an illustrated Western anatomy. But Tôyô's encounter with these foreign pictures of the body did not result in any epiphany; and indeed, he mentions them only once, in passing (see Saigusa, 156). Though they apparently helped confirm doubts that he already had about contemporary views of somatic structure, Western anatomical illustrations had little impact on what he saw in the body and how he depicted it. As we have already noted, Tôyô's *Zôshi* was inspired not by novel European modes of representation, but by his faith in the insight of the ancient Chinese sages, his trust in such classics as the *Zhouli* and the *Book of Documents*.

22. For a careful review of the extant sources on the thought and works of Naotake, Shozan, and Kôkan see Toyama Usaburô, *Tokugawa Jidai no Yôfu Bijutsu. Nihon Yôfu Fûkeiga no Seiritsu*, vol. 2 (Tokyo: Zôkei bijutsu kyôkai, 1977). On Odano Naotake and *Kaitai Shinsho* see Washio Atsushi, *Kaitai Shinsho to Odano Naotake* (Tokyo: Suiyôsha, 1980).

23. Strictly speaking, the Tanuma era corresponds to the period between 1760–1786 when Tanuma Okitsugu served as Grand Chancellor. However, it is commonly used to refer loosely to the entire span of the An'ei and Temmei reign periods, that is, from 1751–1788.

24. For details on the corruption and moral decay in the Tanuma era, see Tsuji Zennosuke, *Tanuma Jidai* (Tokyo: Nihon gakujutsu fukyûkai, 1936), 60–115; Tokutomi Sohô, *Tanuma Jidai* (Tokyo: Kôdansha gakujutsu bunkô, 1983), 390–405; and John Whitney Hall, *Tanuma Okitsugu, 1719–1788: Forerunner of Modern Japan* (Cambridge, Mass.: Harvard University Press, 1955), 106–130.

25. Toyama, *Tokugawa*, 62.

26. *Kôkan Kôkai Ki*. Nihon zuihitsu taisei, vol. I, pt. 2 (Tokyo: Yoshikawa kôbunkan, 1975), 21–22.

27. Toyama, *Tokugawa*, 62.

28. Kôkan presents a virtually identical critique of such uses and of "playthings useless to the state" in *Kôkan Kôkai Ki*, 21–22.

29. On the emergence of a "l'art pour l'art" aestheticism in the literature of this period see Itasaka Gen, *Chônin Bunka no Kaika* (Tokyo: Kôdansha, 1975), 76–85.

30. Toyama, *Tokugawa*, 62. See also Cal French, *Through Closed Doors: Western Influence on Japanese Art 1639–1853* (Rochester, Mich.: Meadow Brook Art Gallery, 1977), 126, for a loose translation of the text.

31. As I have already explained, Gempaku himself does not comment on aesthetics per se. However, it is certain that he, like Shozan and Kôkan, had an acute sense of the decadence of his time—a decadence that he saw primarily in terms of a decline

in martial discipline: "On looking at the condition of the present day military class, I observe that its members have grown up in a most fortunate age of prosperity which has continued for nearly three hundred years. For five or six generations they have had not the slightest battlefield experience. The martial arts have steadily deteriorated. Were an emergency to occur, among the Bannermen and Housemen who must come to the Shogun's support, seven or eight out of ten would be weak as women and their morale as mean as merchants. True martial spirit has disappeared completely." (Cited in Hall, *Tanuma Okitsugu*, 112).

32. Toyama, *Tokugawa*, 106.

33. Indeed, that is what the camera obscura was—the *shashinkyô*, literally, the mirror which copies the true reality of things.

34. Toyama, *Tokugawa*, 136.

35. A. C. Graham, trans., *The Book of Lieh-tzu* (London: Murray, 1960), 73.

36. Wing-tsit Chan, *A Source Book in Chinese Philosophy* (Princeton: Princeton University Press, 1970), 90.

37. *Sugita Gempaku Shû. Asada Sôhaku Shû*, 204.

38. Ibid., 294.

TWO

Epistemological Issues and Changing Legitimation: Traditional Chinese Medicine in the Twentieth Century

Paul U. Unschuld

The British physician Benjamin Hobson published in the 1850s a series of monographs in Chinese on various topics of Western science and medicine. This pioneering attempt to introduce recently developed Western knowledge to China allowed Hobson to comment on what he considered to be the basic conditions for progress in Western medicine, and on what he identified as the backwardness of Chinese medicine. Hobson attributed these divergent situations in China and the West to differences in attitudes toward knowledge of the past. While Westerners saw past knowledge as insufficient, the Chinese, Hobson observed, believed that the wisdom of the ancients required no further additions.[1]

Hobson was unaware that the unconditional reverence for ancient knowledge that he noticed in Chinese medicine was a relatively recent phenomenon. Concomitant with a movement in philosophy known as the return to the "Han teaching," a movement that had emerged during the sixteenth and seventeenth centuries, numerous authors concerned with the current state of China advocated that ideas introduced into medicine during the Sung-Chin-Yüan era of the thirteenth through fifteenth centuries be abandoned again. One prominent example of these "conservatives" is Hsü Ta-ch'un (1693–1771). He and others stated that the Sung-Chin-Yüan ideas falsified the original medicine taught by the sages of a distant but enlightened past.[2] Traditional Chinese medicine was at no time in its documented history dominated by one school of thought, and the "Han teaching" school during the Ch'ing dynasty represented but one of a number of diverging currents. And yet, the sixteenth century appears to have witnessed a final apex in the expansion of traditional Chinese medical knowledge, and it is quite significant that both the most voluminous Chinese encyclopedia of pharmaceutics, the *Pen-ts'ao kang mu* of 1596, and the comprehensive encyclopedia of acupuncture, the *Chen chiu ta-ch'eng* of 1601, had no worthy successors.

When Hobson and other Western physicians entered China in the middle of the nineteenth century, they encountered a situation that was marked, for already more than two centuries, by what might be called general epistemic stagnation. Although numerous contributions were published in the seventeenth and eighteenth centuries on how to move forward in medicine, the latter half of the Ch'ing dynasty saw a declining vitality of medical thought, reflecting a general decline in the vitality of the basic philosophical and political world views of traditional Chinese society.

It is important to keep this situation of Chinese medicine and society in mind lest an erroneous notion emerges to the effect that Western medicine confronted, in the nineteenth century, a flourishing system of indigenous Chinese health care based on a cognitive foundation totally different from that of modern scientific medicine. After an initial phase of reluctance and hesitation, Western medicine was welcomed by a vast majority of Chinese intellectuals, and its fast penetration of all echelons of Chinese society was linked to mainly two circumstances. First, after suffering defeats and humiliations by Western powers, and even by Japan, a country never considered to be a real threat before, many Chinese patriots considered traditional Chinese values and modes of thought, including China's entire sociopolitical structure, unsuited for rebuilding a strong nation. Western science, medicine, and technology were seen by these advocates of fundamental change to be indispensable instruments for regaining dignity and strength in the modern international context. Second, Western medicine did not appear to the Chinese as an altogether alien body of knowledge. Even though Western methods of separating truth from fiction were entirely new to China, certain basic concepts of the emerging Western ontological approach toward illness have also been central to Chinese medicine throughout history. Recent Chinese and Western publications have overemphasized an allegedly all-pervasive antagonism between modern Western and traditional Chinese medical thought while disregarding some basic epistemological parallels. At the same time, one of the most profound discrepancies separating Chinese and Western cognitive approaches—that is the attitude toward truth—appears to have been overlooked.

SOCIOENVIRONMENTAL ROOTS OF CONCEPTUAL SYSTEMS OF MEDICINE

Conceptual systems of medicine are legitimized, first of all, through environmental symbolism. A system of health care concepts and practices is plausible and acceptable when its ideas concerning the emergence, nature, and appropriate treatment of illness correspond to the sociopolitical ideas concerning the emergence, nature, and appropriate management of social crisis adhered to by a social group or by an entire society. It may well be that a social ideology legitimizing a specific conceptual system of health care corresponds to a currently existing social structure, or that it is directed at a future state of society. That is, no historical example exists to demonstrate that mankind could be able to conceptualize health and illness without employing its experiences gained from human interactions in times of harmony and crisis. Historical and anthropological analysis reveals that the encounter with what is considered a state of crisis of an individual organism cannot be conceptualized differently from an encounter with social crisis. A legitimation of conceptual systems of health care through what one might call clinical evidence appears to be, historically at least, of only secondary value.[3] From this it follows that a conceptual system of medicine ceases to be vital and creative when its major legitimizing circumstances, its particular context of social ideology and social structure, vanish, either in reality or in the aspirations of a population.

In China, the social ideology supporting the social system of the Imperial age constituted the epistemological root, that is, the legitimizing context, of traditional medicine. The body of knowledge identified as "Chinese medicine" today emerged as a result of fundamental changes in the social ideology and social structure of China at the beginning of the Imperial age. Its basically unchanged stability over exactly two millennia resulted from an unparalleled permanence of its legitimizing sociopolitical context during this time. With the breakdown of the traditional social structure, and with the demise of the traditional social ideologies supporting the Imperial age, and with the attempts to supply a new ideological basis to a changing social structure in the nineteenth and twentieth centuries, Chinese medicine lost its legitimizing environment. The result may be compared to the removal of a root from a tree. The tree dies but its wood, if preserved carefully, may remain in use for a number of meaningful purposes for a long time to come.

Similarly, the "death" or loss of creative vitality of a conceptual system of medicine does not necessarily entail its immediate disappearance. Satisfied clients, and interest groups profitably employing it, may continue to support and use it for a long time. And yet, the system is unable to develop any further from within itself. It continues to exist "as is," and this is the situation of traditional Chinese medicine since the turn of this century when its two thousand year-long dynamics were brought to an abrupt halt—as feeble as they were at the end.

Traditional Chinese medicine has not received any stimulus from "within" for further development during the twentieth century; all its dynamics during the past eight or nine decades were forced onto it from the outside, on the basis of ideologies closely associated with modern Chinese society— that is, Marxism and Western science. Basically, these dynamics resulted from strategies aimed at legitimizing a continued existence of traditional Chinese medicine in a changing social environment.

These strategies included: (1) a naive idea of combining the best practices of both traditions without realizing the profound historical break that lay between traditional knowledge and modern science; (2) an attempt to revive Chinese medicine by joining it to experimental science and Marxist dialectics; and (3) efforts to present Chinese medicine in a conceptually restructured version adapted to specific cognitive values of Western medicine.

COMPARISON AND THE ADOPTION OF THE USEFUL

By the final decades of the nineteenth century and early into the next, the acceptance of Western medicine by Chinese individuals of all social strata had reached proportions suggesting, to an increasing number of representatives of traditional Chinese medicine, a need to defend their knowledge and legitimize its continued application in clinical practice.[4] Even though a broad coalition of those interested in adapting their country to modern standards rejected traditional medicine along with the old ideologies and social structures, not everybody in China was able or willing to make the dramatic changes and the drastic reorientation this required. Unaware of the dynamic nature of Western science and medical knowledge, and initially condescending toward the foreign element, some early Chinese writers suggested a simple combination of Chinese health-care concepts and practices with those that appeared to be useful from Western medicine.[5] Numerous books and articles were written in China from the 1880s until the 1930s that compared Chinese and Western medicine and attempted to create a union between them. Examples of texts written during that period will demonstrate the arguments they used.

In 1884 T'ang Tsung-hai, acknowledging the dismal state of Chinese medicine, wrote the following in a preface to his book *Confluence of the Essential Meaning of Chinese and Western Medical Classics*:

> Ever since the T'ang and the Sung, [Chinese] medicine has gone astray in many ways. The Western methods that have appeared recently are detailed as far as the morphological manifestations [of illness] are concerned, but they disregard the transformations of the *ch'i* influences. They get a hold of the crude, but they miss the subtle. Both [Chinese medicine since the T'ang and Sung, and Western medicine] are faulty.
>
> This book has been designed for application in practice, and it differs from the old language in all the classic scriptures. In my explanations, I have not distinguished between the schools of the Han and the Sung, and I have refrained from pointing out differences between Chinese and Western opinions. All I intended was to let the message of the classics appear in all its clarity so that it may be put into practice and will benefit mankind.
>
> The organ charts of Chinese [medicine] have all been drawn by people who lived after the Sung-Yuan era. In many instances they do not correspond to the actual shape of the organs of the human body. [In the present book] all charts

have, therefore, been designed in accordance with [the charts used by] Western medicine. In comparison to the old [Chinese] charts they are truly excellent. The Chinese [book] *I-lin kai ts'o* presents a view of the organs that resulted from dissections. [Its statements] correspond, in some respects, to the teachings of Western medicine. This should be sufficient evidence [of the fact] that there is no basic difference between the organs of the Chinese and [those of] Western people. Hence I have adopted their charts to depict reality.

The organ charts of the Western people adopted here do not only correspond to the teachings of the Western people; in fact, they prove that there is not the slightest difference between the morphology outlined by the *Nei-ching* [and that of Western medicine]. To use these charts in order to explicate the meaning of the classics will have the effect that the [physiological doctrines of the] transformations of the *ch'i*-influences [outlined in these classics] will appear even more as a matter of fact.

The five openings of the stomach and the Triple Burner have been drawn in charts neither in China nor in the West. In the present [book] I have drawn [a chart] that is based on the facts related by the *Nei-ching*. There is nothing in Western [knowledge of] morphology that would correspond to [the Chinese knowledge of the five openings of the stomach and of the Triple Burner]. This is sufficient evidence [of the fact] that the Western people, even though they have developed such detailed morphological [knowledge], have not yet reached the sophistication of the *Nei-ching*.[6]

Sylvius, the sixteenth-century teacher of Vesalius, would have enjoyed T'ang Tsung-hai's argument. When Vesalius published his *De humani corporis fabrica libri septem* in 1543, Sylvius called him the worst example of ignorance, "poisoning all Europe with its pestilentious breath" simply because Vesalius had taken the liberty to look into the corpses himself rather than following the custom and reciting only what the ancient authorities had to say on human anatomy.[7] T'ang's scholastic way of reasoning appears in the following paragraph.

Prior to the existence of any person, a male impregnates a female and a foetus develops. This is a fecundation through a union of the *ch'i*-influences of water and fire of heaven and earth. Once a [person] has come to life, he will breathe with his nose, and he will receive the yang [influences] of heaven as a nourishment of his [protective] *ch'i*-influences. He will drink and eat the five tastes, and he will receive the yin [influences] of the earth as a nourishment of his blood. This happens before one is born. After birth, everybody continues his correspondence with heaven [and earth], and this correspondence results from the simple fact that the yin and the yang [influences] of the human body are rooted in the yin and yang [influences] of heaven and earth. Western chemistry states that man lives because he inhales nourishing *ch'i*-influences from the atmosphere. These so-called nourishing *ch'i*-influences are the *ch'i*-influences of heaven. But it is unknown [to Western chemistry] that the five tastes in drinks and food are yin matter of the earth. Although Western books start with a general introductory chapter, the two terms yin and yang are not distinguished.

Hence [these books] lack an understanding of the main forces [governing the existence of man].[8]

In 1918, Mao Ching-i published what may have been one of the first historical accounts of Western medicine in Chinese language. The paucity of data Mao related to his readers resembles the meager information on the history of Chinese medicine available in the West at that time:

> The Origins of Western Medicine
> In the year 460, which was the ninth year of rule of King Chen-ting of the Chou, a Persian named Hsi-p'o-chia was born on Kos. He is the ancestor of the medicine of the Western countries. In the year 1192, which was the third year of the *shao-hsi* period of reign of [Emperor] Kuang-tsung of the Sung, a man named A-da-tz'u-t'i lived in Italy; he studied medical theory, and he was also an expert in astronomy. In the year 1619, which was the 47th year of the *wan-li* period of reign of [Emperor] Shen-tsung of the Ming, the famous English physician Ha-fo realized for the first time that the blood comes out of the heart and revolves through the vessels. In the year 1658, which was the fifteenth year of the *shun-chih* period of reign of the present dynasty, a British named Ha-erh-fei began to study blood circulation by dissecting bodies. Although the principles [of blood circulation] are easy to understand, they represent, in fact, the essence of life. [Ha-erh-fei's] doctrine spread widely; it marked a turning point in medicine.[9]

In 1922, Mao Ching-i included a paragraph entitled "On Differences and Similarities between Chinese and Western Medicine" in a monograph, which read, in part:

> Today's world is a wise and skilled world. Europe, Asia, America, Africa, and Australia—these continents cover an area of altogether seven thousand billion square miles. [Their people] differ in the ingenuity and splendor of their styles, but the illnesses affecting them from the outside or resulting from inner harm are all the same. Just as the colors green, yellow, white, red, and black may appear in as many as one thousand and five hundred variations, human nature may differ in that it can be clever or stupid, skillful or honest. But the abilities of physicians to cure diseases are everywhere the same. Some people say: "Western medicine is much better than Chinese medicine"—I find this hard to believe. Others say: "Chinese medicine is superior to Western medicine"—this is even more difficult to believe! Chinese medicine clings to literature, while Western medicine emphasizes the reality of matter underlying [that what is written in the literature]. Chinese medicine is good in treating the interior [sections of the body]; Western medicine is good in treating [illnesses affecting] the external [sections of the body]. Chinese medicine seeks the essential and disregards the crude; Western medicine starts from the crude to reach the essential. Chinese medicine emphasizes the origin and neglects the consequences; Western medicine starts from the consequences to investigate the origin. In regard to these [differences] it is as difficult to reconcile Chinese and Western medicine as it is impossible to mate horse and ox. However, since we

live in the present time, we should weigh Chinese and Western medicine against each other. Chinese medicine emphasizes vessel diagnosis; Western medicine stresses percussion and auscultation. Chinese medicine emphasizes symptoms manifest in one's appearance; Western medicine emphasizes dissections. Chinese medicine honors theory; Western medicine depends on practice. This being so, [someone might ask]: "That is to say, Chinese and Western medicine are quite different?" The answer to that would be: "There are differences, but there are also commonalities." For example, when [Western medicine] speaks of tubes for blood and air (*ch'i*), this is similar to our Chinese distinction between [the different pathways of the] constructive and protective [*ch'i*-influences]. When they speak of internal membranes and outside skin, this is similar to our Chinese term *ts'ou-li*. When they say that the blood liquid is mastered by the heart, that is similar to our Chinese saying that the heart generates the blood. When they say that the atmospheric air (*k'ung-ch'i*) passes through air tubes into the lung, this is similar to our Chinese saying that the lung masters the *ch'i*-influences, and that the influences of the lung come from heaven. When they say that the gall juice digests drinks and food, this corresponds to our Chinese saying that when the gall moves heat into the stomach, the [resulting illness] is called "emaciation despite eating." We should bring together what is different in order to achieve agreement. Where there is agreement [between Western and Chinese medicine], that may well suffice to demonstrate [in the West] a far-reaching equality [between Western and Chinese medicine], and that there are men of identical mind in our China.[10]

Despite considerable inroads made by Western medicine at the time Mao Ching-i wrote these lines, a lack of knowledge of its epistemology gave rise to stereotypes and half-truths in the same way that stereotypes and half-truths concerning Chinese medicine continue to dominate Western literature down to our own time.

A last example will show that the situation in China had not changed markedly by 1938:

Western medicine came to China about forty years ago. Its treatment of illness is mostly based on scientific methods. Its drugs are splendid. Each day there is something new; each month there is a basic change. And in recent years its progress in essential matters has shown a particular increase because [everybody in Western medicine] focuses his ideas [on this goal]. When [Western medical scientists] treat a serious illness which is difficult [to cure because] one cannot be sure what it is, if [the patient] cannot be healed, they acquire the corpse and dissect it. They take out what is morphologically ill—formless illnesses related to *ch'i*-influences cannot be reached by this approach—and do research on it until they have found a therapy. If they encounter the same illness again, they apply this therapy and, often enough, achieve a satisfying result. After the death of Yüan-hua,[11] anatomy has not been continued in China. For more than a thousand years there was nobody who understood this technique, and, as one can see, the steps undertaken in antiquity were blocked later on.

In all current discussions it is said that, in treating diseases with morphological changes, Chinese medicine is definitely inferior to Western medicine, while, in the treatment of formless diseases, Western medicine is a little less efficient than Chinese medicine. These differences exist because the former argues on the basis of experiments while the latter discusses the transformations of ch'i.[12]

These early attempts to compare Chinese and Western medicine and to combine the best of both were taken up again in the 1960s and 1970s on a more sophisticated level. They were supported then by the paradigm of dialectic materialism. Thesis and antithesis result in a synthesis, and the contradiction between Western and ancient Chinese medicine, it was assumed, should similarly result in a new democratic Chinese medicine. A clinical report published in 1974 by Mao Shou-chung in the Shanghai journal *Nature-Dialectics*, illustrates how Western and Chinese medicine were combined at that time, characterized by political guidelines as well as a quest for clinical success.

In April 1971 a worker-comrade brought his six-year-old child into our clinic for an examination. The child suffered from muscular atrophy. When walking it staggered from one side to the other, and its arms and hands were unable to lift even chopsticks. Our diagnosis stated: "Symptoms of progressive muscular atrophy." In many publications of Western medicine, both in this country and abroad, the opinion is expressed that the causes of this disease are not known, and that there is no method to cure it. We have, therefore, examined the scriptures of our own country's antiquity, and we discovered that the *Nei-ching* contains statements concerning the symptoms and the treatment of this disease. The therapy is similar to the method of "take from a repletion to fill a depletion, and take from an organ/depot to fill an organ/depot." Formerly, those adhering to Western medicine in blind faith considered this method "unscientific"; nobody paid any attention to it. Now, is it scientific or not? Practice is the guiding principle in the search for truth. We are convinced that a therapeutic method that has been transmitted by the people for centuries and millennia until our own time, must have a meaning. The people of ancient times were burdened with the constraints of their historical situation, and they were unable to analyze relationships on the basis of current science. This does not mean, though, that the experiences gained by the working people of ancient times through experience had no scientific foundation at all. We conducted a chemo-analysis of the aforementioned child's urine, and we found an imbalance of creatine and creatinine in its body. Subsequently we attempted to cure the child by using animal cells containing the correct balance of creatine and creatinine. After some initial tests had caused no unwanted reactions, we asked the child to consume the drug that had been decocted in boiling water. After one month there was no effect. Could it be that certain effective ingredients had disintegrated when the drug was decocted in boiling water? Now we had the child swallow the drug with hot water. One month later a clear therapeutic effect appeared. The child was able to rise by itself, and its arms and hands became stronger. While the child took its drug it was asked to do certain gymnastic exercises, and after three months had passed, the child was able to walk a stair up and down without any help. This was the first step toward the child's recovery. . . . The pharmacological analysis of the drug used is still in its beginnings, and in some of the cases treated the old symptoms recurred as soon as the intake of drugs was stopped. And yet, the facts that have been established so far prove that neither the Chinese therapeutic principles nor the Chinese drugs are unscientific—those who adhere to Western medicine in blind faith are marked by prejudice. And it is exactly for this reason that many principles of Chinese medicine and pharmaceutics have remained unknown to us until this day, and cannot be employed in practice.[13]

Today, such dialectic approaches at unification of Chinese and Western medicine find little political support, and the slogan of the "Three Roads" expresses a more realistic perspective in that it encourages Chinese and Western medicine to continue along their respective idiosyncratic lines, and in that it stimulates a cooperation or union between the two only where feasible. The tremendous pressure of the late sixties and early seventies by political dogmatists on physicians of Western medicine to increase the use of acupuncture and other traditional practices vanished almost completely after 1976.

A NEW LIFE-LINE FOR RESUSCITATION

A second approach to restore life to traditional Chinese medicine attempts to "graft new roots to the tree." Some Chinese authors turned to science to provide traditional Chinese medicine with a new vitality. Early attempts of this kind argued that the ancient Chinese classics agreed with many modern insights and that later exegeses of the classics were misinterpretations that had to be revoked, as noted by T'ang Tsung-hai: "Ever since the T'ang and the Sung, [Chinese] medicine has gone astray in many ways." Wang Kung-chen, in 1938, presented a similar view when he published his judgment on his peers in traditional Chinese medicine.

> The *Nei(-ching)*, the *Nan(-ching)*, the *Shang-han (lun)*, and the *Chin-kuei (yao-lüeh)* are revered by all medical experts as the classics of the Sages. Those who wrote commentaries on these [scriptures] were concerned that the people of later times no longer understood the meaning of the original classics, and they provided them with a short-cut for their studies. Occasionally, the [commentators] used terms without applying sufficient diligence, and there were mutual contradictions between the [classics] and the [commentaries]. But nobody would have dared to criticize the original classics. Ch'en Hsiu-yüan was the first to state that Wang Shu-ho, in editing the *Shan-han lun*, ordered the individual paragraphs in the wrong way. And yet, [Ch'en Hsiu-yüan] conceded that, although there were exceptions, [Wang Shu-ho] himself had contributed some valuable ideas.

Now, the physicians of recent times are not acquainted with the ancient classics; they rely on a sharp tongue and they cheat both themselves and others. They show off their own abilities, and they point out the shortcomings of others. They consider it appropriate to be in trouble with those representing different ideas and then to settle their disputes again, and they consider it admissible to push and pull each other, but the [issue of their] patients' life and death is disregarded by them as if they had never even heard of it. Their art does not only fail to be orthodox, it is just false if compared to the writings of the exemplary men of antiquity. Today, the life of this "National Medicine" hangs by a thread.[14]

Authors like Wang Kung-chen considered it their goal to resurrect the message of the classics in all its purity, and to demonstrate that some basic insights as well as therapeutic recommendations of the past could very well be reconciled with the respective knowledge of Western medicine.

The "Sung school" of Chinese medicine had claimed to return to the origins of Chinese medicine while it represented, in fact, an attempt to adapt some basic concepts of the past to the changed world of the Sung era; the "Han school" of the late Ming and of the Ch'ing dynasty discounted the Sung innovations as falsifications of classic knowledge and undertook many efforts to rediscover the original contents of the Chinese medical classics. The new "Han school" of the twentieth century disqualified all developments that had taken place during the Sung, and all the reactions against the Sung during the Ming and.Ch'ing, as "having gone astray in many ways." In fact, this "third renaissance" manipulated basic concepts from the classics to make them appear to correspond to modern science.

Occasionally scientific proof that a drug or a particular treatment had the effects traditionally assigned to it supported this approach, although in the long run this has proved more detrimental to the traditionalists than helpful, because it has suggested the incorporation of scientifically valuable aspects of Chinese medicine into Western medicine and an abandonment of the rest.[15]

Another possibility of re-creating the life-giving relationship between a dominant ideology and social structure and medical concepts also proved to be a short-term illusion. In the 1960s and 1970s when dogmatists held sway, a union appeared feasible between dialectic materialism and traditional practices such as acupuncture and pharmaceutics. The price for this union that promised a permanent legitimation in a socialist society was high. The paradigm of systematic correspondence and the theories of yinyang and the Five Phases were denounced as primitive stages of dialectic and materialistic thought that had blocked development for two millennia. As soon as Marxism was toned down again in Chinese society in the late seventies, this attempt to provide traditional Chinese medicine with a new social vitality proved to be a failure.[16]

THE EMERGENCE OF A RESTRUCTURED "ALTERNATIVE"

A third approach to legitimizing traditional Chinese medicine in a changing social and ideological environment may be called introspective. It aimed at restructuring the conceptual system on which traditional Chinese medicine—at least as far as its literature is concerned—had been based for two thousand years.

Observers like Wang Kung-chen in 1938 pointed out a disadvantage of traditional medicine in comparison to Western medicine in that the latter spoke with one voice, whereas Chinese medicine had never known one dominant school of thought. Wang Kung-chen's concerns about Chinese physicians slandering one another were motivated by insights similar to his complaints about factionalism. Wang Kung-chen wrote:

> Western medicine is learned at schools, and it is transmitted within one line [of thought]. Hence, no matter whether it is in physiology, diagnostics, therapeutics or pathology, there are never two approaches. For example, in case of a given disease, once [the patient] has been examined by a given physician, [the latter] will apply to the disease a given name. And if [the patient] were to turn, then, to a number of additional physicians, they all would [arrive at] the same name. In treatment, in the use of drugs, there may be some minor differences, but, in general, nobody will leave the nest or change the pennon. This is certainly a major advantage of Western medicine, but hardly anybody knows that the disadvantage of Western medicine lies here too.
>
> Medicine has one definite basic principle, but the appearances of diseases are manifold; [diseases] may undergo a thousand changes and ten thousand transformations, and it is difficult to categorize them along any fixed standards. If one were to follow but one pattern, one would barely be able to cure those diseases that take a normal course, but it would be impossible to cure those that appear different [from what is normal]. Hence it is quite possible to apply one and the same name to [all the illnesses resulting from] one disease, but it is impossible to apply one and the same therapy [to all these variations].[17]

The idea expounded here by Wang Kung-chen was not taken up by a majority of authors concerned with the future of traditional Chinese medicine. Chinese publications, especially those of the past three or four decades, as well as virtually all Western authors promoting traditional Chinese medicine as an alternative to Western medicine, have depicted traditional Chinese medicine, in contrast to historical evidence, as a coherent system of thought, basically unchanged since antiquity. They have declared the paradigm of systematic correspondence as the one and only conceptual framework of traditional Chinese medicine. One intention behind this manipulation of historical facts may have been to present a system comparable in its degree of standardization to modern Western medicine. It should be realized, however, that even the "unscientific" and, in modern secondary literature, often neglected demonological and religious traditions of Chinese medicine were transmitted through the centuries as essential facets of traditional Chinese health care in its entirety. They offered, in modern terms, "psychotherapeutic" services that were apparently unavailable through the medicine of systematic correspondence.

SYSTEMATIC CORRESPONDENCE VERSUS ONTOLOGICAL PERSPECTIVES

Very few Western scholars have had linguistic access to the vast resources of Chinese medical literature, and among this small number an apologetic attitude has made some authors unwilling or unable to pursue disinterested analyses. Thus, basic misconceptions generated by Western and Chinese partisans of traditional medicine have come to prevail in the secondary literature.

For example, historically the Five Phases and yinyang theories of correspondence have not been as important as we have been made to believe, even though these theories appear at first glance to dominate medical literature. The entire realm of pharmaceutics, which played and continues to play a far greater role in practice than acupuncture or any other therapeutic technique, was only marginally touched by these theories.[18] Furthermore, diseases like leprosy, in contrast to functional disorders, escaped the logic of yinyang and the Five Phases.[19]

Virtually unknown in the West because publications delineating an idealized picture contain no references to it, Chinese medicine harbors a strong ontological conception of disease. This perspective views health as property given human beings by nature, the gods, or other metaphysical entities. Persons defend this property from their own negligence, and against enemies from outside who attempt to take health from them. Diseases and the pathological agents causing them are viewed in this way as intruders to be eliminated. Militaristic terminology was used in Chinese literature in much the same manner that it was used in Western medicine in the prebacteriological age.[20] Moreover, bacteriological biomedicine continued to be dominated by concepts of attacks and defense. If we literally translate traditional Chinese medical terminology, and look at the ontological perspective it reveals, then we realize that when bacteriology entered China it fell on fertile conceptual ground.

In the eighteenth century, Hsü Ta-ch'un (1693–1771), a prominent representative of the school of Han-teaching in medicine, wrote a "Discourse on the Resemblance between the Use of Drugs and the Use of Soldiers." His essay mixed medical-pharmaceutical statements with quotations from an ancient military treatise, "Master Sun's Military Patterns," written during the middle of the last millennium B.C. by the famous Sun Wu:

Soldiers were introduced to eliminate violence, and if there is no other way, military operations must be started. Similarly, drugs were introduced to attack illnesses, and if there is no other way, they must be employed. The principle is the same. To suffer from an illness means, in minor cases, a loss of one's essential [influences], and in severe cases harm to one's life. It is as if one were confronted with a hostile country. One takes advantage of the unilaterally marked nature of herbs and trees to attack unilaterally dominant depots and palaces. One must know the foreign [territory], and one must know one's own [territory], and if one checks the [enemy] at many places, there will be no grief over a destroyed body or over losses of life afterwards. Hence, where illness is transmitted through the conduits, one occupies, first of all, those locations that have not been reached [by the evil] yet. This way, one interrupts the strategic roads of the enemy. In case of sudden violent illnesses, one must quickly protect what has not fallen ill yet. This corresponds to how we guard our border areas. If an illness results from food remaining [in the body for too long], this food must be eliminated. This way, the enemy's provisions will be burned up entirely. If [a new disease] is about to unite with an old disease, one must prevent their union. This way, the enemy will be cut off from its internal ally. If one distinguishes between those of the transportation channels [that are affected and others that are not], that is called "[employing a] guide." If [someone suffers from] cold or heat, and if one [employs, in such a situation] drugs with exactly opposite effects, that is called "the technique of marching right into [the enemy's] lines."[21]

Near the end of the passage, Hsü writes, "Countries that are rich and strong are in a position to deploy awe-inspiring weapons. However, the [men] chosen [to conduct such interventions] must be appropriate, [just as] the instruments and machines [to be used in war] must be of good quality."

In his voluminous "Statements from Chinese and Western Medicine" of 1918, Mao Ching-i included a paragraph by Yu Feng-pa, who brought therapeutic and military strategies into an even closer relationship. It began, "The use of drugs resembles the use of soldiers. In the military it is important to know the topographic conditions, for the use of drugs it is important to know the location of the conduits."[22]

Beginning with the *Huang-ti nei-ching*[23] and until the early twentieth century, comparisons were drawn in traditional Chinese medical literature between the preservation of peace in the empire and the preservation of health in one's body. Chinese medicine, similar to Western medicine, arose from an attitude not to lose but to fight, an attitude that was criticized by Liao P'ing (fl. 1917), an ultraconservative representative of the "Han"-school of traditional Chinese medicine, who scolded even the first century *Nan-ching* for deviating from the truth conveyed in the *Nei-ching*. In a commentary to the *Nan-ching*, Liao P'ing wrote:

The pattern of the [doctrine of the] Five Phases as outlined in this book implies that everybody's brain is nothing but a battlefield with grace and hatred, generation and destruction, trouble-making and alliances, as well as rivaling doctrines. That is a very great mistake.[24]

Traditional Chinese medicine was characterized by conflicting currents. The paradigm of systematic correspondence, comparable to humoral pathology in Europe, sought to prevent and cure suffering by focusing on the entire human organism, mental and physical, and its relationship with a more encompassing whole, that is, the social and natural environment. Similar to pre-Cartesian health care and even to some later and current European conceptual systems of health care, this perspective may be called holistic, but it was not ecological in the modern sense because it did not accept suffering or those deaths that it considered premature to be the natural result of illnesses. In addition, the ontological current ran through both Chinese and European medical literature for centuries and millennia. When Morgagni (1682–1771), a contemporary of Hsü Ta-ch'un, published his treatise *De causibus et sedibus morborum* (On the Causes and Locations of Diseases), he would have found as many followers and critics in China, had his book been known there, as he did in Europe. The ontological perspective in Chinese medicine was neither ecological nor holistic, and this particular epistemological resemblance to Western medicine probably accounts for its absence from current depictions of traditional Chinese medicine as a preferable conceptual alternative to Western medicine.[25]

CHINESE PATTERNED KNOWLEDGE VERSUS HOMOGENEITY IN WESTERN MONOPARADIGMATIC SCIENCE

In outlining three basic strategies that were developed in China to legitimate a continued clinical application of traditional medicine, I have emphasized the generation of stereotypes which were supposed to demonstrate fundamental cognitive differences between Western and Chinese medicine. A growing knowledge of the historical development of Chinese medical thought makes it increasingly doubtful, though, whether these cognitive differences do indeed constitute a significant division. In particular, the alleged antagonism between a holistic-individualistic Chinese medicine and an ontological-localistic Western medicine is a drastic and misleading historical simplification of both traditions.[26] The issue is far more complex than is usually thought.

A comparison of long-term tendencies in Chinese and Western cognitive culture suggests the possible existence of a fundamental dividing line that shaped the histories of knowledge, including medicine, for the past two millennia in these two civilizations. Western civilization has been and remains a culture searching for, and believing in, the existence of one single truth. This attitude is reflected in Western monotheistic religious culture, and it is reflected in a continuous attempt to build one coherent scientific paradigm, free from internal inconsistencies or contradictions. "Thou shall have no Gods besides me!" is paralleled in secular knowledge by an imperative one might phrase as "Thou shall have no Truths besides one!" Competing paradigms or styles of thought have emerged in China with similar frequency as in Europe. Heated debates about who might be right, and who is wrong, are documented in the history of Chinese knowledge perhaps with similar intensity as in Europe. But in Europe competition was and still is generally expected to give way, ideally, to one single dominant paradigm, accepted by a majority of scholars concerned. Losers are abandoned, or find continued support by outsiders only. Western science is based on an either-or mentality. Contradictions are legitimized only temporarily. Both Marxist dialectics and the Kuhnian idea of scientific revolutions are outgrowths of Western cognitive aesthetics, and it would be very difficult to imagine them emerging from a background of Chinese cognitive culture. Western science primarily relies on logic to find truth. Truth is assumed to exist, and the human mind is asked to discover it. Once it is discovered, it is internalized until it can be replaced with a better truth.

The Chinese search for knowledge followed a different path. Although new opinions and theories were publicized by practitioners and intellectuals at all times, we should not speak of progress in a Western sense. Ever since the Han dynasty, that is, ever since the firm establishment of a unified China, Chinese cognitive dynamics have been marked—an analysis of long-term tendencies suggests—by an expansion of knowledge, adding the new to the old, while Western cognitive dynamics are characterized by a replacing of the old with the new.

The Chinese dynamics entailed the acceptance as truth of even outright antagonistic views, and this resulted in what I tend to call a "patterned knowledge." Patterned knowledge is based on a concept of truth that reveals itself through its usefulness. A knowledge is true when its application leads to a desired end. Different truths may coexist if their application results in a successful manipulation of a perceived reality. Not so much in daily reality but on a level of basic values manifesting themselves in ideals and in long-term developments, a Western dogmatic approach toward knowledge and truth appears to be confronted in China with an instrumental perspective. In China, current evidence suggests, knowledge is treated as an instrument applied to achieve a certain end; it is not a temporary outcome of mankind's search for the one and only final truth. Hence different and even mutually exclusive cognitive "instruments" may coexist if they promise to successfully perform different tasks.[27]

Ironically, the defensive restructuring of Chinese medical concepts in twentieth-century publications aims at presenting traditional Chinese medical knowledge as a coherent and stringent system of thought, matching the coherency and stringency of Western medical thought and terminology. In this process of adapting Chinese knowledge to Western cognitive aesthetics, age-old issues are glossed over as if they had been settled in the meantime, and through a selection of only one pattern from an original context of two or more "contradictory" patterns, the original characteristics of Chinese knowledge are lost in the latter's transfer to a modern environment.

Earlier in this paper, I compared the current state of traditional Chinese medicine to a tree whose roots have been removed. Chinese medicine continues to exist with its traditional cognitive heterogeneity despite recent attempts to transform and revitalize its knowledge from the outside. A creative and balanced union between Western science and Chinese medicine appears impossible, for the moment at least, because traditional Chinese medicine cannot maintain its traditional character and, at the same time, genuinely respond to the "either-or" questions posed by Western logic. Western logic requires definite answers; which of two conflicting statements in the *Nan-ching* and in the *Nei-ching* should be considered authoritative, whether one should follow Li Kao or Chang Tzu-ho, whether blood and ch'i both flow inside the vessels or not, whether "gate of life" refers to one of two kidneys or to a space in between them, and so on. No criteria have existed in traditional Chinese medicine to decide such issues, and Western logic has no basis from which it might step into this situation and identify what is right and wrong. Aside from the overriding political and economic considerations involved in the further development of traditional Chinese medicine, this fundamental epistemological issue has affected the coexistence of Western and Chinese medicine in this century and will most likely continue to do so.

NOTES

1. P. U. Unschuld, *Medicine in China: A History of Ideas* (Berkeley, Los Angeles, London: University of California Press, 1985), 236–238.

2. P. U. Unschuld, *Forgotten Traditions of Ancient Chinese Medicine: The I-hsüeh Yüan Liu Lun of 1757 by Hsü Ta-ch'un.* (Brookline, Mass.: Paradigm Publishing Co., 1990).

3. For a more detailed outline of this hypothesis see Unschuld, *Medicine in China*, 8–15. More recently, see also P. U. Unschuld, "On the reception of acupuncture in early 19th century Europe as reflected in the writings of Francesco Da Camino." *Le Scienze Mediche Nel Veneto Dell'Ottocento. Atti Del Primo Seminario Di Storia Delle Scienze E Delle Techniche Nell'Ottocento Veneto, 2 Dicembre 1989.* Istituto Veneto Di Scienze, Lettere Ed Arti. Venezia (1990): 217–230.

4. R. Croizier, *Traditional Medicine in Modern China* (Cambridge, Mass.: Harvard University Press, 1968), 63–65, 81–104.

5. Croizier, *Traditional Medicine*, 66.

6. Tsung-hai T'ang, *Chung hsi hui t'ung i-ching ching-i* (Shanghai: 1884), chaps. 1, 1a–1b.

7. C. D. O'Malley, *Andreas Vesalius of Brussels* (Berkeley: University of California Press, 1964), 250.

8. Tsung-hai T'ang, *Chung hsi hui t'ung i-ching ching-i*, chaps. 1, 1*a*.

9. Ching-i Mao, *Chung hsi i-hua* (Shanghai: 1922), chaps. 2, 23*b*. The date "460" should be 460 B.C.; Hsi-p'o-chia refers to Hippocrates (who was Greek not Persian). Ha-fo and Ha-erh-fei may both refer to Harvey (1578–1657).

10. Ching-i Mao, *Chung hsi i-hua*, chaps. 3, 4*b*.

11. *Tzu*: name of Hua T'o (110–207), the only Chinese physician of premodern times who is recorded to have performed some spectacular surgical operations.

12. Kung-chen Wang, *Yang-sheng i yao ch'ien-shuo* (Tientsin: 1938), chaps. 1, 7*b*–8*a*.

13. Shou-chang Mao, "Yung chung-i 'i tsang pu tsang' ti fang-fa chih-liao chi-jou wei-su ho nao kung-neng fa-yu pu liang cheng ti ch'ang-shih." *Tzu-jan pien-cheng-fa* 3 (1974): 143–144.

14. Kung-chen Wang, *Yang-sheng i yao ch'ien-shuo*, chaps. 1, 10*a*–10*b*. On the concept of "National Medicine" see Croizier, *Traditional Medicine*, 81–130.

15. This was recognized by some Chinese observers quite early. See, for instance, Croizier, *Traditional Medicine*, 98.

16. For a detailed account of attempts to supply traditional Chinese medical practice with a rationale borrowed from dialectic materialism, see Unschuld, *Medicine in China*, 252–260.

17. Kung-chen Wang, *Yang-sheng i yao ch'ien-shuo*, chaps. 1, 8*b*.

18. Unschuld, *Medicine in China*, 179–188.

19. P. U. Unschuld, "Traditional Chinese medical theory and real nosological units. The case of leprosy." *Medical Anthropology Newsletter* 17 (1985): 5–8. See also, P. U. Unschuld, "Lepra in China," *Aussatz Lepra Hansen-Krankheit. Ein Menschheitsproblem im Wandel*, pt. II, ed. J. H. Wolf (Würzburg: Deutsches Aussätzigen-Hilfswerk, 1986), 163–183.

20. As an example of an ontological pathology with concepts of attack by an abstract evil resembling the Chinese notion of *hsieh* and defense by the human organism prior to bacteriological thinking, see the pathological system developed by Karl Wilhelm Stark in the eighteenth century. A. Bauer, "Die Krankheitslehre von Karl Wilhelm Stark (1787–1845): Ontologische Pathologie als Analogiemodell," *Sudhoffs Archiv* 69 (1985): 129–153.

21. Unschuld, *Forgotten Traditions*, 183–184.

22. Feng-pa Yu, "Yung yao ju yung ping lun," Ching-i Mao, *Chung hsi i-hua*, chaps. 3, 22*b*.

23. See, for example, the paragraph, "Ssu ch'i t'iao shen ta lun" of the *Huang-ti nei-ching Su-wen*. Translation in Unschuld, *Medicine in China*, 283.

24. P'ing Liao, *Nan-ching ching-shih pu-cheng. Liu-i-kuan ts'ung-shu* (1913), chaps. 2, 29*a*.

25. "Militaristic" terminology is occasionally applied thoughtlessly even in a context meant to be an alternative to biomedicine. *Your Health Under Siege: Using Nutrition To Fight Back* is the title of a book distributed by a British supplier of literature on alternative health care.

26. See P. U. Unschuld, "Traditional Chinese medicine: some historical and epistemological reflections," *Social Science and Medicine* 24 (1987): 1023–1029. See also the Prolegomena to Unschuld, *Forgotten Traditions*, 1–41.

27. P. U. Unschuld, "Gedanken zur kognitiven Ästhetik Europas und Ostasiens," *Akademie der Wissenschaften zu Berlin. Jahrbuch 1988* (Berlin and New York: Walter de Gruyter, 1989), 352–366. Some of the consequences of "patterned knowledge" for Chinese diagnostics and therapy are discussed in the prolegomena of P. U. Unschuld, *Nan-ching. The Classic of Difficult Issues* (Berkeley, Los Angeles, London: University of California Press, 1986).

THREE

Time and Text: Approaching Chinese Medical Practice through Analysis of a Published Case

Judith Farquhar

The topic of this essay, a medical case history, is deceptively simple. The English word *case* incorporates Western assumptions about the natural relationship between concrete illnesses and disease categories; a case of pneumonia or Alzheimer's is a more or less "classic" example of an abstracted and named disease. We tend to locate the least necessary material cause of an illness and name a disease "expression" with reference to this agent. In this process the essentialist and reductionist biases of Western scientific thought are clear. When we are successful in understanding a disease in this way, it is purged of temporal and contingent characteristics; the histories both of specific illnesses and of the process through which biomedicine comes to terms with each of them no longer guide daily medical practice.

In the Western relationship between medical practice and bioscientific knowledge there is a productive tension between individual cases and disease nosology: the perception of complex or anomalous cases contributes to a long-term process of scientific revision in disease classification. But most case histories still tell us less than the generalized textbook descriptions of the disease of which any one illness is little more than an example. Consequently publication of case histories in Western medical literature tends to be restricted to strongly anomalous illnesses that challenge or extend existing disease classifications.

A published case history in Chinese medicine must be considered in quite a different light. Cases occupy a much more central place in medical discourse, and they are difficult to understand apart from their emergence *as texts* in a unique social world of scholarly practice. The first idea that must be abandoned about them is that they are examples of eternal fixed categories deriving from the Han Dynasty medical classics. Indeed, in reading them one is impressed with their historical reflexivity and their attentiveness to temporal processes both in the specific illness under consideration and in Chinese medical discourse as a whole. If we read these texts as though they only point backward in time to fixed syndromes or manifestation types named by the early masters, we lose most of their practical richness and didactic force.

I have elsewhere discussed the "epistemological" approach characteristic of many Western studies of Chinese medicine, arguing that such studies create a systematic body of knowledge (implicitly analogous to biomedical science) that has never existed in China.[1] These studies have sought a general, complete, and internally consistent system of medical knowledge in the early classics, a historical displacement of Chinese medicine that obviates the need for understanding concrete social practice. This kind of description is neither anthropological nor historical, and it fails to illuminate the social and intellectual practice of Chinese medicine in any era.

In an attempt to replace this philosophically ethnocentric approach, I have begun to examine the temporal and practical forms of medical life as they are indigenously described and can be observed in the contemporary practice that has been so much expanded in recent years in the People's Republic of China. In the course of my larger study of the temporal forms of the clinical encounter, case histories have emerged as central condensations of the knowledge, agenda, and powers of doctors. Analysis of a case history has the virtue of revealing deep features not of medicine as a system of knowledge but of medical practices, which is to say concrete historically situated healing activity.

Case histories occupy a much more prominent place in Chinese medical publishing than they do in Western biomedical journals and textbooks. Science and technology bookstores in the People's Republic include numerous collections of case histories among the teaching and research texts of Chinese medicine. A rapid review of the professional periodical literature of Chinese medicine reveals many short articles devoted to "discussion of a case" or of a few cases. A great deal of theoretical work revolves around the interpretation of specific illnesses; and the biographies and autobiographies of senior Chinese doctors (the still-powerful *laozhongyi*) focus at length on their famous cases. Advanced students at Chinese medical schools study the cases of their elders as examples of subtle practical mastery of medicine, and practicing doctors read published cases in their specialty as a supplement to their own clinical experience.

As the commentary on the case history translated below partly indicates, published cases (or at least the prescriptions they include) can play an important role in ongoing clinical work. One experienced Chinese doctor of my acquaintance keeps many notebooks in which he records published cases pertinent to his own rural practice; he consults these notebooks in the course of his clinic work, taking prescriptions from them that he modifies to suit the needs of the current patient, who waits while he rummages through these carefully accumulated resource materials. More commonly, the key points of classic or interesting cases are memorized, including the prescription, and clinicians tend to build up an idiosyncratic set of such mental reference materials that they deploy in a wide variety of circumstances. Chinese doctors accustomed to teaching medical students (or foreign anthropologists) can rattle off clinical precedents for their handling of many illnesses while they work, though they may be rather more cavalier in this oral commentary than in published case discussions like that reproduced below. The clinical observations and records of illustrious doctors of the premodern period are more likely to be cited both orally and in publications than are more recently published cases; a few modern doctors are so prominent, however, that their case experience and prescriptions have influence far beyond the relatively small group of their own students. Deng Tietao, who wrote the case discussed here, is one of these.

Case histories and the prescriptions they embody, then, are texts that contribute much to the practical work of Chinese medicine. They are written for and read by experienced clinician-scholars; as a result, especially in translation but to some extent in the original Chinese as well, they read as cryptic and bizarre. This essay attempts to demonstrate how such important but difficult texts might be read and to emphasize the connection of such texts to two central themes in the contemporary discourse of Chinese medicine: practical virtuosity (*ling*) and the accumulation of experience (*jingyan*). Both of these concerns relate to the nature of human agency—the relationship of action to knowledge, individuality to sociality, and the present to the past.

TRANSLATION OF A PUBLISHED CASE

The text to be considered here is "Two Cases of Foetal Death" by Deng Tietao, which appears in a collection of this well-known Cantonese doctor's most famous essays.[2]

TRANSLATION
Two Cases of Foetal Death
[The process of] diagnosis and treatment determination is one of the core components of Chinese medicine. The laboring people of China have for several thousand years undergone countless experiments, generalizing from them a set of theories and methods which, when used to guide clinical [practice], can attain very good results. An example can be seen in the treatment of the following two cases of foetuses dying in the womb.
Case I: Deng X X, pregnant seven months, foetal movement having ceased for 20 days, diagnosed as a missed abortion. After admission the following therapies were used: new acupuncture therapy, castor oil enema, quinine injec-

tions, high-pressure warm water enemas, injection of pituitarin at an acupoint (30 units/day), foetal membrane decollement, and others. In the course of using these various therapies there were minor contractions; by the time she had been in hospital for 10 days, the situation was rather serious; if surgical treatment was used there was a danger of contracting infection to be considered. Therefore Chinese herbal therapy was used.

She was observed to have tongue coating that was both yellow and greasy white, while the tongue itself was red. Pulse sinking and a little rapid but vigorous. These symptoms and pulse indicate excess, thus according to the usual procedure one would use "calming stomach powder" with the addition of mirabilite (Glauber's salt) and the fruit of trifoliate orange.

Drugs used: *cangshu* (*tsang shu*),[3] 9 g; magnolia bark, 12 g; mandarin orange peel, 12 g; licorice root, 4.5 g; dark brilliance powder (magnesium sulphate and licorice-radish powder), 12 g; trifoliate orange fruit, 12 g. Decocted in water as one dose.

Drug was administered at about 2:00 P.M.; at 6:00 P.M. contractions began, delivery commenced around 9:30, and later in the evening the dead foetus was completely expelled.

Patient stated that the cause of the foetus dying was her abdomen having been bumped into by one of the children rushing about.

Case II: Chen X X, pregnant eight months, entered the hospital seven days after foetal movement had ceased. Diagnosed as a missed abortion.

No therapy had been attempted since the patient was admitted to the hospital.

On observation the tongue was pale and tender with a fine white coating, peeling in the middle; pulse full and rapid, but weak under heavy finger pressure. According to analysis of tongue and pulse images, tender tongue and peeling coating indicates that fluids have been depleted, large, rapid, and weak pulse indicates inadequacy at the Qi level, and together these manifestations are classified as "Qi and fluids both deficient." In the course of asking the patient about her condition it was determined that she had had a rather extreme reaction to becoming pregnant, having been severely nauseous, which had induced a depletion of fluids and Qi. But a foetus dead in the womb is classified as a symptom of the excess type, i.e. the illness is overstrong while the body itself is weak. In consideration of this it would be unwise to only use a method of the "assault" type.

First examination: The treatment principle was to nourish fluids, enliven blood, cause Qi to flow, and lubricate the lower processing locus (*xia jiao*). Drugs used: adenophora, Chinese angelica, peach kernel, poncirus, and dark brilliance powder. In addition the "foot-3-inner" and "hegu" points were needled as a concomitant treatment. This procedure went on for two days without producing even the slightest uterine movement.

Second examination: I considered whether a modified "calming stomach powder" would help. So I tried two doses of the prescription used in Case I. The first dose produced two slippery bowel movements after it was administered, the second got no response at all.

Third examination: Switched to use of "fallen petals decoction" (Sichuan lovage, angelica, achyranthes root, plantain seed, and cassia twigs) administered in one dose. The foetus still didn't descend.

Fourth examination: Since I had already used various prescriptions to dislodge it and it hadn't moved, switched to a method of tonifying Qi and enlivening Blood. Drugs used: Cairo morning glory, *dangshen* (*tangshen*), orange peel, angelica, and lovage. But these were also not effective.

Fifth examination: Realizing that the potency of the previous prescriptions for tonifying and moving Qi had been inadequate, switched to use of modified "opening bones powder." Drugs used: *huangqi* (*huang-ch'i*) 120 g; angelica, 30 g; lovage, 15 g; charred human hair, 9 g; tortoise shell, 24 g (less used due to shortage of drug). Administered in a decoction.

Drug was administered at about 4:00 P.M., and at about 6.00 P.M. contractions began (one approximately every 10–20 minutes). At 8:00 P.M. massage and acupuncture were also used, first on the Triple Locus point and the Kidney point in order to put Triple Locus Qi in motion. But after massage the contractions lessened in frequency and became slower. Switched to the use of moxa on the foot-3-inner [point], a particularly efficacious point for bolstering body strength, after which the contractions accordingly gained in strength, about one every ten minutes, the systolic being rather strong. Moxibustion was discontinued after half an hour. Acupuncture was continued on the *zhongji* (Ren-3) point with a rotation every two or three minutes. After needling the contractions were taking place every one to three minutes, with extreme force; altogether the needling lasted fifteen minutes. When acupuncture treatment was terminated at 11:00 P.M., the dead foetus was expelled; it had been strangled by the umbilical cord.

Notes

A foetus dying inside the mother's body has become an illness-inducing entity—a form of heteropathic Qi; and the illness is classified as of the excess type. Since the Song dynasty, in the prescription books of gynecology, "calming stomach powder" with magnolia bark and magnesium sulphate added has been used to cause the foetus to descend. "Calming stomach powder" is mainly a prescription for invigorating and putting into motion clogging of the stomach and bowels due to damp: *cangshu* is a strong invigorating and motivating drug, magnolia bark and orange peel are good for moving Qi and drying up damp, and the addition of magnolia bark and magnesium sulphate can lubricate the lower processing locus. Our forebears considered that "if the Qi of the Stomach visceral system moves then the dead foetus will move of itself, and with the addition of magnolia and magnesium sulphate it cannot but descend."

The Complete Works of Zhang Jingyue from the Ming dynasty recommends using "fallen petals decoction" to cause a dead foetus to descend; this prescription is mainly for moving blood, and is used together with plantain seed and achyranthes to facilitate downward flow. "Calming stomach powder" treats clogged Qi, and "fallen petals decoction" treats blood stasis.

"Opening bones powder" is made from the "tortoise shell" decoction of the

Song dynasty (for treating difficult delivery, foetal death, etc.) with the addition of lovage. The Ming dynasty also had a modified decoction using angelica and lovage to move blood, tortoise shell to press down within, and charred hair to induce flow in the channels while stopping [excess] blood [flow]. This formula doesn't use drugs [of the] "assault downward" or "blood beating" [type], hence it has been widely used since the Ming to treat difficult delivery. Wang Qingren of the Qing dynasty felt that this prescription had both effective and ineffective aspects in the treatment of difficult pregnancy, the reason being that it was only strong with respect to nurturing and enlivening blood, but not specific for tonifying and moving Qi; hence he emphasized a heavy use of *huangqi* on the foundation of "opening bones powder" to tonify and move Qi, thus perfecting and heightening the effectiveness of the prescription.

We knew at the outset that Case II belonged to the class of weak body with overstrong illness, but hadn't come up with appropriate use of drugs, so we got no results. The use of drugs in the second and third examinations was not consistent with this diagnosis, hence ineffective. The treatment principle in the fourth examination wasn't really wrong, but the drugs weren't strong enough, so there was no effect. At last we used "opening bones powder" modified with *huangqi*, using large amounts of angelica and lovage to nourish and enliven blood, a great deal of *huangqi* to tonify and move Qi, and, although it was a little short on tortoise shell, which nourishes yin and presses down within, once Qi had been restored blood was able to flow, orthopathic Qi was able to drive out heteropathic Qi (i.e., the dead foetus), and the foetus descended. This resembled the advice of our forebears, who said, "Attack by building up and stimulating," i.e., use tonifying drugs to get the results of an "assault" drug; this is a typical case [illustrating this principle].

With regard to the acupuncture and moxibustion therapy, we first used moxa on the foot-3-inner [point] to tonify the deficiency, then needled *zhongji* (Ren-3) to drain the excess and lead it downward, this treatment principle being the same [as the above], thus achieving a helpful effect.

PRACTICAL VIRTUOSITY

This text locates itself in the intellectual environment of contemporary Chinese medicine in some obvious ways. Its most overt meaning is as a statement of the continuing efficacy of Chinese medicine in situations where Western medicine falls short, and as an assertion of the appropriateness of some Chinese medical techniques even in cases of acute life-threatening illness.[4] Thus it reflects the continuing importance of distinctions that are maintained between "Western medicine" and "Chinese medicine" and the state of struggle between the institutions affiliated with each approach. Before Dr. Deng took over Case I, for example, a number of therapies classified as either Western or combined Chinese and Western were tried with no success. The ease with which a classic herbal prescription induced labor in this case constitutes another small blow against the hegemony of Western medical methods as well as against a widespread tendency to fragment Chinese techniques within Western-style case management.

But this is only the beginning of the virtuoso performance that can be read in these cases. The commentary, for example, clarifies Dr. Deng's gynecological use of "calming stomach powder" in Case I, a formula primarily intended to treat digestive system disorders: "Our forebears considered that 'if the Qi of the stomach visceral system moves then the dead foetus will move of itself.'" What the commentary fails to mention is the way in which the formula used differs from that of "classic" calming stomach powder. Ordinarily the ruling (*zhu*) drug in the formula would be *cangshu* (Atractylodes spp.), supported (*fu*) by magnolia and orange peel.[5] Dr. Deng has in this case moved the supporting drugs into the ruling position because they are more specific for inducing downward movement than *cangshu*. This is, I believe, a fairly routine form of drug formula customization. Quantities of individual drugs can be altered, alternate drugs can be inserted, and the relations among the drugs, even in a time-honored formula, are tinkered with to adapt the medicine to the illness at hand.

Case II is obviously much more complicated, and its detailed discussion of what appears to be a trial-and-error approach stretching over several days is not likely to connote practical mastery to Western readers. We must first ask, then, why Deng would want to publish a case in which it took him such a long time to hit upon an effective therapy.[6] One can only assume that something important is being asserted about the process of doctoring, and that the way in which Deng gropes toward a therapeutic resolution merits attention in itself.

Table 3.1 schematizes the sequence of therapeutic principles employed in the five examinations of Case II.

TABLE 3.1

	Exam 1	Exam 2	Exam 3	Exam 4	Exam 5
nourish fluids	1				3
enliven blood	1		1	1	2
move Qi	1	1		1	1
ease downward flow	1		2		3
dry up damp		2			
tonify-bolster Yin (blood)					1
stop blood leakage					3

1 = therapy of primary importance
2 = therapy of secondary importance
3 = therapy of tertiary importance

When this table is read in conjunction with Dr. Deng's notes on the case, it is possible to see a pattern in his movement among alternative approaches to the illness. He began with a set of therapies closely connected with the major features of his original description of the patient's condition: depleted Qi and fluids and the patient's general weakness are treated in an effort to improve the wholesome movement of Qi and blood while lubricating the lower processing locus to encourage expulsion of the dead fetus. This approach reflects his careful differentiation between a local excess of heteropathic Qi (*xie qi*) (the dead fetus) and an overall deficiency in the capacity of the patient's normal orthopathic Qi (*zheng qi*) to respond defensively. This is a direct approach in which there is a one-to-one correspondence between each symptom and a specific therapeutic response.

When this procedure fails to induce labor, a new emphasis is introduced. The use of calming stomach powder after the second examination was primarily intended to treat clogged Qi, an attack on problems with yang elements and processes using warm, pungent, and bitter drugs; it is followed in examination three with sweet and pungent drugs that are mainly oriented toward enlivening blood (the yin side of the important blood/Qi dyad). Neither of these approaches proves sufficient, apparently convincing Deng that the problem is not with either blood or Qi but with both. His fourth examination results in a formula designed to treat both aspects, and when this produces no immediate results he chooses the venerable "opening bones" formula, which does the same thing more aggressively with the important addition of more tonic elements. His final intervention is potent partly because of the very large quantity of *huangqi* (*Astragalus membranacea*) used; a drug that both acts as a powerful supplement to natural body Qi and bolsters yin elements (for example, fluids), it makes up for deficiencies of the patient's constitution. It is accompanied by tonic drugs that both bolster blood and enliven its flow. As his notes on the case point out, Dr. Deng has "attacked by building up and stimulating" the body's natural ability to expel heteropathic elements within it.

Clearly, Deng was not just casting about until he happened to hit upon a lucky set of medicines. It could be argued that in an illness such as this, where the heteropathic Qi involved has its origin within the patient's body and consequently has much in common with it, the proper relative weighting of procedures to move Qi and to enliven blood is a delicate matter. In addition, the "failure" of a therapeutic approach, while it demands a modification, does not necessarily result in a fundamental change in the doctor's perception of the illness. (Witness, for example, Deng's argument for using the same procedure after examination four.)

What needs to be understood here is the intimate feedback relationship between perceived syndromes (*zheng*) and therapies. Modern textbooks of

Chinese medicine often explain that therapies arise from the differentiation of a syndrome and constitute the test of that differentiation. This relationship is well illustrated in Case II. Dr. Deng's unsuccessful therapies here are not merely negative information, demanding a whole new approach on each examination. They accumulate information of an increasingly articulate kind, helping him to refine what was finally a highly differentiated response to an illness that could be understood in all its dimensions only after it had been worked with for a while. By supplying an account of a full sequence of clinical encounters for one illness, Dr. Deng makes it possible for us to see the direction in which his understanding develops. His successive approximations to a correct description and intervention are the reverse of the reductionist methods with which we are familiar in the West. He does not rule out causal factors in a process of elimination, rather he adds to them, discovering through a process of elaboration the full dimensions of the problem.

At each step he also takes a certain viewpoint on the illness. Each formula betrays a different emphasis or interpretation of the root (*benzhi*) of the problem. Since it was necessary to avoid drugs of the "assault downward" (*gongxia*) type due to the patient's constitutional weakness, the possibility had to be considered that while her natural motive processes were being supplemented the viability of the heteropathic Qi within might also be enhanced. The various tacks taken on locating the "root" of the illness thus reflect attempts to support aspects of physiological process that can both conceptually and physically separate the fetus from the mother's body.

Examination one resulted in an attack on the symptoms of fluid depletion (seen as a contributing factor) and stasis (failure of the fetus to descend because of sluggish blood and Qi). Examination two focused on moving Qi, while examination three turned to enlivening blood. In examination four the blood/Qi relationship was reasserted, and the successful fifth formula hinged on bolstering and stimulating the body's orthopathic motive forces. When the sequence is read in this way, the large dose of *huangqi*, which bolsters and stimulates Qi, included in the fifth formula is particularly interesting. It suggests that once the mother's body has been strengthened through the benign effect of the previous therapies, it becomes safe to massively stimulate Qi. Presumably strong whole-body yang Qi would act against a dead fetus rather than strengthen its malignant (but relatively yin) force.

The process that becomes visible here is one of centering, of negotiating a path through a number of alternatives in an effort to avoid excess or deficiency, interventions that would be either dangerous or ineffective. Situations like this are repeatedly found as one reads the contemporary literature of Chinese medicine; the virtuosity of senior Chinese doctors is shown to extend far beyond classifying illnesses into static syndrome classes or locating the one appropriate drug formula in the exegetical literature. Rather, one gets an impression of a medical practice that generates complex images of concrete illnesses, and an intellectual process in which abstractions (yinyang, blood/ Qi) are used to characterize the many facets of each specific illness, while never losing the living specificity of the illness itself in generality and abstraction.

This perception is supported by the temporal form of the clinical encounter itself.[7] In the clinical encounter, a collection of drugs that is uniquely structured in a "customized" formula is brought to bear on a collection of illness signs that is comparably structured through analytic methods of differentiation (*bianzheng*). Neither illness nor formula is a foregone conclusion; both are formed and articulated through procedures of description, analysis, and structuring. Thus Deng Tietao's ability to read back and forth between diagnosis and therapy, modifying each in a dialogic process that can only take place through time, is an element of his mastery and one of the important messages to be taken from this published case history.

EXPERIENCE AND TIME

The case history presented here contains elements that are often ignored or devalued by students of contemporary Chinese society. The opening paragraph, for example, refers to the several thousand years of experience on the part of the laboring people of China. If we dismiss this reference as "mere politics," what are we to make of the pervasiveness of the concept of experience (*jingyan*) in contemporary Chinese medical discourse? The rhetorical force of its appearance in this text is clear and typical: the history of Chinese medicine (the experience of the laboring masses) constitutes a privileged foundation for claims that traditional procedures are effective. The weight of experience as an "objective" (*keguan*) justification of Chinese medicine's effectiveness is central to contemporary controversies over modernization and "scientization." The prominence of the term and of the idea can only be fully understood with reference to Chinese medical struggles to resist the increasing hegemony of Western medical knowledge and practice.

This deployment of the concept of experience to justify Chinese medicine involves an obvious and immediate recourse to the voluminous records of the medical practice of the last two thousand years. A Chinese doctor would be foolhardy and arrogant to reject the accumulated healing experience of past generations. The historical record constitutes an important guide to responsible action in the present and, though past procedures never fully determine any therapy, they narrow the possibilities and provide complex options (such as the formulae discussed above) on which doctors can work. Dr. Deng's citation of named formulae used by such luminaries as Zhang Jingyue and Wang Qingren demonstrates this relation to the past. He is not decorating his account with effete classical allusions, rather he is drawing on the scholarly and clinical experience of these forebears. But he puts their insights into play only after he has critically determined that they are appropriate to this specific illness, and he modifies their formulae to increase the degree of correspondence. His modifications, and the reasoning that informs them, then become contributions of the same kind to the accumulated recorded experience of healing practice.

The clinical encounter can be seen as a mode of action in which the doctor masterfully forges a link between a concrete illness and the relevant portions of the medical archive. In doing so he both reanimates the experience of his forebears and makes his own contribution to a continuing process of accumulation. By publishing his own cases with commentary, he adds his experience to the archive, moving gracefully into the past with the assumption that he is making a contribution to the capacity of doctors to act masterfully in the future.

This process of using and generating texts, and the highly selective and individual mode of mastery evident in Deng's handling of this case, suggest that a great many relationships that have been taken for granted in the sinological study of Chinese medicine must be reconsidered. The relationship between contemporary discourse and classic texts must not, for example, be seen as simple and obvious, and texts should not be taken a priori to be authoritative accounts of abstract bodies of knowledge. Knowledge itself must be reconsidered, its specific Chinese forms described, rather than assumed. If the culture-specific uses of textual materials are taken seriously, our tendency to uncritically label the concerns of some classic texts as "theory" in relation to the "practice" of daily clinical work is called into question.

Once the cognitive biases of Western epistemology are abandoned, it becomes possible to see medicine as embodied in the doctor and expressed in his virtuoso practice. Medical action in the present is revealed as a crucial pivot between past experience and future illnesses. Experience is not treated here as an illusion that must be experimentally tricked into yielding factual data through control of variables. Rather it is the only possible ground of responsible action. Consequently, written records of medical experience over the epochs, with all their contradictions and controversies, remain (as Mao Zedong said) a "vast treasurehouse" on which students of medicine and experienced doctors may actively and selectively draw.

Contemporary texts of the kind considered here, then, when read in terms of the practical life of which they are a part, can be seen not as examples of a Chinese version of "scientific knowledge" but as contributions to living experience in a medicine that can only be embodied in its practitioners. The opportunity that a case history provides to study the virtuosity of a senior Chinese doctor is a contribution to the slow increase in the student's own experience. Texts of this kind are thus deeply embedded in the social relations of medicine; even today they have the capacity to teach us much about filiality, creativity, and the ways in which persons are constituted in dialogue with illness, teachers, and the recorded past.

NOTES

1. J. Farquhar, "Problems of Knowledge in Contemporary Chinese Medical Discourse." *Social Science and Medicine* 24 (12): 1013–1021.

2. T. T. Deng, *Xueshuo Tantao yu Linzheng* (Theoretical inquiries and clinical encounters) (Guangzhou, China: Guangdong Science and Technology Press, 1981).

3. Translations for drug names are drawn from S. Y. Hu, *An Enumeration of Chinese Materia Medica* (Hong Kong: The Chinese University Press, 1980). Romanization of those drugs for which Dr. Hu adapts the Chinese name has been changed from Wade-Giles to Pinyin to be consistent with my use of Pinyin romanization elsewhere in this paper. I have, however, included Dr. Hu's spellings in parentheses.

4. In a brief autobiography, Deng Tietao has discussed his lifelong commitment to the use of Chinese medicine in acute life-threatening illnesses. See F. W. Zhou. et al., *Ming Laozhongyi zhi Lu* (Paths of renowned senior Chinese doctors), vol. 2 (Shandong, China: Shandong Science and Technology Press, 1982).

5. The prescriptions of Chinese medicine embody structured relations among the constituent drugs, which are chiefly reflected in the quantities specified. In the usual approach there are four relative positions, those of ruling (*zhu*), supporting (*fu*), assisting (*zuo*), and sending (*shi*).

6. This case is not anomalous for Deng. He has used it often and prominently in his teaching, and his students recognize it as a classic example of their mentor's clinical approach.

7. The temporal forms of the clinical encounter are described at length in my dissertation, "Knowledge and Practice in Chinese Medicine," Department of Anthropology, University of Chicago, March 1986.

FOUR

Winds, Waters, Seeds, and Souls: Folk Concepts of Physiology and Etiology in Chinese Geomancy

Gary Seaman

"You wouldn't know about this," replied Pilgrim. "Our old master fell asleep while listening to Buddha expounding the Law. As he slumped to one side, his left foot kicked down one grain of rice. That is why he is fated to suffer three days' illness after he has arrived at the Region Below" (*The Journey to the West*, Yu 1983*a*, 90).

In this fictional account of a trivial illness suffered by the Buddhist monk Hsüan-tsang, we might easily conclude that because the monk falters in his spiritual quest, he is condemned to suffer a physical punishment for a moral failing:

> This etiology of Hsüan-tsang's illness, to be sure, is expounded and received in the comic mode (witness Pa-chieh's horrified reply: "The way old Hog sprays and splatters things all over when he eats, I wonder how many *years* of illness I'd have to go through!"), but the suffering of the master, here as elsewhere, is not less real or certain. (Yu 1983*b*, 219–220)

We may also imitate old Hog and see the ultimate cause of Hsüan-tsang's illness in a fateful conjuncture: grains of rice fall to earth during the physiological processes of eating. This conjuncture suggests that when a grain of rice is placed on the ground or consumed by a living thing, it thereby not only begins the degenerative process of decay but also initiates the reproductive transformations that are the seeds of existence and ultimately human suffering. As we shall see, the apparent triviality of a grain of rice falling to the ground may indeed suggest ultimate causes to farmers whose existence depends on what happens when grains of rice are planted in the earth. Furthermore, if we view this episode with the appropriate degree of literality, we may perceive in it the basic elements of Chinese geomantic thinking:

74

the nature of human fate is determined by the interaction of heaven and earth, of what is above with what is below.

Taiwan is heir to a tradition of Chinese grave geomancy popularly called *hong-sui*, but known more formally as *Ti-li* or *K'an-yü* (Bennett 1978; March 1968). Geomancy is a way of thinking about the relationship of humans to their environment that has a long history in China, where it informs important aspects of everyday life and consciousness for many millions of people living close to the land. The information presented here was collected from a small, inland Taiwanese township of about one hundred thousand people during 1983 and 1984. The main informants were two Southern Min speakers of Hakka descent, one illiterate and the other with a sixth-grade Japanese education.

Chinese geomancy has at least two faces. One is that of the learned "professor" who uses pseudoscientific texts to articulate a theoretical model relating physical features of the environment to categories of space, time, and energetic forces. This is probably the face referred to by Kleinman: "Geomancers in fact are regarded as akin to 'scientists,' and geomancy is frequently referred to as 'Chinese science'" (1980, 66).

The other face of geomancy is that of the craftsman who applies geomantic principles to common problems. I will examine this aspect of geomancy among the rural Chinese of Taiwan. It concerns the relation between the living and their ancestors' graves from the perspective of the craftsman who actually exumes the bones during the secondary burial. I will show how individual and familial well-being depend on the transformation that the bodies of one's ancestors experience in the grave.

The general public in the West is aware of traditional Chinese medicine and has even adopted some of its practical applications—as demonstrated by the acupuncture clinics found today throughout the United States and Europe. Less well known is the cognate discipline of geomancy, which treats not only the individual but the whole intergenerational family by utilizing theoretical concepts quite the same or closely analogous to those of acupuncture. Geomancy and acupuncture are forms of "medicine" in that they seek to channel or alter natural processes for purposes of curing sickness and securing general well-being. Both are practical applications of "systems of correspondence" and other Chinese cosmological theories (Porkert 1974; Unschuld 1980; Feuchtwang 1974). Both share the troublesome characteristic that the physiological structures at the root of the cures are not always visible to Western techniques of scientific observation (Lu and Needham 1980). This opaqueness is related to the fact that among the Chinese individual fate was derived from a human nature linked to an all-encompassing, "astrobiological" conceptualization of life (Wheatley 1971, 414–419). By medieval times Chinese scholarship had forged a comprehensive worldview based on the macrocosm and microcosm analogy: man . . . mirrored in himself the whole, so that cyclic astronomical, meteorological, climatic and epidemiological factors mattered enormously for physiological and pathological processes (Lu and Needham 1980, 141).

Theories of the correspondence of cosmic cycles with phenomena intrinsic to individual organisms became so important to Chinese thought that during the Song dynasty they were a topic of the imperial examinations (Unschuld 1980, 130–131). Like acupuncture, and Chinese medicine in general, geomancy depends on a doctrine of macrocosm-microcosm analogy. The rhythms and structures of the earth are perceived to parallel those of the human body, and alterations of the earth bring repercussions upon individual human beings (Feuchtwang 1974).

On Taiwan, folk models for transformative processes within the ancestral graves are drawn from ideas about the genesis of plants within the body of the earth. The physiology of the earth is analogous to that of any other living organism, and folk concepts of it are especially interesting in relation to the "systems of correspondence" of Chinese medicine.

Highly trained professionals everywhere distance themselves from both the people who hire their services and from the technicians who perform physical labor. So it is in Taiwan today, where "professors of geomancy" (*Ti-li Hsien-sheng*) advise their clients on the basis of the abstruse theories found in systematic treatises, while "dirt masters" (*thow-sai*) confide the gory details of hundreds of graves they have opened (fig. 4.1). The dirt master's explications and analogies frequently make a lot more sense to the farmer than do the obfuscations of the professor. Most people do not place all their faith in one opinion about where the graves of their ancestors should be placed, and so the learned professor and the dirt master publicly accept each other's special expertise while undercutting each other's reputations in private consulations. The legendary character of this professional rivalry is illustrated by a folktale from Puli, Taiwan. In this tale, Lu Pan is an exemplar of the practical craftsman counterposed to Yang Kung, the "founding ancestor" (*cow-sai*) of professors of geomancy:

Back then, long ago, the geomancer's compass was called the "Original Stone" (*goan-chioh*). It was made from a huge block of stone which was very heavy and required ten or more men to carry it anywhere. Wherever it was taken, as soon as it was set down, the Tiger-Dragon (*how-liong*) would appear at once, and the apertures and excavations (for graves and buildings) were all "alive" (*oah*). Then one time Yang Kung was working as an apprentice for Lu Pan, that's right, working as an apprentice carpenter for him. Since Yang Kung was Lu Pan's apprentice, it was up to him to use the carpenter's plumbline with the inkwell for marking (*bak-tao*). With that plumbline, all you had to do was plunk the string, and planks split off as easy as pie [without having to actually saw them]. But in order to use the plumbline, it was necessary to fill

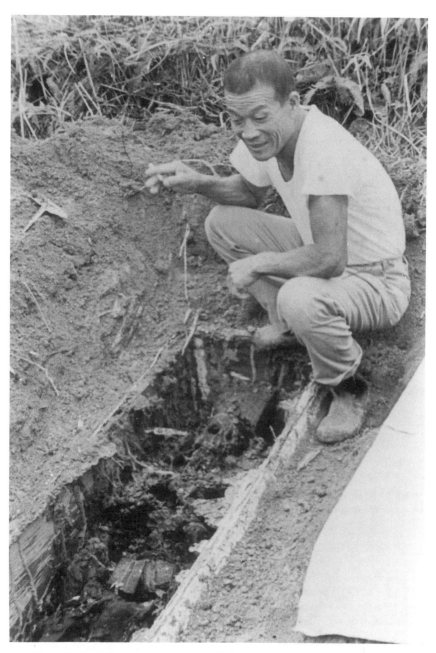

Fig. 4.1. An informant opens a grave in preparation for secondary reburial.

the inkwell with water to color the string. Yang Kung felt that it was far too much trouble to climb [each morning] far into the mountains in order to fetch [the pure spring] water that should be used, so he just decided to piss into the inkwell of the plumbline. Ai-yo! Disaster struck! After he pissed into the inkwell, boards no longer split off by themselves when the string was plunked! [Even though his livelihood was destroyed], there was nothing Lu Pan could do about it. But he thought to revenge himself on Yang Kung and so he said to Yang Kung, "You don't have to cart that heavy stone around and hire all those laborers to carry it. You could save their wages and make more for yourself if you could just keep labor costs from eating up all the profit. I am going to make things more convenient for you by constructing a geomancer's compass out of wood for you to use. Just go ahead and dump that big and heavy old "Original Stone" in the ocean, and I'll make this lighter one for you." After Yang Kung had thrown away his "Original Mother" [the narrator changed *goan-chioh* to *goan-bow* here, presumably the two concepts have some relationship with each other], the Tiger-Dragon turned into the "Tiger Penis Dragon" (*how-lan-liong*) and the true Tiger Dragon appeared no more ["tiger penis" means "a useless thing" in Taiwanese].

At that time when Yang Kung and Lu Pan were playing tricks on one another, carpenters had to worship the carpenter's plumbline-inkwell and offer incense before it, so when Yang Kung pissed in it, the thing was altogether ruined. . . .

Long ago, the carpenters plumbline-inkwell was not like those of today, but rather was carved like a dragon and it had the same shape as a coffin. (Ng A-bang, personal communication, 19 August 1984)

The ability to "summon the dragon" is, according to my informants, the single essential thing that determines whether or not a geomantical site is successful. It matters not how learned the professor of geomancy is, if he cannot "call the dragon" to a gravesite, the family whose ancestor is buried there will not benefit. So how does one call the dragon? Let us compare two versions of how a geomancer proceeds to determine the proper site for a grave. First, consider the learned professor's cogitations, as he sets down his compass with its thirty-eight (more or less) rings of symbols of correspondence that encircle the floating compass needle:

The compass takes the forest and mesh, and makes an order of the things in the world. In the middle of all this is one well, the Heaven Pool, called the Pool of the Great Absolute (*T'ai-chi*) . . . movement and repose working together. Now Heaven first produces water and water is, as the scholar knows, the mother of *Ch'i*. Fix your mind on the water in the pool. . . .

The hard material of the needle enables it to disclose and decide. Moreover, the lodestone was vitalized by earth *Ch'i*. It is earth's offspring, and earth is the central of the five elements. . . .

If it were not for the Heaven Pool, you could not ascertain the direction of the mountains and streams, and the work of the cycles would be uncharted, the

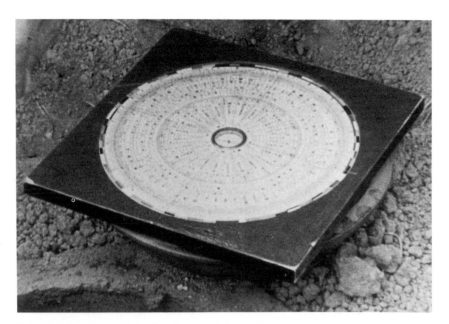

Fig. 4.2. The rings of the geomancer's compass provide a cosmological model that can be fitted to any landscape.

principles of change and movement undivulged and you would not be able to consider the transformations of the spirit or penetrate heaven and earth. . . .

   The secret is in the compass's rows and places, the position of the names opposite the position of the changing [directions of] the streams by which the changes can be investigated. (*Lo Ching Chieh* [Analysis of the Magnetic Compass] trans. in Feuchtwang 1974, 32–33)

As Feuchtwang remarks in regard to this passage, the compass surely functions as a multileveled model of the universe (fig. 4.2), which allows the geomancer, depending on the state of his learning, to relate any particular site to almost all systematized cosmological models extant in the philosophical and speculative literature of China! It is therefore instructive to compare the previous quotation with the way in which my informants view the use of the compass:

   The geomancer's compass was established by Yang Kung, just exactly as Washington established the United States. How did he establish the geomancer's compass? He used one kind of wood, which is called *chhiu-m* or *iang-m-chhiu*, which is the same as *chhi-pho*. That kind of tree blooms at night during the *cu* hour (11 P.M. to 1 A.M.). Rice plants bloom at *gow* hour (11 A.M. to 1 P.M.). The geomancer's compass is supposed to be synchronized with rice. Since rice is synchronized with the *cu-gow* line (north-south) of orientation of the geomancer's compass, this is because *cu* pertains to the North and *gow* pertains to the South, so that is the same as calling the Tiger-Dragon, that is calling the Dragon. If you plant rice and the dragon comes to eat it, only then when the Dragon comes will things prosper. But nowadays everyone is trying to save labor and no one does things right, so I don't know if geomancer's compasses are made of *chhiu-m* wood anymore. (Ng A-bang, personal communication, 14 August 1984)

Here rice is necessary to lure the dragon to its new grave-site lair, and the directions are not associated with abstract cosmological symbols, but with circadian rhythms and the natural processes of feeding animals. According to my informants, nothing in siting graves is more important than "calling the dragon." Other things may affect the fate of those descended from the grave's occupant, but if the first step of "summoning the Tiger-Dragon" fails, then it is ridiculous to treat with other forces.

At the moment when the proper site for a grave is determined, the geomancer sets his compass on top of a plate of polished rice (fig. 4.3). The compass is oriented to the north-south line as it is placed on top of the container of rice, and then is turned to the orientation that has been determined as the optimum one for the grave. Two stakes are erected at the head and foot of the site and a red string is stretched between them along the line of orientation of the gravesite. The event is called "dividing the gold" (*hun-kim*) and with this act, the "posts of Yang Kung are established" (*cai iu*-kong khitta*). The climactic act of selecting the site then occurs. Grains of rice are scraped from the container to fall on the ground to every side. This is "to call the dragon" (*kio liong*) or to "summon the Tiger and Dragon" (*cio how-liong*). After a short wait, the dragon is considered to arrive and "enliven" (*e-oah-tih*) the site. "Dividing the gold" fixes the orientation, and serves as the centerline for construction of further calculations of the site's effects.

According to my informants, if the rice is not thrown onto the ground at the moment of determining the proper site, then the site cannot have the effects it has been selected to produce. As my informant explained, "If you plant rice and the dragon comes to eat it, only then when the Dragon comes will things prosper" (Ng A-bang, personal communication, 14 August 1984).

My informant had in mind a close analogy between planting rice and the dragon's ingestion of the rice "planted" at the grave. This comparison of planting rice with the burial of bodies helps us to understand the analogical thought of my informant. The rice cycle begins with washing the rice selected for seed. Water for this purpose is "bought" from the local Water God (*cui-sin*) by offering him incense and paper spirit money (fig. 4.4). The rice is then soaked *below* the water table until the outer husk begins to split (*thoat-khak*) and sprouting is imminent. It is then planted in built-up seed beds *above* the water table. When the plants have fully sprouted and the fields have been

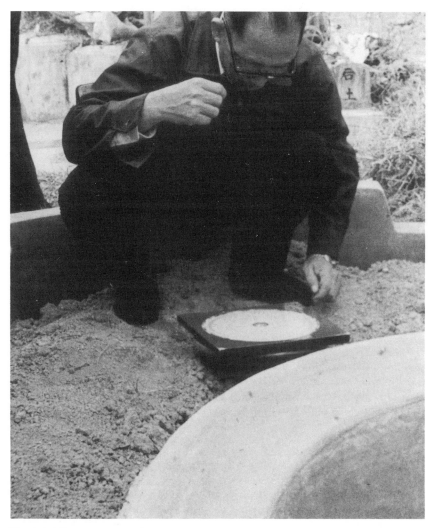

Fig. 4.3. The geomancer places his compass on a plate of polished rice and orients it to the site.

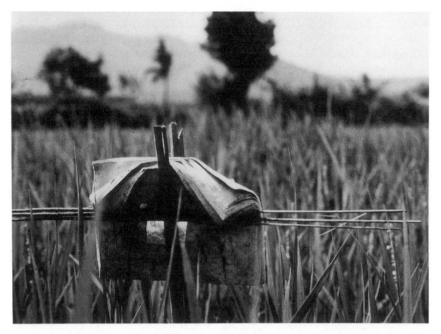

Fig. 4.4. A special kind of "spirit money" is used to buy water from the Water God.

thoroughly manured, the rice shoots are transplanted so that their roots are just *below* the water table when the fields are flooded. This allows the young plants to "eat the filth" (*ciah-lah-sap*) of the newly fertilized fields and thus to grow rapidly. When the plants ripen (*siek*) to a golden yellow they are cut, dried in the sun, and stored (*khng*) in a dry place *above* the water table.

In the course of a burial, the corpse is washed with water "bought" from the local Water God. Although the body is not actually immersed during washing, this act is equivalent to being placed *below* the water table. The corpse is put in a coffin in the main hall of the house on a bed made of boards placed well *above* the ground (fig. 4.5). It is kept from contact with the ground for days or weeks before the funeral rituals are performed. The body in the grave is placed just *below* the water table, and the coffin is pierced at its lowest point so that "the filth can be carried away in the water" (fig. 4.6). The flesh and blood of the body are said to turn into "filth" (*lah-sap*), but this same process of decomposition is likewise thought to "refine the bones" (*lien-kut*) into gold. The funeral rituals end at the grave where one of the last acts of the mourners is to break a duck's egg over the gravestone, so that the dead person can "split the husk" (*thoat-khak*). After one or more years the bones are dug up and if they have ripened into a golden color, then the gravesite is said to have been successful. The bones are dried in the sun, then stored in a

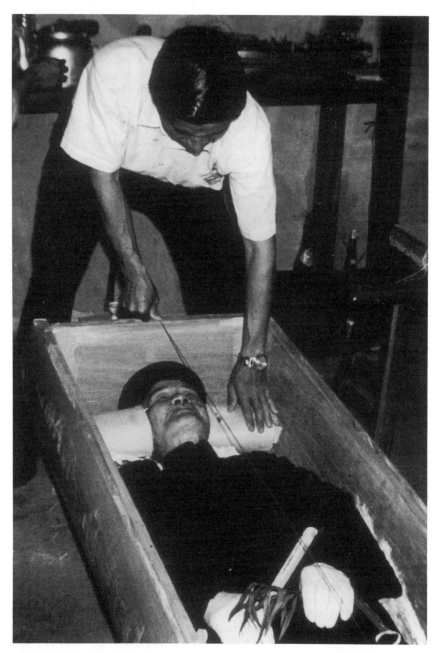

Fig. 4.5. The corpse is laid out in the main hall of the house well above floor level.

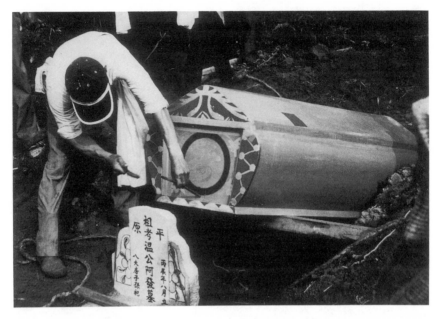

Fig. 4.6. The coffin is pierced at its lowest point, which will be located below the water table.

specially made pot that has much the same shape as traditional rice graneries. This pot is placed so that it rests *above* the water table and is in no danger of flooding (fig. 4.7).

The analogy of planting rice with human burial uses associations that recur in many societies between fertility and death (Aijmer 1964; Watson 1982). The processes that occur within the grave are not only analogous to those that take place in the rice fields but also to human reproduction. The "summoning of the dragon" with the geomancer's compass is not for my informants an abstract calculation of remote cosmic forces. For example, seed grain and semen in Taiwanese are both called *ci*. Even the wood used to make the geomancer's compass suggests a strong sexual and procreational context. The wood is known in Mandarin as *Yang-mei*, the arbutus or "strawberry" tree, *Myrica rubra*. The *Yang-mei* is a broad-leafed connifer that produces fruits with a strawberrylike appearance that are often salted and preserved with honey (Meyer 1911, 275). Because of their similarity to sores from syphilis, the name of the berries has been extended to those sores, and the tree is associated with sexuality. My informants assert that the geomancer's compass must be made from the cross section of a Yang-mei tree trunk, if it is to be truly efficacious.

The classical texts of geomancy also reveal sexual reproductive processes

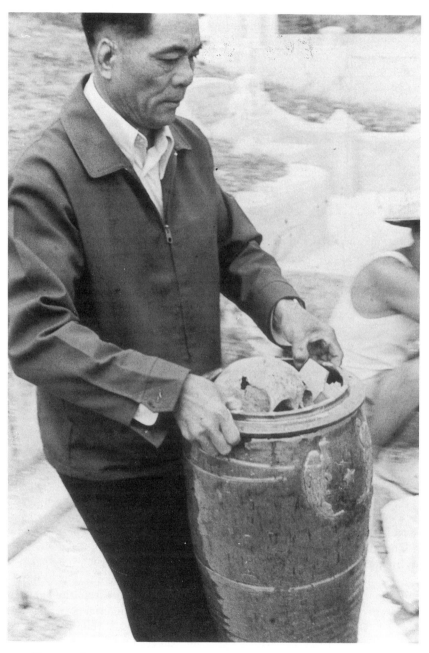

Fig. 4.7. The bones are stored in a specially made pot to keep them dry.

operating at the gravesite. In English, "the womb of the earth" or "veins of ore" refer to geological structures, but geomancy texts use more extensive physiological analogies. In the early seventeenth-century compendium of geomancy, the *Ti-li Jen-tzu Hsü-chih* [What Everyone Should Know About Geomancy], the Hsü Brothers discuss the terminology of geomancy that reveals this analogical thought:

> Q: In geomancy, why do you use the word "artery" (*Mo*)?
> A: In the human body it is the arteries (*Mo-lo*) which transport the pulse throughout the bodily system. In the arteries of a human body, when the arteries are bright, then the person is noble. When they are dull, then the person is base. When the arteries are auspicious, then the person is at peace. When they are inauspicious, then the person is in danger. It is just the same with the arteries of the earth. The good doctor examines the arteries [that is, takes the pulse] of a person and thus knows whether the person is in good health or in danger, whether he will die young or live to a ripe old age. The good geomancer examines the arteries of the mountains and knows thereby whether they are auspicious or inauspicious, beautiful or ugly.
>
> But this is not a simple task. Certainly dragons and arteries have common origins: if there are dragons, then they are characterized by their manifest forms, whereas arteries are characterized by their hidden minuteness. Thus it is said that "It is uncommonly difficult to discern the arteries of the mountains."
>
> As far as the term "aperture" (*Hsüeh*) is concerned, this takes its meaning from being just the same as the apertures of the human body. Master Yang says, "Take for example the moxibustion and acupuncture points on the 'bronze man' (*Tung-jen*), each of these apertures must be fixed in location before they can be used." Chu Hsi says that "the method of determining apertures in geomancy is just like that in moxibustion and acupuncture. There is definitely a fixed position of each aperture and there cannot be the slightest mistaking it." These examples are all good expressions of the meaning of the term "aperture." (Hsü 1970, *kuan* 1, book 2)

Many other technical terms in geomancy have organic connotations. For example, the proposed object of geomancy as put forth by Kuo P'u in his *Tsang Ching* [Burial Classic] was to locate "living breath" (*Sheng Ch'i*) and then bury one's ancestors in the aperture from whence this breath emanated (Kohut 1977).

The use of terminology parallel with or borrowed from that which the traditional Chinese physician used to describe the physiology of his patients is also prominent in the titles of the classical texts of geomancy. For example, the *Cho-mo-fu* [Ode on Pulse Taking] (T'ao 1980), contrary to the expectations that the title raises, explains the effects that mountains of different shapes have upon graves placed on them. There are also a number of titles that use the term *Nang* or "bag" in a manner suggestive of the paraphernalia of the herbal doctor's bag, for example the *Ch'ing-nang-ching* [Blue Bag Classic] attributed to Ch'ih-sung-tzu of the Ch'in dynasty (Chang 1970).

The use of terminology from acupuncture and herbal medicine suggests that the earth is an organism analogous to the human body. As one of my informants put it, "To bury the bones is like planting seeds. Haven't you seen that Chinese graves are made in the shape of a woman giving birth?" In the *Tz'u-pei Hsüeh-ching* [Compassionate Blood Bowl Sutra], one of the texts recited at funerals, the reproductive processes of women are conceived of as the result of worms gnawing at their bone-joints. Because children are generated out of the effluvia of worms feeding within a woman's body, the bones of one's parents and hence one's ancestors create their descendants through the processes of ingestion, digestion, and excretion (Seaman 1981).

The exact nature of the connection between the remains of parents and ancestors is explained in different ways, as for example in a modern manual entitled *K'an-yü yü Ming-hsiang* [Geomancy and Fate Prognostication]:

Q: How is it that the graves containing the bones of the ancestors or one's parents can affect the fortunes of their children and grandchildren?
A: The graves in which are buried the bones of parents and ancestors have various effects stemming from the bones and skeletons which are buried in the graves. Because the bones contain within them a substance, the so-called "basal cause" (*Chi-yin*), this can exert an effect on the "basal cause" of blood relatives. In other words, it is the same principle as that of the transmission and reception of the wireless radio: when the bones of parents or ancestors receive the positive effects of a grave, the "basal causes" contained in their bones stimulate positive effects in the "basal causes" of the bones of their children and grandchildren; thus, the fortunes of the children and grandchildren will take a turn for the good or, on the other hand, for the bad. (Wang 1983, 10).

The "basal cause" (*Chi-yin*) that is given as the tie between ancestors and descendants in the quote above is most frequently expressed colloquially as *kang-kut*, "we are of the same bone." This expressed commonality of substance between parent and child and the analogous handling of corpses and rice give us reason to seek an identity of function for seeds and souls. The gravesite functions as the vessel of transformation in which the material stuff is refined and from which the dead are eventually reborn, that is, returned to the world as newborn infants, thus realizing in a social sense, at least, the goal of Taoist alchemy.

The *Nei-ching-t'u* [Map of the Inner Conduits] is often reproduced as a rubbing from a major Taoist temple in Peking, the Po-yün-kuan. It represents the "internal landscape" of the human body as visualized by the physiological alchemist. In the lower part of this Map of the Inner Conduits, we can see a peasant farmer working the plow behind his ox. Rouselle interprets this graphic representation of the human microcosmos as follows:

One shouldn't just sit uselessly and stare at the wall for nine years, but rather focus on the center of life and warmth in the middle of the body, just about at the level of the navel. Here is found the origin and maintenance of the main pulse and the twelve subordinate pulses. This sinking of thought into the center of life is called "plowing." Therefore one finds in the picture at the level of the navel that the plowman is at his eternal labor in the fields, that is, coordinating the center of life and its power. A short passage is appended to the figure of the plowman—even though somewhat high up by the trees—it goes as follows: "The iron ox plows the earth, in order to produce gold and money." The whole area from the navel through to the kidneys is allotted to the element "earth" and is considered the "elixir field" (*Tan-t'ien*).

The plowing ox of iron serves as allegory for the continuous working of this entire center of life. From the working of the earth comes true blessings; it is the preparation for the seed of a higher life, for the "production of gold and money." This latter is not shown on the engraving but is represented by the painting as beds of cash. (Rousselle 1962, 25–26, my translation)

The imagery in this classical expression of physiological alchemy resembles my informants' ideas about the similarity between processes occurring in the grave, rice fields, and the human body. When I asked how graves were connected with the descendants, one informant explained:

Dragons are really worms and snakes that gather in a place to eat things. Some of these turn into flies and these can lay eggs in things that people eat. If there is a "karmic relationship" (*na u ian*), then a woman can eat this and she will get pregnant. Then there is the "water god" (*cui-sin*, which is the same thing as "water energy" (*cui-khi*). The water god can carry "energy" (*khi*, Mandarin *Ch'i*) from the grave to people's houses if the house is built where there is a "live aperture" (*hiet e oah*). (Ng A-bang, personal communication, 27 July 1984)

House sites are selected by a geomancer in much the same way as a gravesite is fixed upon. Since both my informants are of Hakka origins, it is also noteworthy that the "lord of the lot site" (*te-ki-cu*), the god worshipped with incense below the altar table of the main hall of the house, is called the Dragon God (*liong-sin*) by Hakka people, and indeed this god's place is often marked by a painting of a dragon or the written character for dragon. The god's place beneath the table is exactly the point where the geomancer sets down his container of rice and places his compass upon it. It is the point of orientation for building the house, and from which all the activities of the inhabitants find their starting point. Thus, the house is linked with the grave and living descendants with their dead ancestors.

The Map of the Inner Conduits provides yet another link between decay in the grave and fertility of the fields and of the family. At the bottom of the Map of the Inner Conduits, male and female figures are mounted on a water wheel at the edge of the water which trails off into the unrepresented part of the cosmos. This wheel is called the Mysterious Waterwheel of Yin and Yang (*Yin Yang Hsüan-t'a-ch'e*). It is the driving force for the waters that flow uphill

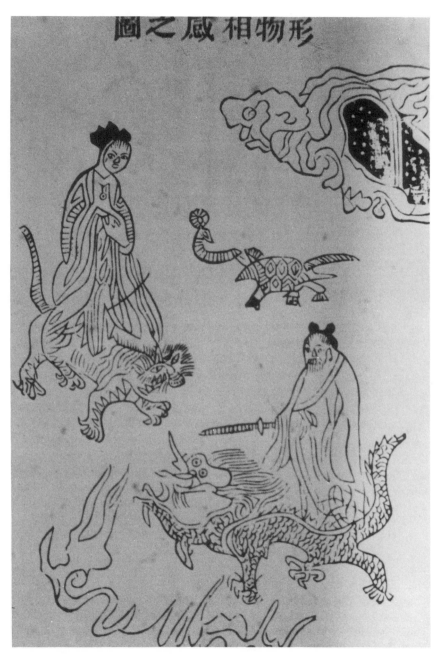

形物相感之圖

Fig. 4.8. An "alchemical marriage" as illustrated in a medieval Chinese text (Needham 1983: 103).

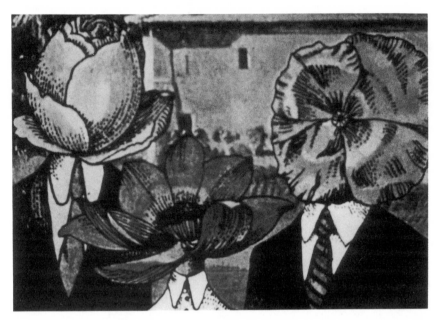

Fig. 4.9. The cover of a modern geomancy text represents decendants as having plantlike characteristics.

through this imagined microcosm of the human body, powering the combination of fire and water that is the source of life's energy (Rousselle 1962, 27). This wheel is sited at the margin of the water table, and if we pursue earlier versions of this imagery, the man and woman first ride upon and then lose their identities in figures of a tiger and a dragon (fig. 4.8). The vision of the dirt masters, who emphasize the importance of summoning the "Tiger and Dragon" to the gravesite, can be extended beyond the grave to the sources of the social cosmos and human fertility. As Schipper puts it:

> It is therefore in the womb of everyday life that one can realize the insertion into the rhythm of the cosmos. The return to one's origins is to be found by way of the kitchen, where one prepares the food to nourish one's ancestors and descendants. The perfect regularity required for the realization of nonaction must be through the integration, at every instant, of the phases of physical existence with those of one's social body. Hence with restored equilibrium, thanks to harmony with ceaselessly changing time, we find restored to us a silence, a "pure blankness." At the center of a world that advances inexorably toward death, there operates a way of return, a passage to *another time*. (Schipper 1982, 273–274, my translation)

The tombs of the ancestors in the view of my informants literally represent this passageway to another time. Death is not the end of existence, but the

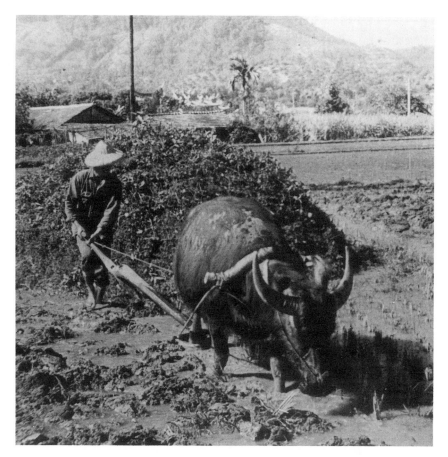

Fig. 4.10. A farmer plows his field; a grave mound is in the background.

means whereby one becomes an ancestor and thereby transforms oneself into a new expression of another time. It is through the daily and yearly round of laboring in the fields, through growing and preparing food and eating and feeding, that the ancestors are transformed into descendants. Within the grave the processes of decay refine them into the object of the alchemist's quest: the bones of the ancestors turn into gold, immutable and infinitely precious. Yet paradoxically the processes of decay also nourish their descendants, and thus create a true immortality: the corporate Chinese family spanning the generations (fig. 4.9).

For the people of South China, both individual and social existence have long hinged upon the processes that take place when a grain of rice is placed within the muck of the rice fields (fig. 4.10). By some miracle this act does not result in corruption but the generation of new life. Old Hog shows no surprise at the illness resulting from Hsüan Tsang's clumsy handling of a single grain of rice, but is moved to consider his own bodily functions as containing the seeds of karmic fate. Mixed with our perception of Old Hog as a comic figure should also be an appreciation of the cosmic forces contained within a single grain of rice.

CHINESE CHARACTER INDEX

bak-tao　墨斗
cai iu*-kong khitta　裁楊公杙仔
Chang Ming-feng　張鳴鳳
chhi-pho　？
chhiu-m　樹梅
Chi-yin　基因
Ch'i　気
Ch'ih-sung-tzu　赤松子
Chin-t'ai In-shuai-ch'ang　金台印刷廠
Ch'in [dynasty]　秦
Ch'ing-nang-ching　青嚢経
Cho-mo-fu　捉脈賦
Chūgoku Chūsei Kagaku Gijitsu-shi no Kenkyū
　　中国中世科学技術史の研究
Chu-lin Ch'u-pan-she　竹林出版社
ci　種
ciah-lah-sap　吃拉☆
cio how-liong　招虎龍
cow-sai　祖師
cu　子
cu-gow　子午
cui-khi　水気
cui-sin　水神
e-oah-tih　会活得
goan-bow　元母
goan-chioh　元石
gow　午
hiet e oah　穴会活
hong-sui　風水
how-lan-liong　虎屧龍
how-liong　虎龍
Hsin-chu　新竹
Hsüan-tsang　玄藏
Hsüeh　穴
hun-kim　分金

I-wen Ch'u-pan-she　宜文出版社
iang-m-chhiu　楊梅樹
Kadokawa　角川
K'an-yü　堪輿
K'an-yü yü Ming-hsiang　堪輿与名相
kang-kut　仝骨
Kao-kuo Shu-chü　高国書局
khi　気
khng　攄
kio liong　叫龍
Kuei　鬼
Kuo P'u　郭璞
lah-sap　拉☆
lien-kut　練骨
liong-sin　龍神
Lo-ching-chieh　羅経解
Lu Pan　魯班
Mo　脈
Mo-lo　脈絡
na u-ian　那有緣
Nang　囊
Nei-ching-t'u　內経図
oah　活
Pa-chieh　虸蜡
Po-yün-kuan　白雲觀
Qi　気
Sheng-ch'i　生気
siek　熟
T'ai-chi　太極
Tan-t'ien　丹田
T'ao K'an　陶侃
te-ki-cu　地基主
thoat-khak　脫殼
thow-sai　土師
Ti-li　地理
Ti-li Hsien-p'o-chi　地理仙婆集
Ti-li Hsien-sheng　地理先生
Ti-li Ren-tzu Hsü-chih　地理人子須知
Tsang-shu　藏書
T'ung-ren　銅人
Tzu　子
Tz'u-pei Hsüeh-p'en-ching　慈悲血盆経
Wang Yü-teh　王裕德
Wu　午

Yabuuti Kiyoshi　藪內清
Yang Kung　楊公
Yang Mei　楊梅
Yin-yang Hsüan-t'a-ch'e　陰陽玄踏車

REFERENCES

Aijmer, Goren
　1964　*The Dragon Boat Festival on the Hupeh-Hunan Plain, Central China: A Study in the Ceremonialism of the Transplantation of Rice.* Monograph Series, Publication No. 9. Stockholm: The Ethnographical Museum of Sweden.
Anderson, Eugene N., and Marja L. Anderson
　1973　Feng-shui: ideology and ecology. In *Mountains and Waters: Essays on the Cultural Ecology of South Coastal China,* ed. Anderson, Eugene N., and Marja L. Anderson, 127–146. Taipei: Orient Culture Service.
Bennett, Steven J.
　1978　Patterns of the sky and earth: a Chinese science of applied cosmology. *Chinese Science* 3: 1–26.
Bloch, Maurice, and Jonathan Parry, eds.
　1982　*Death and the Regeneration of Life.* Cambridge: Cambridge University Press.
Chang, Ming-feng, ed.
　1970　*Ti-li Hsien-p'o-chi* (The fairy crone's collection on geomancy). Taipei: Chin-t'ai In-shuai-ch'ang.
Ch'ih-sung-tzu.
　1970　*Ch'ing-nang-ching* (Blue bag classic). In *Ti-li Hsien-p'o-chi.* (The fairy crone's collection on geomancy), vol. 5, ed. Chang, Ming-feng. Taipei: Chin-t'ai In-shuai-ch'ang.
Feuchtwang, Stephen
　1974　*An Anthropological Analysis of Geomancy.* Vientiane: Vitahagna.
Freedman, Maurice
　1958　*Lineage Organization in Southeastern China.* London: London School of Economics.
　1967　Ancestor worship: two facets of the Chinese case. In *Social Organization: Essays Presented to Raymond Firth,* ed. Maurice Freedman, 85–104. Chicago: University of Chicago Press.
　1968　Geomancy. *Proceedings of the Royal Anthropological Institute of Great Britain and Ireland for 1968,* 5–15.
Groot, J. J. M. de
　1892–
　1910　*The Religious System of China.* (Reprint 1969). Leyden: Brill.
Harrell, C. Stevan
　1979　The concept of "soul" in Chinese folk religion. *Journal of Asian Studies* 38 (3): 519–528.
Hsü, Shan-chi, and Hsü Shan-shu, eds.
　1970　*Ti-li Jen-tzu Hsü-chih* (What everyone should know about geomancy), preface, 1567–1573. Hsin-chu: Chu-lin Ch'u-pan-she.

Keightley, David N., ed.
1983   *The Origins of Chinese Civilization*. Berkeley, Los Angeles, London: University of California Press.

Kleinman, Arthur
1980   *Patients and Healers in the Context of Culture: An Exploration of the Borderland between Anthropology, Medicine, and Psychiatry*. Berkeley, Los Angeles, London: University of California Press.

Knapp, Ronald G.
1977   The changing landscape of the Chinese cemetery. *The China Geographer* (Fall): 1–14.
1982   Chinese vernacular burial. *Orientations* 13 (7): 28–33.

Kohut, John
1977   Translation of the *Tsang-shu* [Burial book]. A.B. honors thesis, Harvard University.

Leslie, C., ed.
1972   *Asian Medical Systems*. Berkeley: University of California Press.

Li, Hui-lin
1983   The domestication of plants in China: ecogeographical considerations. In *The Origins of Chinese Civilization*, ed. David N. Keightley, 21–63. Berkeley, Los Angeles, London: University of California Press.

Li, Yih-yuan
1976   Chinese geomancy and ancestor worship: a further discussion. In *Ancestors*, ed. William Newell, 329–338. Mouton: The Hague.

Lip, Evelyn
1979   *Chinese Geomancy*. Singapore: Times Books International.

Lu, Kuei-djen, and Joseph Needham
1980   *Celestial Lancets: A History and Rationale of Acupuncture and Moxa*. Cambridge: Cambridge University Press.

March, Andrew L.
1968   An appreciation of Chinese geomancy. *Journal of Asian Studies* 27 (2): 253–268.
1978   The winds, the waters and the living *Qi*. *Parabola* 3 (1): 28–34.

Needham, Joseph
1983   *Science and Civilization in China*, vol. 5, pt. 5. Cambridge: Cambridge University Press.

Pasternak, Burton
1973   Chinese tale-telling tombs. *Ethnology* 12 (3): 259–273.

Porkert, Manfred
1974   *The Theoretical Foundations of Chinese Medicine: Systems of Correspondence*. Cambridge, Mass.: MIT Press.

Potter, Jack M.
1970   Wind, water, bones and souls: the religious world of the Cantonese peasant. *Journal of Oriental Studies (Hong Kong)* 8 (1): 139–153.

Rossbach, Sarah
1983   *Feng Shui: The Chinese Art of Placement*. New York: Dutton.

Rouselle, Erwin
1962   *Zur seelischen Führung im Taoismus*. Darmstadt: Wissenschaftliche Buchgesellschaft.

Ruitenbeek, Klaas
1986   Craft and ritual in traditional Chinese carpentry. *Chinese Science* 7: 1–24.
Saso, Michael R.
1978   What is the Ho-t'u? *History of Religions* 17 (3–4): 399–416.
Schafer, Edward H.
1977   *Pacing the Void: Tang Approaches to the Stars*. Berkeley, Los Angeles, London: University of California Press.
Schipper, Kristofer M.
1978   The Taoist body. *History of Religions* 17 (3–4): 355–386.
1982   *Le Corps Taoiste: Corps Physique-Corps Social*. Paris: Fayard.
Seaman, Gary
1981   The sexual politics of karmic retribution. In *The Anthropology of Chinese Society on Taiwan*, ed. Emily Ahern and Hill Gates, 381–396. Stanford: Stanford University Press.
Sivin, Nathan
1968   *Chinese Alchemy: Preliminary Studies*. Cambridge, Mass.: Harvard University Press.
Skinner, Stephen
1982   *The Living Earth Manual of Feng-shui: Chinese Geomancy*. London: Routledge and Kegan Paul.
Strickmann, Michel
1979   On the alchemy of T'ao Hung-ching. In *Facets of Taoism*, ed. H. Welch and A. Seidel, 123–192. New Haven: Yale University Press.
T'ao, K'an
1980   *Cho-mo-fu* (Ode on pulse taking). In *K'an-yü Lei-fan Jen-t'ien Kung-pao* (Vast treasures of men and heaven, a collection of geomancy texts), vol. 5. Taipei: I-wen Ch'u-pan-she.
Unschuld, Paul U.
1980   *Medizin in China: eine Ideengeschichte*. Beck: Munchen.
Wang, Sung-hsing
1974   Taiwanese architecture and the supernatural. In *Religion and Ritual in Chinese Society*, ed. Arthur Wolf, 183–192. Stanford: Stanford University Press.
Wang, Yu-teh
1983   *K'an-yü yü Ming-hsiang* (Geomancy and fate prognostication). Tainan: Kao-kuo Shu-chu.
Watson, James L.
1982   Of flesh and bones: the management of death pollution in Cantonese society. In *Death and the Regeneration of Life*, ed. M. Bloch and J. Parry. Cambridge: Cambridge University Press.
Wheatley, Paul
1971   *Pivot of the Four Quarters*. Chicago: Aldine.
Wolf, Arthur M.
1974   Gods, Ghosts, and Ancestors. In *Religion and Ritual in Chinese Society*, ed. A. Wolf, 131–182. Stanford: Stanford University Press.
1976   Aspects of ancestor worship in northern Taiwan. In *Ancestors*, ed. W. Newell, 339–364. Mouton: The Hague.

Yabuuti, Kiyoshi
1963   *Chūgoku Chūsei Kagaku Gijutsushi no Kenkyū* (Studies in the history of medieval chinese science and technology). Tokyo: Kadokawa.
1973   Chinese astronomy: development and limiting factors. In *Chinese Science*, ed. S. Nakayama and N. Sivin, 91–104. Cambridge, Mass.: MIT Press.
Yoon, Hon-key
1975   An analysis of Korean geomancy tales. *Asian Folklore Studies* 34 (1): 21–34.
1976   *Geomantic Relationships Between Culture and Nature in Korea*. Taipei: Orient Cultural Service.
Yu, Anthony C.
1983*a*   *The Journey to the West*, vol. 4. Chicago: University of Chicago Press.
1983*b*   Two literary examples of religious pilgrimage: the *Commedia* and *The Journey to the West*. *History of Religions* 22 (3): 202–230.

FIVE

The Fragile Japanese Family: Narratives about Individualism and the Postmodern State

Margaret Lock

One has the impression these days when talking to Japanese people, reading their newspapers, watching television, and looking over the vast array of Japanese books on "school refusal syndrome," "apartment neurosis," "the kitchen syndrome," "moving-day depression," sleep disorders, family violence (which refers to children attacking their parents), and so on, that despite its relatively calm and rather opulent exterior, Japan has paid a price for its economic "miracle" in the form of a toll on the health of individual people.

The plethora of syndromes and neuroses said to be of recent origin and thought to abound in the urban centers of Japan are a delight for the news-hungry mass media and are often described as diseases of civilization, *bunmeibyō* (Kyūtoku 1979, 19). Of course Japan has a long history and civilization of its own, but this particular blight is associated with the new postwar "civilization": the Westernized, "high-tech" culture, source of prosperity and material comfort, and typified by urban nuclear family life and a loss of traditional values.

It is well known that Japan now has the second largest economy and the greatest longevity in the world. It also has the most literate population, relatively little poverty, and a long-established socialized medical system. All ingredients for a smoothly running, salubrious society, one would assume, but a glance through a few newspaper headlines tells another story: "More Girls, Housewives Becoming Drug Addicts"; "Schools Reverting to Corporal Punishment"; "More Middle-Aged Men Killing Selves"; "Continuing Fight for Women's Rights"; "Stress: Serious Problem of Japanese Work Force"; "Japanese Youth Unhappiest (among eleven industrial countries polled), in Spite of Economic Growth." This last article concludes by saying that youth are "like a floating generation, without any sense of purpose. *And the real problem lies in the family*" (emphasis added, *Asahi Evening News*, 1984).

The Health and Welfare Ministry of Japan has recently launched a number of projects, including the establishment of counseling services and the introduction of regular public lectures with such titles as "Neurosis and Other Stress-related Problems," in order to combat what they see as the "increasing incidence of mental illness arising from the pressures of modern life-styles." Liaison panels are being formed to improve links between local governments, health centers, educational boards, and mental hospitals, and the Japan Medical Association has pledged its support for these projects (*Mainichi Shinbun*, 1985*a*).

The issue I wish to take up in this essay is the remaking of a cultural identity in postwar Japan, in particular the part that the nuclear family, and most especially the pivotal figure in the family, the mother, is assigned in this endeavor. A postulated relationship between the behavior of family members and their individual physical health is couched in explicitly moralistic terms and forms one part of the cultural debate about identity. Included is a stereotype in which women are said to be vulnerable to experiencing one of several syndromes and neuroses especially associated with their gender. Popular medical and psychological literature contributes to this rhetoric, in which links are made between certain styles of family life, personality traits, interpersonal dynamics, and the occurrence of specific syndromes and neuroses. It is characteristic of this literature that concern is expressed about the effects of modernization, in particular, urbanization, on the health of individuals and families. Among the many changes associated with modernization, two are of particular concern: a loss of contact with nature due to urbanization, and the decline of the *ie*, the traditional extended Japanese family, the seat of moral and religious education.

One of the new diseases of civilization associated with middle-aged women has recently received official recognition. Members of the Japanese gynecological association asked to have the group of symptoms that they label as "climacterium syndrome" included among the list of diseases recognized by the government. Their request was granted, and physicians can therefore receive reimbursement under the socialized medical system for the care and treatment of women placed in this diagnostic category. The following description of the rhetoric associated with menopausal women will be placed within a broader discussion about the modern Japanese family, which in turn is part of the national debate about cultural identity and the place of Japan as an economic and political force in the world today. Results of survey research and interview data are presented in order to demonstrate that there are large discrepancies between the rhetoric broadcast about menopausal women, and their actual experiences during midlife.

The attempt to medicalize menopause and its lack of success to date will also be discussed in order to clarify the relationship between the cultural debate, the interests and concerns of the medical profession, and middle-aged Japanese women. It will be shown that, although popular medical literature in Japan is potentially a powerful tool through which a dominant discourse can be imposed upon selected subjects, there is no neat fit between the rhetoric and the lives of the women it is aimed at. Middle-aged women are well aware of the gist of the argument contained in the rhetoric, which has, therefore, permeated everyday consciousness. However, despite the fact that the literature predicts a difficult time at menopause for many modern Japanese women, and suggests that medical treatment would be of help, its effect so far has been neither to ensure that the majority of women submit themselves to gynecological examinations, nor to stimulate a high rate of reporting of menopausal symptomatology. The mythical menopausal woman bears very little relationship to her living counterparts who, for the most part, do not find this part of the life cycle to be particularly trying.

THE "MEDICALIZATION OF LIFE"

Medicalization has traditionally been depicted in the literature as a process in which the medical community attempts to create a "market" for its services by redefining certain events, behaviors, and problems as diseases (see, for example, Freidson 1970; Illich 1976; Merkin 1976; Zola 1978).[1] The institution of medicine, which serves to legitimize professional knowledge and power, is said to be the agency by which physicians can justify the process of medicalization. According to Zola (1978), the medical profession is "a major institution of control . . . nudging aside law and religion" in which ordinary people lose their rights of control and autonomy over their own lives. He believes that this tendency is reinforced by the haste with which many people bring everyday troubles to the care and attention of a physician.

Studies on medicalization have frequently been criticized for their apparent lack of attention to the fact that both the institution and the practice of medicine itself reflect the social organization of the society in question. This line of argument states that medicine serves to express and reinforce the social relations of society at large including those of class, race, gender, and age (Ehrenreich 1978; Frankenberg 1980; Krauss 1974; Stark 1982). Epidemiological studies have demonstrated that the incidence of distress and illness is reflected in these same social relations.

Among the limitations common to several of the studies cited above has been the assumption that both state and medical interests are monolithic, moved largely by self-interest, and are virtually independent of pressures for change that originate, for example, with the public, out of developments in medical knowledge or technology, or with a new political leadership. A second assumption has been made of a gullible and vulnerable public, lacking in skepticism, willing to sit in doctors' offices and submit readily to medical procedures. Through an analysis of the actual process of medicalization, this essay reveals a gap between the aspirations of possessors of power and knowledge and the patients they seek to produce and act upon; the process is not simply one in which the public is made the passive victim of the latest medical trends.

It has been pointed out that when physical disorder is conceptualized as a biological problem this serves to divert attention from the larger social issues involved (Comaroff 1982; Young 1982). The language of biomedicine, couched in the supposedly neutral terms of science, is theoretically amoral and asocial. The occurrence of disease is assumed to be entirely predictable and explainable with reference to biology, and hence, in principle, all other variables are irrelevant. Biomedicine, therefore, serves in part to maintain a status quo in connection with social relations.

Numerous ethnomedical studies have emphasized that in "traditional" medical practice an understanding of the social and psychological origins of illness is often made use of in diagnosis and therapy (Evans-Pritchard 1937; Janzen 1978; Lewis 1975; Manning and Fabrega 1973), an observation that is also true of some disciplines of modern medicine, most notably psychiatry. There has been a tendency to assume (although not by those cited above) that the broadly conceived, multivariable approach characteristic of traditional medicine is clearly more humanistic, more socially committed, and hence superior to the reductionistic and mechanistic methods said to be typical of biomedicine. The ways in which inequalities in the distribution of power relations are reproduced in the "traditional" therapeutic encounter have, with a few notable exceptions (for example, Glick 1967) been downplayed, and an inclination to romanticize rituals of healing has held sway in anthropology. However, medical explanatory systems of all kinds, biomedical or otherwise, make statements that have bearing on the moral and political order, and establishment medicine, whether it be shamanism or biomedicine, can serve equally to uphold the existing social order.

In the particular case of menopause, it is open to question, I believe, whether an explanation that limits itself to statements about changes in the endocrine system is potentially more or less misleading and reactionary than statements that claim that women in certain social roles and with certain psychological dispositions are at risk for distress (Lock 1982*a*). In Japan, specific social and psychological variables are very frequently cited as causal. Survey research indicates that these statements are erroneous, but they are nevertheless apparently believed by most women. No doubt this causes unhappiness, guilt, and probably enhances physical distress in a vulnerable few; a purely biomedical explanation would be less likely to produce this result. Both the moralistic menopausal rhetoric and a biomedical model of menopause have recently become subjects for much discussion and debate in Japan, partly as a result of the attempt to medicalize this part of the life cycle. So far the debate has functioned principally to subject to scrutiny what had been taken as "common knowledge" and "natural" about middle-aged women. If this trend leads to a heightened awareness of the discrepancy between personal experience and rhetoric, then the medicalization of menopause will have had a dual function of producing a new disease, while at the same time sowing the seeds that ensure that this particular disease category will not be made much use of.

THE GOOD WIFE AND WISE MOTHER

Women are fools, but mothers are wise;
Women are weak, but mothers are strong.
Japanese saying quoted in *Onna no Imeeji (The Image of Women)*

Contemporary Japanese feminists usually trace the origins of the inferior position women have officially occupied throughout much of Japanese history to Shinto ideas of pollution and, of even more importance, to Buddhist doctrine about female inferiority (Uchino 1983). The concept of *danson johi*, the "natural" subjugation of women, is claimed by some to have come originally to Japan by way of India (Hirano 1984). In postwar years the middle-class housewife has become the representative of a "typical" modern Japanese woman and her role is thought to embody *danson johi* along with a second, newer view of women as "homebodies" *(katei seikatsusha)*. This latter image was consciously fostered during the Meiji era at the end of the last century, and is modeled after European ideas current at that time. Until then, the official image of women had been one of a "borrowed womb," a vehicle for the production of offspring to continue the patriline. Over the past one hundred years, that vision has been transformed into one in which the role of nurturing rather than mere fertility has become central. Women have been encouraged to become, within the confines of the domestic sphere, the guardians and educators of their children since, it is claimed, a woman's nature equips her best to nurture others (Nakamura 1976[1875]). The idea of a mothering instinct, *bosei honno*, forms the core of this argument. Popular literature of the Meiji era was replete with articles on how a woman should behave in order to become the ideal "good wife and wise mother" *(ryōsai kenbo)* (Kameda 1984), a subject which is still discussed today in magazines directed at housewives. Meiji women were gradually granted a certain degree of autonomy in the home, largely in order to fulfill their duties as educators of their children. The creation of a homebody role with associated rights and duties has been refined throughout this century, and in postwar years the autonomy associated with this role has become so marked that it is very common for women to regard their husbands as an extra child around the house. In the world at large, however, the majority of women apparently remain subservient, and it is customary to ask permission from one's husband before undertaking any form of activity outside the home, including going to PTA meetings (Higuchi 1985, 55).

Recent surveys indicate that most middle-class women are largely satisfied with their roles as housewives and mothers of two (Kokumin Seikatsu Hakusho 1983; Lebra 1984; White and Moloney 1979), despite the mixed images that are associated with this role, which has disparagingly been described as *san shoku hiru ne tsuki* (implying an easy, permanent job with three meals and a nap thrown in). This negative view is strongly countered by a belief in the value of running a harmonious household, and especially in the nurturing and training of children. Numerous studies have shown that even when a woman does have a role outside the home, the homemaking role is ranked highest in importance (Imamura 1987; Lebra 1984).[2] It is also clear that, even in households with every modern convenience, being a housewife is a much more time-consuming job than it is in the West, largely because of demands that are made upon one's time in connection with children and their schooling (Imamura 1987, 19).

Central to the task of being a housewife is the discipline and early moral training of children. This is expected to be achieved in part by setting up oneself and one's husband as good examples to follow. Appropriate "womanly behavior" (*onna rashiisa*) is partly based, even today, upon rules originally laid down for the wives of samurai. The Confucian-dominated government of premodern Japan encouraged discipline in women, not for military service, but in order that they would practice unquestioning submission and obedience to their husbands. Modern Japanese women were taught by their mothers to believe, like their predecessors in feudal times, that patience, diligence, endurance, even-temperedness, compliance, gentleness, and a positive attitude all contribute to womanliness. A Kobe housewife has this to say on the subject:[3]

> Women have delicacy and gentleness. You know, they have talked about *onna rashiisa* since the old days in Japan, and I think it's best to live in accord with that. Of course there are some women who are special, who can work the same as men, but even they are best at being things like nursery-school teachers and nurses.
>
> Young girls have lost their *onna rashiisa*, they have no consideration for others; equality and freedom are being misinterpreted. They drink and smoke and if you criticize them they say, "It's my body, I can do what I like." But a woman's most important job is bearing and raising children, so their body is not their own; it's meant for leaving descendants.

This woman, in common with many others, prides herself on getting up at 5:30 each day in order to prepare breakfast and elaborate boxed lunches for the family, and she retires to bed at midnight every evening once she has finished clearing up after everyone else. She claims that she never openly expresses an opinion contrary to that of her husband, but she admits that she goes ahead and acts on her own initiative about many things her husband never hears about.

This womanly style of behavior should be accentuated by discipline of the body and feminine language usage (Lebra 1984, 46). The existence of female language forms, associated with gentleness and submissiveness, still goes virtually unquestioned by anyone (Ide 1982). Courteous greetings, good posture, a neat appearance, good manners, elegance in the handling of things, an orderly house, and established routines in one's life-style are all connected with womanly behavior (Lebra 1984, 42). These traditional values are reinforced in the mass media where images of "foolish" young women, who will perhaps eventually become "wise" mothers, are the norm.

> Young, cute, smiling and apparently mute girl-women are on every genre of [TV] program at any hour of the day or night.
> Why does this phenomenon exist? Television personalities reflect the ideals and values of any given society, and the women that appear on television are therefore only "ideal" women. . . . In Japan, women, in order to fit the definition of the ideal woman, must not only be youthful and pretty, but they should also be sweetly silent.
> According to Tomoyo Nonaka, a newscaster . . . "People think of women as flowers and if there were no women on TV it would be a bit bizarre. So they think, 'O.K., let's put a nice flower on the table.'"
> These televised blossoms do not only represent idealized women but they also act out the ideal role between women and men. The reason that these women are not outspoken is that they must be properly deferential towards men. (Itazaka 1984)[4]

The middle-class housewife is associated particularly with several of the syndromes and neuroses of modern Japan, including "the kitchen syndrome" (in which a variety of severe somatic symptoms are experienced every time one enters the kitchen to prepare the evening meal), apartment-living neurosis, childrearing neurosis, menopausal syndrome, and so on. In addition to being "professional" housewives (*sengyōshufu*), women who suffer from these problems are believed to have other things in common, most notably certain personality defects. Menopausal syndrome[5] is described, for example, as a luxury disease (*zeitakubyō*), a problem that occurs in women with too much time on their hands, who are selfish and concerned only with their own pleasures. Women like this are said to lack a real identity (which in Japan is bound up inextricably with one's social role [Lebra 1976]); they have no sense of self (*jibun ga nai*), and are deficient in the willpower, positive attitude, and endurance that was characteristic of their mothers. Such

women, it is said, are likely to raise children who are undisciplined or deviant.
A second set of etiologies associated with physical distress in housewives, including menopausal symptomatology, focuses less on inadequate role playing and more upon personality defects. Women who are "oversocialized," overcontrolled, too concerned about tidiness and order, and of nervous temperament (*shinkeishitsu*) are vulnerable. These women are thought to produce children who suffer from psychosomatic ailments or problems such as "school refusal syndrome" (Lock 1986). The stifling atmosphere they create in the home and its effect on their children is described as follows by one commentator: "The roots of even a healthy plant confined in a pot will rot if given too much water" (Higuchi 1980, 90). When asked if he thought that all women experience trouble at menopause, a Kyoto gynecologist answered this way:

> Not necessarily. Women who are busy, who don't have much leisure don't complain about menopause. It's a sort of luxury disease (*zeitakubyō*), it's "high class" [said in English]. Women with lots of free time are the ones who say it's so bad.

A Tokyo physician had this to say:

> These women have no *ikigai* (purpose in life). They have free time but can't think of anything to do, so they get a psychosomatic reaction; they can't complain openly so they use "organ language" [said in English]. They find that there is no reward today for all their sacrifice and suppression and they're lonely. Working women have fewer symptoms and in any case do not notice them; housewives can't control and master their symptoms like they used to.

A physician who specializes in the practice of traditional herbal medicine focused on family dynamics in addition to individual shortcomings.

> Being in a nuclear family affects women very much. There is no one to teach life's wisdom to the children and everything falls onto the shoulders of the housewife. She often becomes neurotic, obsessed with trying to create a good child. Her husband doesn't talk to her. Also women have changed, they used to *gaman* (persevere, endure), but they've lost all that since women's lib. They have low self-control now.

Japanese physicians debate about whether the physical symptoms that they most readily associate with social and psychological origins such as headaches, shoulder stiffness, and dizziness, for example, are indeed all "true" symptoms of menopause. In contrast, when they discuss changes in endocrine function and in the autonomic nervous system, these changes are said to be clearly menopausal. Of the thirty physicians interviewed, with only one exception, all agreed that the specific hormonal changes associated with menopause make women more vulnerable to distress as they pass through the social transformations characteristic of midlife. They *all* agreed that men have to go through a phase similar to menopause (the term simply means a midlife transition in Japanese), and that they too experience many of the same general symptoms as women. The belief is that whenever the homeostatic mechanisms of the body are out of balance, then one is prone to experience a whole range of somatic symptoms, a loss of balance is likely to occur at times of "stress" (a Japanese term), and that the midlife transition is one such time (Lock 1980). Women are unfortunate because the endocrine changes they undergo put a special toll on the body and increase the likelihood that they will have some physical discomfort that men do not experience. Middle-class housewives are especially unfortunate because the traditional midlife female role is in jeopardy with the rise of the nuclear family, and hence they are more vulnerable to stress.

MIDLIFE AND THE MIDDLE-CLASS WOMAN

It's the forty year olds you have to worry about, they have nothing to do but perfect their game.
Comments by a young woman, member of a Kyoto tennis club, 1984

In 1940 the average age at death of Japanese women was 49.6 years, just seven years after their average youngest child entered school for the first time (Imamura 1987, quoting Foreign Press Center of Japan Statistics 1977), whereas in 1983 life expectancy for Japanese women was 79.78 years (Keizai Koho Center 1984). It is not surprising, therefore, that there was little concern about menopause until recently, and the term that is used to express this concept was created at the turn of the century under the influence of German medicine. It is probably fair to say that an interest in the symptomatology of menopause is largely a postwar phenomenon, although one or two physicians, whose work is clearly indebted to German writing on the topic, took up the subject in the prewar years (Yamada 1927; Furuya 1940).

Not only are virtually all Japanese women living through what has now come to be described as middle age, but the present generation of forty-five to fifty-five year olds are the first postwar group of women to reach this stage in the life cycle who will for the most part live out their days in a two-person household with their husbands. Whereas the average household size in the 1940s was 4.98, by 1980 it had decreased to 3.33 (Fukutake 1982, 124). This particular group of women, who were raised before and during the war, were usually steeped in traditional values as children, but they have taken part in the rapid transformation of their society into one in which there is a constant debate about individualism, and where urbanization has changed from its earlier "villagelike" model (Dore 1958), into one in which there are more metropolis-like centers characteristic of *Gesellschaft* (Fukutake 1982).

These women are the first generation who have no obvious role once they become middle-aged: their extended family tasks as conveyor of a cultural tradition, minder of children, extra farmhand, or store-minder no longer exist. As younger women, their community involvement was in all probability limited to PTA work. Imamura's research shows that women at this midlife stage see themselves as "shut in" and experience problems of isolation: "They feel their usefulness to society is gone, through no fault of their own, and they blame society" (Imamura 1987, 87). Housewives expect under these circumstances to have physical problems.

> My family doctor told me to take up another hobby when I went to see him complaining about headaches. He said it was my menopause and that I needed to do something with my time. I'm tired of flower arranging and tea ceremony—that's for young girls who have to catch a husband. I tried doing water colors for a time. . . . My life has no purpose. My sole job is to look after my husband but he's never at home and anyway we just avoid talking to each other. I thought about going out to work, but I can't do anything, and anyway it doesn't look right if a professor's wife works.

Both women and physicians believe that because middle-class women have time on their hands they are less likely to be able to practice the self-control that is necessary to avoid or ignore the physical symptoms associated with menopause. Lack of a clear social role, basic to the development and maintenance of individual identity in Japan, is considered to be the major contributory factor to trouble at menopause, and is cited much more often as causal than is sadness about the end of fertility, concern about loss of sexuality, or even fears about aging and death.

Ambiguities associated with this time in the life cycle are layered one upon another: hard work, perseverance, and self-discipline are valued; but running a small modern household where one's husband is absent most of the time does not require of these virtues. Nevertheless, women are said to be the pillar of the family (and apparently accept this image [DeVos and Wagatsuma 1959; Lock 1982*b*]); they should, therefore, devote themselves fully to the care of family members. However, many agree that today they become bored and lonely in a nuclear family; but seeking employment outside the home for middle-class women is unseemly and unnecessary (Imamura 1987, 47). Frequently these contradictions are summed up by saying that housewives are victims of modernization and of the isolation inherent in the nuclear family; they have been pushed into a structural position that actually encourages selfishness and unwomanly behavior. The anomalous position that middle-aged women find themselves in is, however, just one part of a much bigger story, a nagging concern about the "health" of the nation at large and all its people. This larger issue will be discussed briefly in order to set into context the debate about middle-aged women.

MODERNIZATION AND MORAL PANIC

An ark drifting alone an a rough sea is an apt metaphor for the contemporary [Japanese] family.
                    Keiko Higuchi, "Changing Family Relationships"

Unlike most societies undergoing industrialization today, Japan was able to orchestrate its own entry into the international market and its acceptance or rejection of values and commodities perceived to be foreign and threatening to traditional order. This relatively gradual transformation since the middle of the last century was brought to an abrupt halt by defeat at the end of World War II and the ensuing economic and spiritual crises.

After an initial period of numbed shock, there followed for the next twenty years or so what appeared superficially to be an all-out embrace of Western values, including the idea that the nuclear family is the "natural" primary unit for modern times and that individual rights and freedom should be given much more consideration than was formerly the case. These ideas were congenial at that time since traditional group-oriented values were thought to be responsible for the nationalistic regime that had brought Japan to its crushing defeat and crippling poverty.

Today, Japan finds itself in an embarrassingly strong economic position in the world, so much so that it is at times driven to accusing other capitalist societies of laziness. However, numerous books and articles, many of them written by foreigners, claim that Japan's "economic miracle" was in fact based upon a mobilization of traditional values (Dore 1973; Vogel 1979) and not upon a Western-derived ethos, and it is now generally accepted that modernization does not by definition necessarily involve an abandonment of tradition. Shattered postwar egos have been glued together, national confidence restored, and the dominant theme in the current internal cultural debate (Parkin 1978) is a search for a modern, uniquely Japanese identity, in which traditional values figure prominently and the dry rot of individualism is firmly contained. The government, including the former prime minister, have been active and very visible participants in this debate (Pyle 1987).

Being part of a culture infused with a tradition of self-reflection and introspection, the Japanese have themselves cast this rhetoric into a genre known as *nihonjinron*: essays on being Japanese. Ideas about the concept of self, the relationship of individuals to the family and to the state, and about health and illness are all central in this literature.

At the core of *nihonjinron* is a concept of racial (genetic) homogeneity, which leads "naturally" to language and cultural unity. The line between insiders and outsiders is sharply delineated and notions of separateness, uniqueness, and of certain irreducible "essences" that make one Japanese are taken for granted. This type of rhetoric is not unique to the Japanese, of course, nor is it new to Japan (it has been traced back to at least the early eighteenth century [Kawamura 1980]), but the specific way in which the uniqueness is defined and redefined, the "invention of tradition" (Hobsbawm and Ranger 1983), changes through time, and is recast around topical themes that provoke anxiety. Almost seven hundred monographs in a thirty-two-year period have been officially identified as part of this genre, and, if journal articles are added to this number, the total must be many thousands (Befu 1983).

The outpouring of *nihonjinron* represents a state that Cohen (1972, 28), writing about Britain, has termed a "moral panic," when, during times of social and political unrest, self-appointed public moralists air their views about the supposed breakdown of morality and the collapse of social control in the media, courtrooms, and in popular literature.

Contemporary observers believe that the recent internationalization of Japan has precipitated this current crisis of national identity on a massive scale (Befu 1983; Mouer and Sugimoto 1983). Paradoxically, it has provoked a response of a reassertion of uniqueness, coupled with a marked increase in a sense of national self-esteem, which has been demonstrated statistically and published in government documents entitled, "The Survey of the National Character," which are carried out every five years (Hayashi et al. 1975).

Winston Davis (1983) has noted five characteristics of *nihonjinron*. First, the uniqueness of Japan is assumed, and pure fantasy or random data is cited to demonstrate its specific characteristics. One example is the story, which virtually everybody I asked in Japan knew well, about the differences between Japanese mothers and Western mothers when they are attacked by a big bear while out with their child. The Western mother puts her child behind her and faces the bear aggressively, while the Japanese mother turns her back on the bear and shelters her child by drawing it to her breast and encircling it with her arm. This is cited as an example of the way in which masculine principles dominate in the "West," while feminine ones dominate in Japan (Kawai 1976).

Second, the Japanese essence is usually summed up by a broad appellation: recent examples are the society of protean man, or moratorium man; the maternal society; the society of the everlasting child; the hollow onion; the vertical society. Lists of characteristic attributes common to the entire genre are created under these headings: Japanese are hard-working, tenacious, persevering; they understand one another best by nonverbal communication; they foster dependent relationships with one another; harmonious interpersonal relationships are valued above all; they have a vertically structured society where groups and not individuals are of prime importance.

Third, no sampling procedures are used in creating these images, which despite the recurrence of certain themes, are ambiguous and vague. *Nihonjinron* is not designed for dissection and debate; on the contrary, it is like a collection of "Just-So" stories. Authors take an openly moralistic stance, and the litany of who the Japanese are becomes, at the same time, a broadsheet for how one *should* behave. Fourth, *Nihonjinron* functions as a "civil" religion; no one can escape its pull, and it serves to provide a legitimation of modern Japanese society. Last, frequent exposure to other cultures stimulates an author to produce his version of "theory Japan" (this genre is almost completely male dominated).

The sociologists Mouer and Sugimoto state that "one might simply dismiss the literature [of *nihonjinron*] except for the heavy involvement of the academic community and of the political and business establishment in promoting such images not only at home but abroad." They point out the similarity between contemporary rhetoric and that of prewar Japanese nationalism, and also indicate how it tends to become a self-fulfilling prophecy, and hence serves the interests of various elites in preserving the status quo.

Although well-known people from all walks of life contribute to *nihonjinron*, popular medical literature is particularly prominent in this genre. One of the best known is the work of a Jungian psychiatrist, Hayao Kawai (1976), entitled *The Pathology of Japan's Maternal Society* (which includes the story of the big bear). In it Kawai states that reform or rebellion is essentially futile since one can never escape the lap of the "Great Mother," the eternal feminine principle of Japan: a profoundly conservative vision that is typical of most variations of *nihonjinron*.

Another is a best-seller entitled *Bogenbyō* (Illness Caused by Mother), in which the author states that mothers were formerly good at childrearing, but in the past twenty years they have become very poor at it. Industrialization has, he says, distorted the "natural childrearing instinct" into something that satisfies the mother's "narcissistic ego" but does not produce a healthy child. Mothers are described as too bossy or too overprotective (Kyūtoku 1979).

It is characteristic of this type of medical literature to indicate that people just one generation ago, that is, those raised in prewar Japan, were stronger in spirit and physically tougher. Modernization, the "thinness" of traditional values, poor junk-food diets, and so on have, it is alleged, combined to produce a nation of weaklings suffering from mental and physical pathologies of all kinds (Ikemi and Ikemi 1982; Iino 1980; Kyūtoku 1979).

Nihonjinron tends to focus on what is uniquely Japanese, but comparisons, either latent or explicit, are also very evident. Traditional Japan, a group-oriented society, is contrasted with the individualism thought to be characteristic of Western societies. It is also contrasted with Westernized, modernized, and urbanized Japan (Moeran 1984), in which the nuclear family is usually selected out for special critical attention. It then takes only a small conceptual leap to account for the "stress" and plethora of "neuroses" that medical practitioners, traditional and modern, report as rampant and on the increase in the workplace, schools, and the home. This is accomplished by conjuring up the spectres of modernization, the nuclear family, individualism, selfishness, and a lack of group spirit, tenacity, and endurance, which are thought to be the source of "the increasing incidence of mental illness arising from the pressures of modern life" (*Mainichi Shinbun* 1985*a*).

THE "PATHOLOGICAL FAMILY"

Today the home is expected to provide an environment for the pursuit of personal happiness. It has to be an enjoyable place promising happiness to each individual member of the family. We should be thankful that the home has been transformed from a place of strict control to a place for the pursuit of happiness. Yet, should the home be considered a panacea promising complete happiness? Both the government and the public seem to think that all is well if home life is stable. We should rather be aware of the danger of becoming preoccupied with family happiness, for this may divert our attention from the problems of society, which underlies the family. (Higuchi 1980, 93)

Part of the recent debate in Japan has been devoted to the question of whether a new national holiday known as "family day" should be instituted. Those supporting the campaign complain that despite a "healthy" economy, the "spiritual health" of the country is poor (Mochida 1980). The traditional household, the corporate unit known as the *ie*, has certainly been eroded almost beyond recognition, largely because of a decline in the rural population and a rise of urban nuclear families living in a confined space. Throughout the feudal period in Japan the *ie* became established as a distinct unit among the privileged classes, but with democratization instituted by the Meiji government (1869–1912) the ideology associated with the *ie* became generally accepted throughout Japan, including the concept that the *ie* is the most fundamental of social units and that individuals should be totally identified with and subordinated to it. The economic function of the *ie* has always been of prime importance, but apart from this function it is also the center of religious activities, since the ancestors are enshrined there and *ie* members are in regular communication with them. The *ie* is, therefore, a source of moral and spiritual education (Smith 1974, 151), the training of which is inculcated in young members by their parents, who make use of the presence of the ancestors to legitimize their authority beyond mere parental rights into a sacred mission. The participation of both parents is thought to be essential in order to provide a balanced training, but while the role of the mother demands her complete attention and active physical presence, that of the father can be performed in large part in absentia; his dedication to his various social tasks is pointed out (usually by his wife) as a good example to be emulated.

A small research project presented on Japanese television a couple of years ago showed children living in Korea, Taiwan, and Japan, who were asked to draw a picture of the evening meal in their family. The majority of the Korean and Taiwanese depicted a family sitting together around the dinner table, but many of the Japanese children drew a single child holding a bowl of instant noodles sitting in front of the television set. These results reinforced the idea, already present in the minds of many Japanese, that the nuclear family is in danger: a family with no core, where "all its members are turned away from one another," as one educational administrator put it (Lock 1986).

Compared with the *ie*, the nuclear household, lacking in enshrined ancestors and composed of distinct individuals, is often characterized as a fragile, "pathological" system, in which sexual equality, liberalization of parent-child relations, and egalitarian inheritance laws have disrupted the traditional forms of control, leading to the deviance that is said to be rampant in modern Japan (Mochida 1980). Other analysts disagree, among them Yuzawa (1980), a psychologist at the Tokyo Family Court, who uses statistical analyses to support his point that a "pathological evolution of the Japanese family" has not taken place in recent years. He states that the mass media, by giving undue coverage to deviancy, divorce, and so on, has convinced the Japanese public that the family is an "ailing" system. He believes the reverse to be true: "The family has thrown off the shackles of the traditional family system, freed itself from poverty, and eliminated inhuman relationships" (1980, 85).

Like many women, Keiko Higuchi, a sociologist, does not have so rosy a view. She is very concerned about absent fathers, the school system, and especially about the isolation of women, who are held responsible for any failures in their children and because their "very love" is being criticized as the source of the child's problems (1980, 90). She believes that too great a burden is being placed upon the family at the expense of examining the goals of society at large.

The basic ingredients in the discussion of the modern Japanese family and its members are accepted by virtually everyone: changing demography, urbanization, loss of contact with "nature," limitations of space in the Japanese archipelago, postwar reform of the family system, the rise of the nuclear family, and the widespread acceptance in theory of the concept of individualism. These ingredients are combined to create various discourses, some of which consider the family in a positive light but, more often, and particularly in official documents and the mass media, the family is viewed as ailing and in need of help. One version or another of *nihonjinron* is almost inevitably drawn upon in order to buttress arguments for the ailing family.

Medical practitioners, traditional and modern, have both responded to and helped to create this unruly rhetoric, which includes statements about each family member.

THE "ABSENT FATHER"

It is usual in Japan today for businessmen to be transferred at the whim of their companies all over the country for extended periods of time, often several years. This phenomenon is on the rise and is thought to be the result of the customary lifetime employment system. It is believed that the chance of promotion will be lost should one refuse to move.

The family with an absent father has become a central theme in the rhetoric produced about the modern Japanese family that is frequently summed up in the phrase *otōsan no kage wa usui* (father's shadow is thin), implying that he does not exert paternalistic discipline over his family.

> Are the fathers of Japan the men they ought to be? The government seems to be having doubts.
>
> In a new guide for parents of three-year-olds, authorized by the Health and Welfare Ministry . . . fathers are urged to take a more independent role in the upbringing of their children to demonstrate their masculinity and to teach them to be brave and strong-minded.
>
> The new guide apparently stems from anxiety about recent social changes within the Japanese family structure which have made father only a fleeting figure if not nonexistent, and where not father but mother "knows best."
>
> An overdominance [sic] of the mother in the child's upbringing, experts fear, is leading to the "feminization" of Japan, since many children are growing up without sufficient masculine influence to provide the balance they need. (*Mainichi Shinbun* 1985*b*).

Other articles feature the working life of Japanese men: a report on a cross-cultural survey reveals that, comparatively speaking, Japanese are "worker bees" and that many put work before their homes. Training on the job it is said produces "company-centered people" (*Mainichi Shinbun* 1983*a*), particularly when employees can be subjected to all-night training sessions (*Mainichi Shinbun* 1983*b*). "Stress" at work is thought to be severe because of the lifetime employment and seniority system used in Japan in which everyone is advanced up the ladder to executive jobs. According to one psychiatrist, "Sober, diligent but mediocre managers" who possess a "weak character and have few hobbies, [who] do not drink with colleagues after hours nor play mah-jongg or golf during weekends" are particularly vulnerable to physical ailments (*Japan Times* 1984). When surveyed, 72.8 percent of male workers reported that they suffered from "nervous tension" (*Mainichi Shinbun* 1983*c*). "Stress-related ailments" include vomiting, heart attacks, loss of appetite, rheumatism, impotence, insomnia, and depression: the leading cause of these ailments is cited as overwork (*Mainichi Shinbun* 1985*c*).

The Japanese salary man is frequently depicted in comics today as a sad figure fit only for ridicule (Skinner 1979), disciplined by his employers for the life of a worker bee, and labeled as incompetent as a husband and father. Largely because of his temporal and spatial removal from his family, the shadow of controlled samurai masculinity as a model for future generations has certainly worn thin.

THE "CEREBRAL CHILD"

Prekindergarten Institutions Flourish

A group of one-year-olds is seated on tiny chairs made just for them, their faces showing dazzlement as they listen attentively to their teacher.

These toddlers, barely weaned, are attending a prekindergarten tutoring institution. They take to school not books and pencil boxes but bottles and diapers.

"There are many children still on the waiting list . . ." the chief instructor said . . . the institution teaches mainly three things to the children: basic manners in a group, cultivating memory, and creativity. (*Japan Times Weekly* 1985)

Japanese education is theoretically designed today to be egalitarian. It is possible for a child from the most humble of families to enter the best universities, and this does in fact happen at times. The majority of children go to public schools where everyone in the same age-grade proceeds at exactly the same pace; there is no streaming or acceleration of students, and textbooks, course materials, and examinations are standardized by the Ministry of Education. Despite this standardization, some schools are known to have better academic success than others. University places are limited, and in 1980, for example, 58 percent of high school seniors decided to apply for advanced education and it was estimated that only one in four succeeded at the first attempt in finding a place in college or university (Rohlen 1980). A financially rewarding career is virtually guaranteed if one graduates from one of the better public or private universities. These universities select a large proportion of incoming students from those high schools best known for their academic successes, which in turn draw upon middle and primary schools with which they have close affiliations. In some cases primary schools take the majority of their students from what have come to be known as elite kindergartens. It now appears that a privileged adult life with a good income can be secured by attending the right pre-kindergarten (see the quotation above). Of course, this jostling for material success can only be assured finally if one passes the required examinations, regardless of the school one attends, but one's chances are greatly increased by starting early training in one of the educational institutions known for its successes and then being passed through the relatively secure conduit from one academically re- nowned school to another, to the opened gates of the best universities. The education system therefore creates a paradox: a fiercely competitive system, which is said to be based upon principles of equality.

An Ad Hoc Council on Education formed during 1984 calls for basic re- form in the Japanese educational system. It recommends that the "fostering of individuality" in students should be a key to the reform process (*Mainichi Shinbun* 1985*d*). Recently, serious discipline problems have been acknowl- edged in many middle and high schools, and the media has documented cases of delinquency, violence, bullying, and vandalism with increasing reg- ularity. A resumption of corporal punishment has been reported simul- taneously with the increase in school disruption (*Mainichi Shinbun* 1983*d*).

The Ministry of Education, teachers, and parents have all stated at var- ious times that intense competition in the school system is partly to blame for the perceived breakdown in discipline. Rohlen sums up contemporary Japanese education very bluntly:

> The facts of life are that competition decides success and that all Japanese want educational success because it leads to better employment, higher status and more power. Society is seen as "naturally" hierarchical, but the top is open to those who through special effort struggle upward. Opportunities narrow radi- cally with time, however, and closure comes early. . . . No rationalization about individual freedom or equal opportunity or the joys of childhood changes this fact. (1980, 235)

Japanese physicians claim that there has been a dramatic rise in postwar years in the incidence of "psychosomatic" complaints in children, including asthma, ulcers, and heart disease (Ikemi et al. 1980). These illnesses are attributed most frequently to urbanization, the weakness of "character" of the children, lack of group spirit, changing family dynamics, and especially to the behavior of mothers, but it is also acknowledged that pressures in the school system could conceivably have a poor effect on health. The phe- nomenon of "school refusal syndrome" in which middle-school children stay at home in their beds for extended periods of time is also a cause of consider- able national concern and thought to have the same origins as psychosomatic illnesses (Lock 1986).

Contradictions are rife in connection with each member of the nuclear family. While the purported stress associated with a "modern" life is ac- knowledged in connection with the respective roles of salary man, housewife, and schoolchild, at the same time it is generally agreed by those commenting on the nuclear family and the illnesses associated with it that it is those family members who do not uphold traditional values who are particularly

vulnerable to distress, and that these people help to create a family environment that is not conducive to good health. While all members of the family
are to some extent responsible, it is the pivotal member of the family, the
mother, who is most explicitly to blame, since she is held accountable for the
health and care of husband and children and, in addition, is also responsible
for the formation of the moral character and behavior of her children (Hendry 1986; Lock 1987). During the earlier parts of her life cycle, the "inept"
and "selfish" mother of an urban nuclear family is associated with health
problems related to childrearing and the running of a household: she is
"at risk" for "childrearing neurosis," "high-rise apartment neurosis," "the
kitchen syndrome," and "moving-day syndrome." As the family gets older
and the woman is left with no acknowledged work other than the caretaking
of her husband, she becomes particularly susceptible, it is believed, to menopausal syndrome, which is associated with a lack of role rather than a failure
to carry one out.

RHETORIC AND "REALITY": DISJUNCTIONS BETWEEN BELIEF AND THE BODY

It has been pointed out by Kelly that the New Middle Class (which over 90
percent of Japanese when surveyed claim to belong) is in fact a "folk sociology" (1986, 605) in which a "new glossy projection of a socially and physically nuclear unit of ricewinner husband, homemaker housewife, and two
samurai-student children; full-time, lifetime, large organization employment
(*sarariiman*) has become the workplace norm: and mass public education,
relentlessly meritocratic and entrance exam oriented, now links home and
work, child and adult" (1986, 604).

That the majority of people do not, despite their claims to the contrary,
participate in the New Middle Class is very evident: over 50 percent of married women work (Cook and Hayashi 1980). It is estimated that 68 percent of
the elderly, many of whom are bedridden, live with their children (Higuchi
1985, 53), only between 30 and 40 percent of workers have lifetime employment benefits, and only about half the younger population succeeds in
obtaining a place in a college (Rohlen 1980). As Higuchi puts it, "Hidden
behind the superficial glamour . . . the prewar family system lives grimly on"
(1985, 53).

While statistics indicate that the incidence of illnesses of all kinds is on the
increase in Japan, it is impossible at the moment to assess if this is due to
changes in the health care system, physician attitudes, the number of physician visits, or in actual health status. It is also difficult to ascertain if certain
types of illnesses are especially associated with people living in "typical"
nuclear families. The results of the cross-sectional survey I carried out with
over 1,700 women between ages 45 and 55 reveal very clearly, however, that

while, comparatively speaking, Japanese women report very few symptoms at menopause, it is the "professional housewives" who report the fewest among three occupational subsamples. Women working on and running farms and women working in factories report more symptoms than do housewives, despite their shared stereotype to the contrary (Lock, Kaufert, and Gilbert 1988). Neither are housewives more likely to visit a physician in connection with midlife changes than are women with other occupations. Only 12 percent of the entire sample had visited a gynecologist in the past two years even though 53 percent reported that they were going through menopause; less than one-third of this group were housewives. Only 2 percent of the entire sample had taken prescribed estrogen replacement therapy (the usual medication given by gynecologists for "menopausal syndrome" in the last two weeks, and only 3.2 percent had taken prescribed tranquilizers.

It seems, therefore, that there is a large discrepancy between the rhetoric used in connection with menopause and the subjective experience of middle-aged women. It is remarkable how little the rhetoric is subjected to questioning, and this is perhaps due to the fact that it is just one part of the much larger, oft-repeated mythology about the nuclear family, modernization, and the loss of traditional values that many middle-aged women, together with the majority of Japanese, appear to accept as reality.

MEDICALIZATION OF MENOPAUSE

The attempt to medicalize menopause seems to be a response on the part of the medical profession to two principal factors: first, an influence from American and European professional literature in which menopause is portrayed as either a deficiency disease or a syndrome treatable, it is said, by physicians; and second, a reduction in gynecological business in Japan. Japanese gynecologists in private practice are usually also practicing obstetricians. They obtain most of their income from three sources: obstetrics, performing abortions, and prescribing medication. Two of these sources have declined recently: Japanese women now usually opt to have their babies in large hospitals with full technological backing, and birth control is more widely practiced through the use of contraception than by means of abortion, as was formerly the case (Coleman 1983). There is, therefore, considerable incentive for gynecologists in private practice to create new sources of income, and the promotion of the concept of menopausal syndrome and associated counseling for distressed women are recent innovations.

That women with no well-defined role are an anomaly in a society dominated by the work ethic is clearly a further incentive for attempted medical intervention. Flourishing middle-aged women who play tennis every day, make plastic flowers, and decorate cubes of sugar with delicate traceries of pink icing for their European-style tea represent a national wastage and are a cause for great concern; because of changes in living arrangements, these women have been forced into a structural position where they cannot participate properly as Japanese citizens. Since it is believed that a healthy body can only be fully maintained through an active cultivation of one's assigned social role, it is not surprising that middle-aged women are regarded as likely candidates for distress and ill health.

Despite the incentives, professional, financial, and cultural, to create a medical problem out of menopause, by no means do all gynecologists participate in this trend. Some regard it as essentially a social problem, and although they are often very sympathetic with the women involved, they believe that it is a matter into which physicians should not be drawn. Others are already too busy with a thriving practice in which surgery, for example, is central. Among those physicians who do have an interest in the problems, some choose to focus on research-related issues and "experiment" (legally) with the administration of hormone therapy to patients; these physicians use an essentially biomedical model in which social dimensions of the problem do not loom large. Others choose to add counseling to their repertoire and turn over two afternoons a week to this activity for a small fee. At least one physician, who has an interest in spiritual matters, has set up a shrine beside his clinic where women can pray to the souls of the fetuses they have aborted, since both he and his patients believe that guilt in connection with abortions causes trouble at menopause.

In the process of making menopause into a disease, therefore, representatives of the institution of medicine do not act uniformly, neither do they necessarily act only in their own self-interest. Nevertheless, a considerable number of physicians have taken it upon themselves to write about and publicize menopause. Some of this literature is highly stigmatizing to middle-aged women since it lists supposed personality defects and an inadequate life-style as causing physical distress at menopause, and it is frequently suggested in this type of literature that professional help is the only satisfactory way to resolve one's problems. Moreover, statements of a similar nature, referring not only to menopause but to a wide range of "new illnesses" appear in the general literature of *nihonjinron*. In this type of writing, explicit links are made among the bodies politic, social, and physical, and the ills of today are contrasted with an idealized, nostalgic image of traditional Japan and its people. Thus far, however, the effect has not been to encourage women to seek out help in great numbers. In contrast, what appears to be slowly gaining momentum is the creation of self-help and discussion groups by women in which the contemporary problems associated with middle age in Japan are discussed in detail.

The popularity of tennis-playing among middle-aged women has not passed unnoticed by the conservative government in Japan. Defense and the aging society are pressing issues, and there is a perceived need to increase revenues, but an unwillingness to upset the business world by raising taxes. In their recent report based on the findings of the special Commission on Administrative Reform, the Liberal Democrats put forward their plans for the new "Japanese Style Welfare State," in which it is suggested that a return to the *ie* should be considered (McCormack 1984). At the heart of the modern *ie* will be the Japanese housewife, no longer free to play tennis, her hands full, providing social services for her extended family (and hence avoiding government expenditure). She will look after her aged parents-in-law until they die, provide care for any family member with a chronic illness or a disability, practice frugal home economics, and produce savings to supplement meager old-age pensions. In short, she will become, once again, the "good wife and wise mother" of turn-of-the-century Japan, who endures the unendurable, controls her emotions, does not express selfish desires, is fully occupied with caring for the family, and hence is not troubled by petty illnesses and complaints such as menopausal symptoms; nor will she have the time or inclination to seek work outside the home. Once this paragon is reinstated, the body politic, it is believed, will be in better shape and the "English Disease" (that is, a welfare state) will have been avoided. The elderly and the sick will be taken care of, while at the same time, in one ingenious move, middle-class women will continue to stay out of the permanent work force, which will therefore remain in a relatively stable state with little unemployment.

CONCLUSION

The cultural construction of "menopausal syndrome" in Japan is a comparatively haphazard affair: refractions created out of snippets taken from an idealized history of the nation, from medical mythology originating in the West, from current concerns over the future direction of Japanese society and the economy and, in particular, its international image, and from more local concerns about the lack of a role for middle-aged women. Paradoxically, although it makes reference to physical discomfort, virtually none of this rhetoric is grounded in the biological transformations that take place in connection with midlife and the natural process of aging (Lock 1986). Moreover, this rhetoric touches the lives of only a few Japanese women directly.

With some notable exceptions (Aoki 1982), very few Japanese women question what Western observers regard as their second-class citizenship. By far the majority believe that the work of running a household and raising children is not only indispensable but of outstanding importance. Furthermore, to many middle-class women who have the freedom to make a choice about participation in the work force, there does not appear to be anything very inviting about the punishing work routines that most Japanese men endure. The effectiveness with which the female body is still "disciplined" to accept its assigned place in Japanese society must also contribute to an outward acceptance of the status quo. There are, nevertheless, some signs of unrest. The divorce rate of middle-aged women is soaring (Madoka 1982), for example, and there is a small but active feminist movement.

It would be premature to draw any firm conclusions, but the heightening awareness in connection with menopause, stimulated to a large degree by the attempt to medicalize the problem, appears to have functioned to break down some of the isolation experienced by women living in urban environments in Japan. Where formerly public meetings of women were most frequently in connection with children, their health, and education, now in addition women have begun to discuss their own problems. Health and female biology are ostensibly the subject of such meetings, but they often turn into a forum for debate about family relationships, social roles, and even politics. It may be that medicalization can serve indirectly as a means for the heightening of political consciousness. If, through discussion, it is gradually revealed that both the biomedical and the psychosocial explanations for distress at menopause are mythologies that women are inappropriately encouraged to adopt as natural and inevitable, then, in the long run, medicalization will not have been all bad.

ACKNOWLEDGMENTS

The research on which this paper is based was supported by a grant from the Social Sciences and Humanities Research Council of Canada (grant no. 410-83-0175 R-1).

NOTES

1. The "medicalization of life" is an expression coined by Ivan Illich and first used in his book *Medical Nemesis* (1976).

2. Interviews conducted by the author in 1984 with thirty women running farms in Nagano prefecture produced contrary evidence. Since these women are farm managers, they believe this role to be crucial to the survival of the family and rank it above homemaking and childrearing.

3. The quotations cited in this paper were obtained from open-ended interviews conducted in 1984 with 150 Japanese women in their homes; one-third are housewives, one-third have rural occupations, and one-third work in factories.

4. The *Mainichi Shinbun* is a daily newspaper, one of three with the largest circulations in Japan.

5. This information was obtained from fifteen gynecologists, fifteen general practitioners, and six practitioners of traditional medicine whom I interviewed in 1983–1984, and from popular literature and articles written by medical practitioners.

REFERENCES

Aoki, Yayohi
  1982   *Josei: Sono Sei no Shinwa* (*Women: the myths about their sex*). Tokyo: Origin
            Shuppan Senta.
Asahi Evening News
  1984   Japanese youth unhappiest, in spite of economic growth: poll. 22
            February.
Befu Harumi
  1983   Internationalization of Japan and Hihon Bunkaron. In *The Challenge of
            Japan's Internationalization: Organization and Culture*, ed. H. Mannari and
            H. Befu. Tokyo: Kwansei Gakuin University.
Cohen, Stan
  1972   *Folk Devils and Moral Panics: The Creation of Mods and Rockers*. London:
            MacGibbon and Kee.
Coleman, Samuel
  1983   *Family Planning in Japanese Society: Traditional Birth Control in a Modern
            Urban Culture*. Princeton: Princeton University Press.
Comaroff, Jean
  1982   Medicine: symbol and ideology. In *The Problem of Medical Knowledge*, ed.
            P. Wright and A. Treacher. Edinburgh: Edinburgh University Press.
Cook, Alice, and Hiroko Hayashi
  1980   *Working Women in Japan: Discrimination, Resistance, and Reform*. Ithaca: Cor-
            nell International Industrial and Labor Relations Report No. 10.
Davis, Winston
  1983   The hollow onion: the secularization of Japanese civil religion. In *The
            Challenge of Japan's Internationalization: Organization and Culture*, ed. H.
            Mannari and H. Befu. Tokyo: Kwansei Gakuin University.
DeVos, G., and H. Wagatsuma
  1959   Psychocultural significance of concern over death and illness among ru-
            ral Japanese. *International Journal of Social Psychiatry* 5: 5–19.
Dore, Ronald
  1958   *City Life in Japan*. Berkeley, Los Angeles, London: University of Califor-
            nia Press.
  1973   British factory and Japanese factory: the origins of national diversity. In
            Industrial Relations. Berkeley, Los Angeles, London: University of Califor-
            nia Press.
Ehrenreich, John
  1978   *The Cultural Crisis of Modern Medicine*. New York: Monthly Review Press.
Evans-Pritchard, E. E.
  1937   *Witchcraft, Oracles and Magic among the Azande*. Oxford: Clarendon.
Frankenburg, Ronald
  1980   Medical anthropology and development: a theoretical perspective. *Social
            Science and Medicine Bulletin* 14: 197–207.
Freidson, Elliot
  1970   *Profession of Medicine*. New York: Dodd and Mead.

Fukutake, Tadashi
    1982   *The Japanese Social Structure: Its Evolution in the Modern Century.* Tokyo: University of Tokyo Press.

Furuya, Kiyoshi
    1940   General advice for examining women in menopause. *Chiryō oyobi shohō* 21: 35–38.

Glick, Leonard
    1967   Medicine as an ethnographic category: the Gimi of the New Guinea Highlands. *Ethnology* 6: 31–56.

Hayashi, Chikio, et al.
    1975   *Nihonjin no Kokuminsei (The national character of the Japanese).* Tokyo: Tōkei Sūri Kenkyujō Kokuminsei Chōsa Iinkai.

Hendry, Joy
    1986   *Becoming Japanese: The World of the Pre-School Child.* Manchester: Manchester University Press.

Higuchi, Keiko
    1980   Changing family relationships. *Japan Echo* 7: 86–93.
    1985   Women at home. *Japan Echo* 12: 51–57.

Hirano, Tankako
    1984   Gendai no Joseikan (The present-day image of women). In *Onna no Imeeji* (The image of women), ed. Joseigaku Kenkyūkai. Tokyo: Keisō Shobō.

Hobsbawm, Eric, and Terence Ranger
    1983   *The Invention of Tradition.* Cambridge: Cambridge University Press.

Ide, S.
    1982   Japanese sociolinguistics, politeness and women's language. *Lingua* 57: 357–385.

Iino, S.
    1980   *Tōkōkyohi no kokufukuhō.* Tokyo: Bunrishoin.

Ikemi, Y., and A. Ikemi
    1982   Some psychosomatic disorders in Japan in a cultural perspective. *Journal of Psychotherapy and Psychosomatics* 38: 231–238.

Ikemi, Yujiro, Yukihiro Ago, Shunji Nakagawa, et al.
    1980   Psychosomatic mechanism under social changes in Japan. In *Biopsychosocial Health*, ed. S. B. Day, F. Lolas, and M. Kusinitz. New York: International Foundation for Biosocial Development and Human Health.

Illich, Ivan
    1976   *Medical Nemesis: The Expropriation of Health.* New York: Pantheon.

Imamura, Anne
    1987   *Urban Japanese Housewives: At Home and in the Community.* Honolulu: University of Hawaii Press.

Itazaka, Kikuko
    1984   The main dish—sweet and silent. *Mainichi Shinbun.* 26 November.

Janzen, John M.
    1978   *The Quest for Therapy in Lower Zaire.* Berkeley, Los Angeles, London: University of California Press.

Japan Times
1984   Employment, seniority systems cause mental depression. 16 February.
Japan Times Weekly
1985   Pre-kindergarten institutions flourish. 14 December.
Kameda, Atsuko
1984   Shūzoku ni Miru Joseikan (Conventional images of women). In *Onna no Imeeji* (The image of women), ed. Joseigaku Kenkyūkai. Tokyo: Keisō Shobō.
Kawai, Hayao
1976   *Bosei shakai Nihon no byōri* (The pathology of Japan's maternal society) Tokyo: Chūō Kōrō, N.
1980   The historical background of arguments emphasizing the uniqueness of Japanese society. *Social Analysis* 5/6: 44–46.
Keizai Koho Center
1984   *Japan 1983: An International Comparison.* Tokyo.
Kelly, William
1986   Rationalization and nostalgia: cultural dynamics of new middle-class Japan. *American Ethnologist* 13: 603–618.
Kokumin Seikatsu Hakusho
1983   *Keizai kikakuchō.* Tokyo: Ōkura Insatsu Kyoku.
Krauss, Elliot
1974   *Japanese Radicals Revisited: Student Politics in Postwar Japan.* Berkeley, Los Angeles, London: University of California Press.
Kyūtoku, S.
1979   *Bogenbyō.* Tokyo: Sanmaku Shuppan.
Lebra, T.
1976   *Japanese Patterns of Behavior.* Honolulu: University of Hawaii Press.
1984   *Japanese Women: Constraint and Fulfillment.* Honolulu: University of Hawaii Press.
Lewis, Gilbert
1975   *Knowledge of Illness in a Sepik Society.* London: Athlone.
Lock, Margaret
1980   *East Asian Medicine in Urban Japan: Varieties in Medical Experience.* Berkeley, Los Angeles, London: University of California Press.
1982*a*   Models and practice in medicine: menopause as syndrome of life transition? *Culture, Medicine and Psychiatry* 6: 216–280.
1982*b*   Traditional and popular attitudes toward mental health and illness in Japan. In *Cultural Conceptions of Mental Health and Therapy*, ed. A. Marsella and G. White. Dordrecht: D. Reidel.
1986   Plea for acceptance: school refusal syndrome in Japan. *Social Science and Medicine* 23: 99–112.
1987   A nation at risk: interpretations of school refusal in Japan. In *Biomedicine Examined*, ed. M. Lock and D. Gordon. Dordrecht: D. Reidel.
Lock, Margaret, Patricia Kaufert, and Penny Gilbert
1988   Cultural construction of menopausal syndrome: the Japanese case. *Maturitas* 10: 317–332.

Madoka, Yokiko
1982   *Shufushōkōgun.* Tokyo: Bunka Shuppan Kyoto.
Mainichi Shinbun
1983*a*   Japanese are "Worker Bees" after all. 2 November.
1983*b*   Education by order. 2 November.
1983*c*   Office work breeds tension, study says. 20 November.
1983*d*   Schools reverting to corporal punishment. 26 December.
1985*a*   Projects to combat stress under way. 24 August.
1985*b*   Dad playing weak role in bringing up offspring. 14 March.
1985*c*   Stress: serious problem of Japanese work force. 3 October.
1985*d*   Big changes in education called for. 27 June.
Manning, Peter, and Horatio Fabrega
1973   The experience of self and body: health and illness in the Chiapas Highlands. In *Phenomenological Sociology*, ed. George Psathas. New York: John Wiley.
McCormack, Gavin
1984   Beyond economism. In *Democracy in Contemporary Japan*, ed. G. McCormack and Y. Sugimoto. New York: M. E. Sharpe.
Merkin, D. H.
1976   *Pregnancy as a Disease: The Pill in Society.* Port Washington: Kennikat Press.
Mochida, Takeshi
1980   Focus on the family. *Japan Echo* 3: 75–76.
Moeran, Brian
1984   Individual, group and seishin: Japan's internal cultural debate. *Man (NS)* 19: 252–266.
Mouer, Ross, and Yoshio Sugimoto
1983   Internationalization as an ideology in Japanese society. In *The Challenge of Japan's Internationalization: Organization and Culture*, ed. H. Mannari and H. Befu. Tokyo: Kwansei Gakuin University.
Nakamura, M.
1976   *Creating Good Mothers. Meiroku Zasshi: Journal of the Japanese Enlightenment*,
(1875)   trans. W. Braisted. Cambridge: Harvard University Press.
Parkin, David
1978   *The Cultural Definition of Political Response.* London: Academic Press.
Pyle, Kenneth
1987   In pursuit of a grand design: Nakasone betwixt the past and future. *The Journal of Japanese Studies* 13: 243–270.
Rohlen, T. P.
1980   The Juku phenomenon: an exploratory essay. *Journal of Japanese Studies* 6: 242.
Skinner, K.
1979   Sarariiman manga. *The Japan Interpreter* 12 (3–4): 449–457.
Smith, R. J.
1974   *Ancestor Worship in Contemporary Japan.* Stanford: Stanford University Press.

Stark, E.

1982   Doctors in spite of themselves: the limits of radical health criticism. *International Journal of Health Services* 12: 419–457.

Uchino, Kumiko

1983   The status elevation process of Soto sect nuns in modern Japan. *Japanese Journal of Religious Studies* 10: 177–194.

Vogel, Ezra

1979   *Japan as Number One: Lessons for America.* Cambridge: Harvard University Press.

White, M. I., and B. Moloney, eds.

1979   *Proceedings of the Tokyo Symposium on Women.* Tokyo International Group for the Study of Women.

Yamada, Kazuo

1927   Clinical aspects of the menopause. *Rinshōigaku (15th year)* 9: 1095–1102.

Young, Allan

1982   Anthropology of sickness. *Annual Review of Anthropology* 11: 257–285.

Yuzawa, Yasuhiko

1980   Analyzing trends in family pathology. *Japan Echo* 7: 77–85.

Zola, Irving

1978   Medicine as an institution of social control. In *The Cultural Crisis of Modern Medicine*, ed. J. Ehrenreich. New York: Monthly Review Press.

PART TWO

Āyurveda, Cosmopolitan Medicine, and Other Traditions in South Asia

Margaret Trawick's essay provides a good beginning for this section because she outlines the systems of thought in four Indian healing traditions, showing variations in their conceptions of gender, nuturance, death, and immortality. She writes that they form a "loosely woven paradigmatic set" on the theme that life, pain, and death arise from the union of body and soul. This creates the problem of "how to have the good part, life, without also pain and death," since birth entails death and "for one thing to be fed, another must be eaten." This set of indigenous traditions coexists with biomedicine, homeopathy, astrology, and so on, to form the structure of medical pluralism in South India. Trawick addresses the epistemology of pluralism directly, showing the structural complimentarity and paradoxes of the traditions she analyzes. Other aspects of medical pluralism are in turn analyzed by Mark Nichter and Charles Leslie in essays that follow Trawick's. However, the subject matter and structuralist analysis in her work are most closely related to Gary Seaman's description of Chinese geomancy. The conceptual systems of humoral science, religious thought, and ritual practice are intimately related to one another. Outside the present volume, these essays by Seaman and Trawick add to the tradition of studies on comparative religion in *Death and the Regeneration of Life* (1982).

The scientific character of learned Āyurvedic practice is Gananath Obeyesekere's subject. His essay provides an ethnographic mirror of Judith Farquhar's essay on Chinese medicine. What he describes from observing and tape recording consultations in the clinic of an Āyurvedic physician in Sri Lanka, and in analyzing "samyogic experimentation," resembles the process Farquhar identifies in medical literature. The two essays seem to describe exactly the same kind of clinical reasoning and practice. But if this is so, what are we to make of the fact that publishing and studying case histories like the one Farquhar analyzes is a central path to knowledge in Chinese medicine, while this is not true for Āyurvedic literature? Francis Zimmermann writes that Āyurveda is part of the Indo-European universe, but the Hippocratic Corpus and subsequent literature in this tradition contain historical descriptions of particular patients for which there is no parallel in Āyurveda. What have been the changing functions of literacy and of libraries in these traditions? Reformers in nineteenth- and twentieth-century India criticized traditional restrictions on access to Āyurvedic knowledge that they attributed to customs and sentiments related to caste, religion, and the secrecy of practitioners. This contrasts greatly with Farquhar's image of physicians drawing continuously over several thousand years upon a cumulative archive of medical wisdom created by "the laboring people of China."

The extended descriptions of practice in the essays by Obeyesekere and Farquhar are complemented by Trawick's transcription of an Āyurvedic consultation, and by her characterizations and comparisons of various Āyurveda and Siddha physicians. The practitioners in all these essays belong to the class of learned professionals that is further described in Charles Leslie's essay. He analyzes the intellectual confrontation between Āyurveda and biomedicine acted out by leading Indian scholars and politicians. While Trawick and Obeyesekere focused on historical continuities in modern Āyurveda, the essays by Leslie and Zimmermann analyze the epistemological break in contemporary thought. Zimmermann traces the consequences of commodification as Āyurvedic companies and sanatoria modify theories and practices to exploit a market for alternative forms of health care.

Finally, Mark Nichter's description of Tuluva interpretations of epidemics of a new tick-born fever show a kind of bricolage on the part of laypeople that complements Obeyesekere's contrast between bricolage and samyogic experimentation on the part of Āyurvedic physicians. Most important, he shows us one of those "diseases of development," in this case brought on by clearing forests for new plantations, and the awakening political awareness of environmental issues that it entailed.

REFERENCES

Bloch, Maurice, and Jonathan Parry, eds.
  1982   *Death and the Regeneration of Life.* Cambridge: Cambridge University Press.

SIX

Death and Nurturance in Indian Systems of Healing

Margaret Trawick

INTRODUCTION

This essay describes the tenets of four indigenous systems of healing in India, as they were taught to me by practitioners and as they appear in the texts that these practitioners used.[1] The statements of practitioners often went beyond the texts, and in these cases, I have been more concerned with their understanding of the texts than I have been with the texts themselves.

The four systems are:

(1) Āyurveda, "the science of life," the classical Sanskrit system of medicine based on texts composed in North India between the time of Christ and A.D. 1000.[2] Āyurveda is now practiced throughout India, and more recent texts exist in several languages, but the original texts are believed to be of divine origin, and their truth to be eternal and complete.

Unlike other healing systems considered here, modern Āyurveda is not strongly associated with any particular deity or "religion," but is said to have been originally given to humanity by Śiva. Neither the personality of Śiva nor the philosophy of Śaivism, however, seems to play much part in Āyurvedic theory or practice. In the bodily processes with which Āyurveda deals, the willful intervention of spirits and deities is not generally invoked as a cause of illness or of healing.

In modern South India, Āyurveda—because of its Sanskrit textual basis—is linked with Brahminic tradition. The most prestigious Āyurvedic institution in the south is run by a family of Nambudiri Brahmans who jealously guard their medical and pharmacological practice as part of the family tradition. Before the establishment of Āyurvedic medical colleges, Āyurvedic practice was normally passed on from father to son or from uncle to nephew. Since the establishment of Āyurvedic colleges, the transmission of the tradition has become more open, but the Sanskrit component remains central, and the modernization of Āyurveda, like its traditional transmission, remains largely in Brahman hands.

Āyurveda is thus the most authoritative of the various healing systems considered here. Its texts are also the most "scientific" in that their authors' principal concern seems to have been the development of a coherent general theory of one aspect of the natural world—namely, the human body. Āyurveda is not, however, a fundamentally closed or exclusive doctrine. Rich and poor men and women of high and low castes resort equally to Āyurvedic physicians for treatment, and the basic categories of Āyurveda—the names and activities of the humors, the qualities of different times and places and types of weather, the categories of food and their effects upon the body—are common knowledge in Tamil Nadu as elsewhere.

(2) Tamil Śaiva *bhakti*, the devotional worship of Śiva in Tamil Nadu, is inspired by the poetry of the Tamil Śaiva saints, most notably the poetry of the tenth-century saint Māṇikkavācakar and the spiritual evolution he describes in the long poem *Tiruvācakam*. Modern Śaiva gurus are often approached for solutions to life problems, including illness. Solving such problems through both mystical and rational means is their service to the world. The sacred ash they distribute, their blessings, their glance, their touch, and above all, their words are believed to have healing powers.[3]

Śaiva bhakti is at the opposite extreme of Āyurveda in that Śaiva bhakti is known to Westerners and thought of by them as a "religious system" and not as a "medical system." The essence of Śaiva bhakti is the emotional relationship binding the worshipper to the deity. The state of a person's body is only of concern to the extent that it expresses, impedes, or enables this relationship. Weeping and trembling express bhakti, the desires of the body such as hunger and sexual attraction impede it, quiet meditation enables it. Ultimately the well-being of the body is not a goal of Tamil Śaivism: one may blind oneself or do worse out of love for Śiva.

However, I think it may be truthfully claimed that in Indian thought, "religion" and "medicine" are not separate categories, any more than "body" and "soul" are contemplated independently of each other there. The soul may of course (with great difficulty) be extracted from the body, but then so (with much greater ease) may a heart or a tongue.

Like Āyurvedic and Western doctors as well as spirit mediums, Śaiva gurus are considered important because they are bearers and conduits of *śakti*, invisible power that may effect great changes upon people. Like doctors, Śaiva gurus may convey this power through some material substance (such as sacred ash), but their principal display of śakti is in their conduct and in their words. They are teachers as well as moral exemplars. Through skillful explication of the Śaiva canon, the hymns of the Tamil Śaiva saints, they change their followers' conception of themselves, and move them to change their lives.

(3) Siddha medicine is a system of medicine in Tamil Nadu based on the writings of certain yogis who, in their quest for physical immortality, discovered various life-prolonging and medicinal substances. These yogis are called siddhars (Tamil *cittarkaḷ*) because of their achievement of miraculous powers called siddhis. The siddhis include the ability to make oneself invisible, to move from body to body at will, and so forth. The Tamil siddhars wrote a large body of poetry that overlaps with the Śaiva devotional poetry. Tirumūlar's *Tirumantiram* of around the eighth century is regarded as the earliest extant Siddha text. The collected work, *Tiruvarutpā*, of the nineteenth-century saint, Rāmalingar, is perhaps the second most important corpus in the Siddha group.[4]

The moral status of the siddha yogis is ambiguous. By some accounts,[5] their exercise of miraculous powers is a consequence of their inability to resist the temptations of the world as they travel on the road to enlightenment. Instead of preserving their hard-won *tapas* to propel them toward spiritual liberation, they stop before they reach this goal and use their power for lesser purposes. Popular stories of siddhars portray them as secretive, miserly alchemists, as makers of fairy gold, as dangerous tricksters, as producers of nightmares, as voyeurs who use their powers of invisibility to spy on married couples.[6] The medicines they produce may be derived from foul substances that no self-respecting person would knowingly consume, such as head lice. Some Siddhars are said to rejuvenate themselves through Tantric-style sexual and gustatory "perversions."[7] Indeed if one goes by their advertisements, sexual rejuvenation potions appear to be one of the great fortes of Siddha medical shops.

Yet in more scholarly accounts of the great "eighteen siddhars" and in the Tamil siddha poetry itself, the siddhars come through as stern, ascetic prophets, railing against the futility of worldly life.[8] Basing their arguments on this body of poetry, proponents of Tamil ethnic pride claim Siddha medicine as a distinctly Tamil medical system, set apart from Āyurveda.

(4) Trance healing by mediums of the smallpox goddess Māriamman is a tradition that claims no written texts as its own, priding itself instead on its grass-roots character. But it has associated with it a set of myths and a clearly expressed philosophy concerning human nature.

In modern South India, worship of Māriamman and of other "village goddesses" is coming to have a strong political import, for it is associated with nonvegetarianism, with ecstatic religious practices such as alcohol-induced trance, and with downtrodden people of low status and of little means. The origin story of Māriamman suggests defiance of caste and sexual hierarchies. The goddess is born of a merger of Brahman and untouchable bodies, and she separates herself from her husband and sons and lives independently of them. The goddess is believed to selectively inflict diseases that she controls according to the purity of people's hearts and the strength of their belief in her; she will protect only those of pure heart and strong belief, and she will give her power only to such people. The wealthy and the educated are said to have too much pride to be capable of pure belief, and the goddess is said to be especially fond of people of untouchable castes, and of women.[9] In villages and cities of modern Tamil Nadu, festivals to the goddess may form an arena for the intense expression of conflicts between classes (for example, between landowners and laborers), between political factions, or even between the two sexes.[10]

There is evidence that in precolonial times, the practice of variolation formed part of the worship of the smallpox goddess.[11] Discharged material from the pustules of people who had undergone mild cases of smallpox was collected and applied to a scratch on the skin of the worshipper, essentially as a vaccine. It would not be unreasonable to surmise that this practice was related to a religious ideology permitting the goddess-mediated mingling of bodily fluids of people of different communities. Under British rule, variolation was outlawed and knowledge of the technique was lost.

Each of these four systems of thought and healing flourishes in modern Tamil Nadu. In the conceptual systems of particular individuals, they sometimes occur in commingled form, yet they are separately named and are in principle distinguishable from one another. They could perhaps be regarded as ideal types, altered in their realizations by context and by one another. Considered together, the four of them appear to form a kind of loosely woven paradigmatic set, or a group of variants on a single theme. Though they differ from one another in many ways, they share the idea that life as it is known to most creatures, with pain and death, arises from the union of body and soul, and the problem that they all try to solve is how to have the good part, life, without also having the bad parts, pain and death. Beneath this philosophical problem lies the idea that from death arises birth, or (stated more strongly) that there cannot be birth without death, or (more specifically) that for one thing to be fed, another must be eaten. For one occupying the status of female this means that since she is the nurturer, she must also be the consumed, and since she is the bearer of life, she must also be the bearer of death.

If it is true, as I will try to show, that these four separate and competing healing systems, with their different views of life, fit together into a coherent overall pattern, then new questions arise that must be answered: For whom do these different systems fit together to form a set, and how and why do they?

Here, I would argue that it is primarily for the patient, and to a lesser extent for practicing healers, that different healing systems mesh on a fundamental level in meaningful ways. While it is true that there is often a gap between the knowledge of the patient and the knowledge of the healer, and yet another gap between the perspective of the healer and the broader perspective of the ancient texts or myths upon which the healing tradition is based, in the case of a successful healer these gaps are bridged by the healer's communication with the patient. Part of the talent of the healer is his or her ability to bring the ancient and general knowledge to bear upon the patient's present and particular problem, giving this problem a place in the overall scheme of things. The patient comes away from the successful healing session not only with a changed body but with at least a slightly changed cognition—with physical health and with mental satisfaction. Hence the most trusted healers, whatever their persuasion, are those who explain things to the patient, or in some way communicate powerfully in a medium that the patient can understand.

Even when there are great differences between the knowledge of an indigenous healer and that of a patient, from the point of view of an outsider, areas of common understanding between healer and patient are enormous.[12] In a complex civilization, as culture changes and innovations are introduced, healers and patients must continually adapt their perspectives to one another. Thus, for instance, since the introduction of cosmopolitan medicine to India, laypeople have fitted injections and antibiotics into their overall understanding of how medicine works, have instilled these elements with new meanings, and now demand them even from healers belonging to noncosmopolitan traditions. Indian cosmopolitan doctors, in turn, have learned to prescribe more or less elaborate dietary restrictions to accompany medication, because patients in their experience with other modes of healing have come to expect this. In such ways, healing systems adjust to the conditions imposed by the general culture and by one another.[13]

It has been said that medical pluralism is a desirable state of affairs because it allows for the presence of modes of healing especially suited to local cultures, in a way that a worldwide, thoroughly standardized "scientific" medical system could not.[14] But in South Asia, this advantage appears to take a peculiar twist. Several analysts have argued that medical pluralism itself, almost regardless of the particular variety of healing systems that it comprises, is uniquely suited to the radically pluralistic cultures and societies of South Asia. Nichter (1980) describes medicine *masala* (mixed to taste and pocketbook) as a basic strategy pursued by villagers seeking medical treatment in the city, and by pharmacists catering to them. Beals (1976) suggests that, as an Indian villager is used to contradiction and does not expect to get a consistent total picture of the universe, so he feels comfortable in the presence of mutually contradictory medical systems. Obeyesekere (1977) says that, even within the single healing system of spirit exorcism, a person may "choose" from among many demons and deities any one or several to possess her, and having been possessed by a demon of complex personality may choose which of its character traits to emphasize. This allows for great individualization of spirit possession and exorcism as a mode of psychotherapy in a culture where personality "types" are extremely diverse. Finally, Amarasingham (1980) has shown that in the context of Sri Lankan medical pluralism, the prognosis for patients diagnosed as schizophrenic is more optimistic than in the West, where schizophrenia is seen as incurable. She suggests that schizophrenia in Sri Lanka may be healed because each medical system diagnoses the patient's illness differently. In effect, the disease disappears because it has no consistent definition. Strangely, it seems that in a society with plural medical traditions, sometimes the very lack of congruence among these traditions, the lack of a single meaning expressed by all of them together, accounts for their culturally satisfying quality and sometimes even for the healing of the patient.[15]

In this essay I will argue that more positive kinds of symbolic relationship also exist among diverse medical traditions in South Asia, and that this kind of relationship also may contribute to the process of healing. I follow Lévi-Strauss's (1963b) assertion that one of the principal functions of the healer (someone possessed, in Lévi-Strauss's terms, of an excess of imagination) is to substitute meaning for the apparent meaninglessness of sickness and death, and so lend courage to the sick and dying (those possessed of an excess of experience). I follow Lévi-Strauss also in supposing that the most fundamental problems of meaning, such as those posed by illness and death, are never approached directly or solved completely, but rather, through a series of incomplete symbolic formulations, as for instance a set of myths, are at least given patterned expression.[16]

Here, the incomplete symbolic formulations are not myths—that is, they are not stories—but are messages developed and relayed in the practice of healing traditions. Although the four traditions have not always formed a mutually complementary set, practitioners' interpretations of these traditions to themselves, to patients, and to other practitioners have molded the different traditions to one another, so that, for the sufferer who visits all of them, a basic message emerges, a message that gives meaning to the experience of suffering and to the inevitability of death.[17]

THE FOUR SYSTEMS

Āyurveda

The Āyurvedic cosmology consists of a modified synthesis of several of the orthodox systems of Hindu philosophy, most notably Sāṁkhya and Yoga. According to the model adopted by these systems, the cosmos and each person are formed of two components: a female component, or *Prakṛti*, which constitutes the body, and a male component, or *Puruṣa*, which is the soul.

Puruṣa is indivisible, atomic, and immutable, but Prakṛti has parts and is subject to change. Prakṛti in Sanskrit means "she out of whom it is made." Puruṣa means "husband" or "man."

The cosmos comes into existence when Puruṣa impregnates Prakṛti with his essence. Then Prakṛti, who previously had been in a state of internal balance, is thrown into disequilibrium, and proceeds to evolve the universe (and the body) from varying combinations of the different components (the three *guṇas*) of herself. Puruṣa, being unchanging, is also nonproductive. Prakṛti creates out of her own substance; her ability to change (become other) is her ability to create. Puruṣa does not participate in the evolution of the body/cosmos, but only observes it, as a prisoner within it.

Although Puruṣa is conscious and Prakṛti is not, the Āyurvedic texts tell us that Puruṣa, being a nonparticipant in the life process, is indifferent to pleasure and pain, whereas Prakṛti is not. Puruṣa only thinks he feels pleasure and pain inasmuch as he is bound to Prakṛti and identifies with her. According to the philosophic text *Sāṁkhya-kārika*, when creation is completed and Puruṣa has watched Prakṛti evolve the body around him, he sees himself in her mirror and realizes he is different from her. Then Prakṛti, having fulfilled her function, returns to her original undifferentiated state, and Puruṣa is free again.

This return is not automatic, however. The practice of yoga (as described in Patañjali's *Yoga-sūtras*) consists of a deliberate effort to isolate Puruṣa from Prakṛti, and to achieve for him a state of total changelessness and singleness liberated from her.

The Āyurvedic idea of physical conception and birth is roughly parallel to the idea of cosmic conception and birth sketched above. Just as the body exists for the purpose of the soul only, to contain and finally to show it to itself and liberate it, so in the classic Āyurvedic texts, *Suśruta Saṁhitā* and *Caraka Saṁhitā*, woman is treated as existing for the purpose of producing a (male) child only, and the female body is discussed only in connection with pregnancy.

In the Āyurvedic description of this process, when a woman becomes pregnant, and as the pregnancy advances, her body loses its health. The fetus draws its substance from the mother, and as it absorbs her flesh and blood, she grows thinner. The mother's body is said by the texts to contribute many substances to the body of the fetus, while the male contributes only semen. The female is able to create an offspring without the aid of a male, but the male substance is necessary in order for the substances of the fetal body to differentiate. The male element produces in the fetus the heavy, hard, and enduring parts of the body—bones, hair, nails, and semen itself (the male impregnates the female with his own essence, which thus endures, like the soul, from body to body). The softer, lighter, and more perishable parts of the fetal body come from the mother.

A person's bodily constitution is called his prakṛti, and consists of a particular combination of what are called the three *dōṣas: vāta, pitta,* and *kapha* (usually glossed in English as "wind," "bile," and "phlegm"). These dōṣas are responsible for all bodily processes, good and bad. Vāta drives all movement in the body (breath and bowels as well as convulsions), pitta is present in all light and heat (the healthy glow of eyes and skin, as well as fever), and kapha stabilizes and facilitates cohesion (binding lungs with phlegm as well as holding the joints together). But unqualified, the word dōṣa means fault, illness, or suffering. Thus the body, the protean substance of prakṛti, though producing both pleasure and pain, seems primarily a locus of pain.

For the unchanging puruṣa or soul, the prakṛti or body is the locus of change, and by implication, of death. For the texts of Śuśruta and Caraka, any change (of season, diet, place, and so on) causes sickness. But further, they say time is change, and time is what leads all beings to destruction: and any change in the temperament of a man is to be regarded as a harbinger of death. Long lists of the signs of impending death are given, and most of these signs consist of changes, including seemingly positive ones, from the person's normal state. Thus, though death is not defined by the texts, it seems that one of the defining features of death, and perhaps the most important one, is change.

But life also is change, and is called, in one definition given by Śuśruta, "the flux." The body is imaged, not in terms of anatomy, which receives scant description in these texts, but in terms of the flow of substances through channels, and the transformations of these substances into one another. The practice of Āyurveda is concerned with keeping physiological process going. Each substance flows in its own channel, according to Āyurvedic theory; sickness occurs when a channel gets blocked—when normal process is interrupted—and the substance in that channel flows over into the channels of other substances.

But what is normal physiological process? It consists in the derivation and purification of essential substances (*dhātus*) one from the other, in a chain of substances running from the least pure to the purest, each preceding and less pure substance containing the succeeding and purer ones, as ore contains gold. The goal of physiological process is the liberation of the heaviest, innermost, least mixed, and purest substance of the body, semen. Each substance before semen contains three parts: a waste substance, which is discarded, an essence, and the succeeding substance, which is purified from the preceding one. So for instance the first substance *rasa* (food in the stomach) contains (1) the essence of rasa; (2) the waste substance, feces; and (3) the next element, blood. Blood, having been purified from rasa, contains the essence of blood, the waste substance urine, and the next substance, muscle. In all, say the texts, there are seven essential substances or dhātus: rasa, blood, muscle, fat, bone, marrow, and semen. The seventh dhātu, semen, alone is indivisible, "like gold a thousand times purified," says Śuśruta: semen produces no excrement, and no purer element is derived from it.

Within semen, however, is something called *ojas*, which means strength or light. This is, say the texts, the element of consciousness. It is interesting that although semen is categorized as hard and heavy, ojas is called soft and light, and described in terms that place it just on the border of what we would call the material and the immaterial. It is "light," "consciousness," "strength," but it is also "fat" and "oily." Ojas is said to be what gives female bodies their supple quality. Ojas is also the substance connecting the heart of a pregnant mother to the heart of the baby within her, making them competitors for life itself (the ojas is said to go back and forth dangerously between their two hearts), but also making their desires and their feelings one. Ojas, then, is intriguingly similar to the notion of *śakti*, spiritual power or life energy, personified in India as any goddess. But although semen is purified of its substrates and so liberated as part of the natural course of things, ojas remains locked within semen, and if it is lost, the loser will die.

In sum, the classic Āyurvedic model of life and death takes this form: the changeless soul is male, impregnating and existing within the changing body, which is female. The coming of the male/soul into the female/body is what initiates the changes that the body undergoes. The soul witnesses and is the cause of these changes, but they occur within the body only. Change is inherently painful and leads to death, but it also leads to liberation of the soul. Within the body itself, the enduring parts are male and the perishable parts are female, and bodily process, leading though it inevitably does to the death of the body, occurs for the sake of the production and liberation of the male substance from its female substrate—a good and necessary liberation. The dichotomy male-soul/female-body seems clear-cut, but at the end of the description of the basic life process are hints of a different view: a female life force locked within the male, the bond of consciousness between mother and child, equal to light and strength.[18]

An Interview Between an Āyurvedic Physician and a Patient   Āyurvedic philosophy must seem, in this context, arcane and abstract, and it may be hard to imagine how such a set of ancient speculations has any bearing upon the life of some poor, illiterate villager of the twentieth century visiting her local vaidya for foot problems.

But real life, if we look at it closely, is at least as subtle as books. In simple conversation about mundane things, the most complex ideas may be conveyed. Earlier I suggested that an important skill exercised by certain kinds of healers is the bringing to bear of abstract philosophies upon the concrete experience of patients. The patient's illness is given meaning within the general frame constructed by the physician. Consider the following translated script of an interview between an Āyurvedic physician in a village of southern Tamil Nadu and a patient who has come to visit him.[19]

> *Doctor:* What village?
> *Patient:* Kaḍalnallūr.
> *D:* Let's see your eyes. Let's see your pulse. Is your age over sixty?
> *P:* Probably.
> *D:* You don't know your age exactly, do you? But I think you are sixty, judging from the condition (*amaippu*) of your body. Is there chest pain?
> *P:* A little (*lēcā*).
> *D:* Does your heart flutter (*paṭappaṭakkiṟatā*)?
> *P:* It flutters.
> *D:* At night does sleep come to you?
> *P:* For ten days good sleep comes, and then for ten days good sleep won't come.
> *D:* Does urine pass okay? Is hunger and all good? From time to time, does weariness come?
> *P:* Yes.
> *D:* Does weariness come alone or does it come with dizziness? Is there obstruction of the ears, blurring (*mayakkam*) of the eyes? Is there obstruction of the ears?
> *P:* Yes.
> *D:* Do your eyes see well?
> *P:* Somewhat diminished.
> *D:* Is there pain in the joints?
> *P:* Yes.
> *D:* Is this pain always there, or does it come more in the day and less at night?
> *P:* In the day it is felt; at night it is not felt. I sleep well.
> *D:* Are you a woman who is able to work every day?
> *P:* I am idle.
> *D:* You are just in the house eating.
> *P:* Yes.
> *D:* Very good. Do you bathe daily?
> *P:* I don't bathe daily.
> *D:* How often do you bathe?
> *P:* I bathe once every two or three days.
> *D:* Have you taken any treatment for this?
> *P:* I have taken no treatment at all.
> *D:* So you have just kept it, letting it be however it wants to be?
> *P:* Whatever. . . . A person from our village came to you and got well. I came because of that boy. If you make me well many people will come from there.
> *D:* Are your feet and all numb?
> *P:* They feel very numb (*matamatamatamataṇṇu*). They feel as though they have sandals on.
> *D:* I will give you medicines and all. Your blood is ill (*kuṭṭapaṭṭu*), and your age

too is sixty, isn't it? Your body and the skin on your feet has lost its feeling and is in the condition that between it and the flesh there is no connection. Therefore it is as though a thing were stuck on the outside. The blood that it needs is in a turbulence in all places in the body. At night your hands and feet and all become cold; they become very much like sticks. For that I will give an oil to rub on the body and bathe. Rub the oil on and then pour warm water. For the head, all the nerves of the brain, eyes, ears, nose, tongue—all of these are feeling nerves, aren't they? The strength of all these has decreased. I will give an oil to keep it from decreasing even faster. To keep vigorous what hunger you have, for feces to move when you have eaten, for urine to separate properly, for the body to be light, I will give medicine. You take that regularly, and with the medicine it will get better.

What is called food is an important matter. That important matter . . . if you eat whatever you feel like and take medicine it is useless. Therefore I will tell you a diet. If you eat according to that discipline it will become better. Are you in the habit of drinking coffee?

P: I drink coffee.

D: Drink two coffees, in the morning a coffee and in the evening a coffee. Add palm sugar to the coffee, filter it and remove the dirt, add cow's milk and drink it. Buffalo milk will not be digested—it is not good for vāta diseases. If you want feeling to return to your nerves you should not eat very heavy things. So you eat this and return. Afterwards, in the morning what you eat, you may eat *idli* (rice cake). When I say idli, you are capable of eating five idlis. But you must not eat more than two idlis. If you eat more they won't be digested. Then if the undigested food goes and joins with this food it will become poison. That is the poison that first will create evil for your body, will create evil liquids, and will pervade the whole body. Therefore you must eat as I tell you. Don't eat differently.

P: Okay.

D: Don't eat very many sweet items. Things made of rice, *dōsai* (rice pancake), idli, oil, pepper powder you must not eat much of. You must eat correct, orderly foods. Eat wheat grain made soft. In the afternoon, eat it with spices without tamarind. The sourness of lemon, tomato *rasam* (spicy soup), cooked *pappadam* (deep-fried rice tortilla), chutney, pickle, *ciruparuppu* (a legume), *nāraṅkāy* (a vegetable), cow's buttermilk, *pulikkut* (very sour) buttermilk, add these and eat. Add cow's ghee and eat.

At three o'clock drink only one cup of coffee. Eat more food than coffee. In the evening, if you are hungry eat two idlis. Otherwise, take rasam and filter it and drink it. Or eat *rava uppumā* (steamed cracked wheat with spices). When it is time to sleep, when it is cool, heat some cow's milk mixed with water and drink that milk. Don't drink it with coffee. Good sleep will come. It will be good and correct to rise in the morning. It seems as though dung is stuck (on your feet), doesn't it? All that will go away.

The perceptual power of the nerves of your brain has diminished, eyesight has diminished, your ears don't hear sound, your nose is without good feeling, without smelling well, your tongue is as though you had eaten a lot of hot spice. All this will change and your regular body will return. For all this to get better, it will take fifteen days. You eat this and return, or send a person to tell me.

I will give you a medicine. In the time of age, at this age of sixty, if the strength of the body has diminished it is difficult for it to return. Therefore you must carry with you your existing strength without its diminishing still more quickly. You must carry it without evils coming and without making room for other diseases. Don't show your head and mix in noisy places; don't get caught in the crush of a crowd; don't go to common places and take the air for long. You must go to mountain places refreshing to the mind, and seeing the plants and trees there be happy. Or else go to the temple and worship God. From that your mind will be pure. A good refuge for your body will be found.

Comments on the Interview　　Āyurveda is a naturalistic healing system and Āyurvedic physicians are inclined to emphasize the rightness of material life processes and in their treatment of disease to facilitate these processes rather than to oppose them. Āyurvedic theory says that the body evolves through changes that are necessary to purify and liberate the essences within. The flow of life within the body, as long as it is orderly and unobstructed, produces naturally this purification and liberation of essences. It is important, therefore, that the channels of flow remain open, clear, and free. The culmination and termination of the flow of life is death, when the soul itself is purified and liberated from its bodily prison.

In the dialogue recounted above, the doctor, a highly educated man in his mid-eighties who is, by his own estimation, himself approaching death, through his questions, diagnosis, and prescriptions communicates these basic tenets of Āyurveda to the patient, a lower caste laboring woman from a remote village. He inquires about the various channels and processes of flow in her body and about different points of connection: the eyes and ears, through which emanations from perceived objects are believed to travel; the heart, which Āyurvedic theory regards as the center of all channels of flow in the body; the passage of urine and feces; hunger, which spurs the digestive process; the regular activities of life that purify the body, render the channels clear, and keep things moving through: work, sleep, bathing. Such questions tell the patient what the doctor views as significant.

He finds that several of the processes he asks about are indeed blocked—the heart is not functioning properly, the joints are painful (so that the patient cannot move freely), the eyes are dim, the ears are blocked, the skin of the feet is numb. The final complaint is the one that the doctor and patient both focus on. Her most serious problem, as he sees it, is that the connection between the skin of her feet and her flesh has been severed; consequently, the flow of both feeling and blood is blocked and the blocked blood is poisoning her body. He prescribes a medicine that will get everything moving again.

In a subsequent discussion with a woman patient who comes the same morning, the doctor says this: "The feet must always be hot. The feet must always be running. The head must always be cool. Judgment (*putti*) must always be cool. The feet must always be hot. If the feet become cool it is very bad for the body. [In English] It is an indication of some serious nervous disorder. It is the direction among aged people. [Back to Tamil] As for young people, they can even lie down in the street."

What he seems to be saying is that coolness in the body starts at the top and over the years flows downward. So the best state, the prime of life, is the state in which the head is cool and the feet are warm. In young people, even the head is hot, so they can lay their heads in the street where warm feet have stepped without suffering the illness that would result from heating an ordinarily cool head. In old people, the coolness of the head has flowed all the way down to the feet. It is the natural "direction" for the old, but it is a bad sign, because it indicates that the process of life is nearing its end. For this reason, coolness and numbness of the feet are of special significance.

Having made his diagnosis, the doctor makes his prescription. "Orderly" food, he believes, is the key to health; medication is secondary. The dietary restrictions that the doctor sets forth are directed toward quickening (in both senses) the body of the patient. For instance, tamarind is not permitted the patient because it is believed to cause "dullness" (*mantam*), from which condition she is already suffering. The doctor advises the patient to eat lightly. Food must not get crowded and stuck inside her. "Heavy" food will keep feeling from flowing' back into her nerves. Undigested food will block up digested food and cause it all to turn to poison.

From time to time throughout the interview, the doctor has made reference to the patient's age. Finally, he gently tells her what he regards as the most important aspect of her condition: she is growing old. The changes she is experiencing can be slowed somewhat, but they cannot be stopped. However there is a benefit to this process—she herself may become free. Just as materials in her body should not be crowded and obstructed, she also must not become crowded and obstructed. She must leave the crush of common places and go to peaceful mountaintops or temples. Thus unshackled, her body will find its proper resting place and her soul will be purified.

Tamil Śaivism

In Tamil Śaiva *bhakti*, the aim of life is not isolation of the soul, as in Āyurveda, but union of the soul with its lord Śiva.[20] Each person consists of a soul, *uyir*, contained within a body, *mēy*. But the Tamil concept of uyir differs sharply from the Sanskrit concept of puruṣa. In the first place, the Tamil uyir, to the extent that it is ascribed a sex, is regarded (addressed and described) as female, rather than as male. In the second place, it is not changeless; the ability to change is what enables it to move from union with the world and body to union with Śiva. Nor is it free from its own suffering. The Tamil Śaiva body, like the Āyurvedic body, has certain more masculine and certain more feminine parts. Masculine and feminine, in Indian thought, are not binary opposites, but ends of a spectrum of infinite shades and degrees, like light and dark. As in the Āyurvedic body, the Śaiva body's masculine parts are harder and the feminine parts are softer. But in the Āyurvedic body, the transition from the most exterior, most mixed substance, food in the belly, to the most interior, purest substance, semen, is a transition from light to heavy, from more mutable to less mutable, and (implicitly) from feminine to masculine. Conversely, in the Śaiva body, the transition from the outermost, "grossest" body, the body of food, to the innermost, most subtle body, the soul itself, is a transition from harder to softer, from less mutable to more mutable, and from masculine to feminine. The imagery used to describe this structure is multifarious: the hard and rough and less generative male contains and protects the soft and vulnerable and more generative female; the hard outer shell of a seed contains and protects the soft, generative, and edible kernel. The soft inner part is more valuable because it is more able to be used: in the case of food, only soft food is able to be eaten and digested; in the case of earth, only soft earth is able to yield produce; in the case of hearts, only a soft heart is able to melt and give itself to another heart. The softer something is, the more subject it is to further softening: a soft heart melts more easily than a hard one, butter melts more easily than stone.

This softening, melting, and being used involves suffering and loss of self, and this is precisely what happens to the human soul in its ultimate union with Śiva. Just as a fruit must mature to be ready to be eaten (says Ramalingar), just as a girl must mature to be ready to be loved by a man, the soul must mature, or ripen, or soften, to be ready for union with Śiva. When this happens, it is destroyed completely. The canonical poet Māṇikkavācakar is quite unambiguous on this point. "The realizing soul softens, frays, and melts," he says, "the black rock heart will melt. . . it will tremble, scream and dissolve. . . the river of love will overflow its banks and the body too will soften and will stand rotting."

Union with Śiva is described as Śiva's planting his feet in one's heart, almost as though one's heart were the earth from which the deity can grow. The soul of the worshipper seeks the "flowerlike" feet of Śiva.

Āyurveda and Śaiva bhakti are both concerned with the relation between male and female and body and soul, and life and death are seen by each system to result from the union of, and differences between, the members of each pair. Death and liberation both are processes continuous with the processes of life—softening for Śaiva bhakti (the transformation from hard to soft), purification for Āyurveda (the purification of male from female). In

Śaiva bhakti, death and liberation seem almost to be the same end of the same process of melting until the self is lost completely. (For the Śaiva bhakta death is only loss of self to the world; loss of self to Śiva is something else. Nevertheless, the two processes are parallel, just as final release of the spirit is parallel to sexual release, though each excludes the other.) In Āyurveda, the changeless is liberated from the changeable, which is discarded. In either case the female component, whether soul or body, changes while the male does not, and gives up herself for something beyond her, which is male; and if death is change, death is hers.

Siddha Medicine

The Siddha yogis (according to modern Siddha doctors) had a different approach to the problem of death. They believed that the soul was dependent upon the body: "Without the soul, the body is a corpse, but without the body, the soul is only steam," says Tirumūlar; elsewhere he likens the body to a trellis on which the soul grows like a vine. If the trellis falls down, the vine does, too. Hence the only way to make the soul immortal is to make the body immortal also, and this is what the Siddha yogis aimed to do. Thus, whereas Āyurveda and Śaiva bhakti sought to foster the flow of life which led ultimately to the dissolution of the body, the Siddha yogis aimed to stop this flow.

First, the sexual flow was stopped. Semen, rather than being emitted, was to be kept inside the body and pumped up into the head, in classic yogi fashion. Stopping the flow of semen meant, of course, avoiding women. Thus we have the story of Ramalingar, who, pressured into marrying, ignored his wife, so that shortly after the marriage, overpowered by the saint's saintliness, she (conveniently) died. Tirumūlar, finding himself with a wife, entered a trance, in which state he spent the remaining three thousand years of his life, coming out of the trance only once a year to compose a verse of poetry.

But not only does the Siddha yogi stop the flow of sex, he also does not eat—he has no need for food because his body secretes a special liquid that drips from the roof of his mouth onto his tongue, and this sustains him. And finally, claims Tirumūlar, the accomplished siddhar does not even breathe.

This brings us to the topic of nurturance. Let nurturance be defined as one living thing flowing into another (as milk into a child's mouth) or out of another (as plants from the earth) or more generally as one thing being changed into another, such that the first thing diminishes as the second grows.

In one sense, death is a denial of nurturance, for it is the cutting off of one thing from another. It is for this reason, I was told, that the god of death in Tamil is called *kūṭṭavan*, "the separator," and it is easy to find other associations between the concept of severance, or cutting off the flow, and the concept of death in Tamil culture.

But in another sense, death is just an extreme case of nurturance, for it involves one thing changing completely into another. So when a person dies, they say he has gone to the elements, the earth in his body merging with earth, the water with water, the wind with wind, the soul with Śiva. As one person put it, death makes good manure. The most fertile earth is full of corpses.

Partly, this seeming contradiction in the conception of death is just a problem of different points of view. Separation from one thing may mean merger with another. Or death may be seen as existing at the two extremes of the flow of life—absence of flow on the one hand, unbounded flow on the other. (We have seen that Āyurveda regards sickness in this way—the normal flow of a substance is blocked, and as a consequence of this it swells up and flows over its boundaries).

But when there is an attempt to deny death categorically, as in the Siddha system, the ambiguous, liminal character of death comes into full focus.

The act of the Siddha yogi involves a denial of nurturance in the most absolute and general sense. Nothing flows into him and nothing flows out of him and he does not change. Stories of the siddhars show them isolating themselves from the world in every possible way. Some hide in caves, some lock themselves up in rooms, some go into deep trances and refuse to be disturbed. The siddhar is not dead in that he has undergone a change or lost himself, for he is changeless and perfectly self-contained. But he is lifeless in the sense that nurturance, the life process, is not there. This lifelessness is what gives him immortality. For the siddhar, denial of nurturance means the denial of death. The contrapositive of this statement is that death is nurturant (the converse of the Āyurvedic and bhaktic idea that nurturance feeds into death), and this is seen in the type of medicine that the Siddha medical system regards as uniquely its own, namely, mineral poison.

It is congruent with the naturalism of Āyurveda that its medicines are said by practitioners to come only from living things, nowadays from milk and plants, which as one Āyurvedic doctor pointed out are seasonal medicines and locality-bound, as opposed to minerals, which are not seasonal and can be shipped long distances without deteriorating. Minerals possess just that lifeless-deathless quality that the Siddha yogi seeks.

But the Siddha doctors are careful to emphasize that, more than just being minerals, their medicines are mineral *poisons*, and this quality gives them a special medicinal power. In short, that which has the power to inflict death also has the power to restore life—to heal.

The depth of this idea is illustrated by the mythology of the Murugan temple at Paṟani, the town that is regarded as the center of the Siddha medical system. The story is that a certain Siddha yogi named Pōkar traveled to China and then returned to Tamil Nadu. He came to Paṟani and there in the mountain temple belonging to Murugan, the youthful god of war, beauty, and the sun, he made a statue of Murugan out of nine mineral poisons (*nava-pāśaṇam*). The substance of the statue is supposed to have great healing power; sick people come and drink of the offerings poured over it, for these offerings are thought to have some of the substance of the statue. The name of this particular image of Murugan is Sri Daṇḍāyudapāṇi, "Lord with a punishing weapon in his hand."[21]

Pōkar, at the end of his life, crawled into the mouth of a cave inside the temple at Paṛani, and never came out. The place into which he crawled is referred to as Pōkar's *samādhi*. But samādhi also (and originally) refers to a state of deep trance, such as the one Siddha yogis go into. So it is uncertain whether Pōkar died in the cave, or entered a deathless trance there, and people I asked about this were vague in their answers. In whatever way it occurred, after Pōkar crawled into the cave, the hill in which the cave was set burst forth with medicinal plants, and this is why Paṛani is now a medicinal center.

This popular myth expresses the womb-tomb idea with a directness that the more philosophical texts seem to avoid. It also merges in an interesting way, like the highly erotic imagery of these life-negating poets, the quest for lifelessness with the inescapability of life.

From what I have seen of the Siddha poetry, negation appears to be its most pervasive theme. First there is a negation or reversal of the natural, which contrasts with the naturalism of Āyurveda. For instance, Pāmpāḍḍi ("Snake-Charmer") Śiddhar sings: "We will make the pillar appear a splinter and the splinter appear a pillar; we will make male into female and female into male . . . we will make the bright-rayed sun into the cool-rayed moon; we will make this great world cease to be. Spewing up the poison, dance, snake, dance!"

Second, Siddha poems are often bitterly antiritualistic, as for instance Sivavākkiyar's verse: "Vedas are spit, mantras are spit, spiritual teachings are spit, semen is spit, the moon is spit, sound is spit. In what is there no spit? Nothing!"

Third, where Āyurveda is much concerned with typology, Siddha poetry tends to be powerfully anticaste and in general antistructural. And fourth, where the Āyurvedic writers seem to find a certain beauty in the life process, Siddha poetry sees with anguish the fruitlessness of it. "Running, running, they go in twilight, / Seeking, seeking, the days passing, / Drying, drying human corpses, / Dying, dying countless millions," writes Sivavākkiyar.

Finally, just as the siddhars are said to have isolated themselves from women especially among all creatures, their poetry is deeply misogynist. Tirumūlar describes women in a series of meaning-laden images: they are like the beautiful *eḍḍi* tree, whose shining fruit is deadly poison; they are like a clear mountain lake filled with whirlpools; they are like a sweet dream that turns to bitter waking; they are like a tank pond covered with moss that those who enter get tangled and caught in.

Sivavākkiyar identifies woman with the perishable body: "If another man sees the body of my woman and wants her, knowing her beauty, will I let him take her? I will say I should have cut him down before. But when death comes and calls her, I will take that fine stinking body to the burning ground, and leave it in the hands of the scavenger."

Akappēy Siddhar, whose name means soul-demon, addresses his inconstant soul as a vagrant female who will not be tamed. (*Akam* is interior, heart, or soul; *pēy* is the restless, bodiless spirit of someone who has died. It is apparently a literary convention in Tamil for the male poet to address his own heart as a willful wife or mistress, so a bhakti poet writes, "Your home, your master, the children that you've born—forget all these, you innocent fool heart.")

More subtle verses of Tirumūlar's identify woman with the life that the dying man leaves behind, that gluts him with love and thereby kills him, that feeds him delicious things as long as he lives but feeds him to the crows the minute he dies, that weeps for his loss, then has a ritual bath, turns away, and forgets him.

Wherever she is seen, woman represents to the siddhar the changefulness that he is so bent upon avoiding, unlike the Āyurvedic and Tamil bhakti writers, who sought to work *through* this change to final release. Tirumūlar's poetry suggests that when we try to "enjoy" a woman (which is to consume her as a fruit in Tamil idiom), she instead consumes us. Her nurturant body is poisonous; *because* it is nurturant, death is in it.

Differences of Opinion between Āyurvedic and Siddha Doctors　　　Modern Āyurvedic physicians interpret the biocosmology of their ancient texts according to their own experiences and understandings, but in general it can be said that Tamil Āyurvedic physicians, in keeping with the tone of their texts, show a positive valuation of the external, feminine, diverse, and changing material of life. This is so even though most Āyurvedic physicians in Tamil Nadu are Brahmans, whose contact with the substances of life is highly regulated and restricted. These physicians are aware of their paradoxical situation: they represent a Sanskritic tradition that is symbolic to many of status, purity, and disengagement from the grosser side of physical being; they are themselves strict vegetarians; yet the texts that are the source of their authority are unabashedly carnivorous, worldly, and unconfined.[22]

Dr. M., a village practitioner in his eighties (the one engaged in the dialogue given above) often said to women and to nonvegetarian patients, "There is nothing wrong with eating meat. We are none of us true vegetarians for we all drink our mother's blood for ten months before we are born and then for ten months after we are born we drink her blood again in the form of milk." To a woman sick from grief over the death in childbirth of her daughter, he said that only women have the power (*śakti*) given by God; "Man has not a single power." This power, he said, would enable a woman to be healed of a disease that would kill a man. The same power was also in the belly of a woman and in her milk. "Letting down her heart (*manam iranki*) she gives milk. What the child drinks is that power itself. . . . Great, great souls and wise people and lights of the house, women give milk to children. . . . The power of the mother is important. . . . The wife must be given equal power in the administration."[23]

In Dr. M's words was respect, even love, for the multiform matrix of life, combined with a desire to escape it. Yogis, he said, were people who had learned to live on air and light. They were the purest of beings, greatly to be envied. But he also told me, "The world is nature. Nature is in the form of feminine character," and, "it is the female part of the world that protects the people." Surely the Āyurvedic *mūla-prakṛti* ("root-prakṛti," the original substance of existence) was on his mind.

Dr. N., a leading urban Āyurvedic practitioner, emphasized his belief that Āyurveda is an objective, externally verifiable tradition, not spiritual but material, not subjective but objective, not religion but science. "Science you can prove," he said, "religion is only a feeling." Because their tradition is grounded in material reality, he said, "Āyurvedic physicians do not as a rule treat mental illness, only physical." He stressed the idea that people should, for the sake of their health, lead a natural life, and that villagers were for this reason more healthy and long-lived than urbanites. In the villages, people do not suppress their natural urges, and "they defecate anywhere," he said. He felt that this was not so in the cities. "If these *vehas* (natural urges, to urinate, defecate, sneeze, belch, and so forth) are controlled, you get diseases. If they are not controlled, you don't get diseases," he said. In *Suśruta Saṁhitā* there is a section entitled, "On the Nonsuppression of Natural Urges," which expresses precisely the sentiments that Doctor N. was here paraphrasing for me. The *vehas* should not be suppressed, says the ancient text. People living in urban environments, such as courtesans, politicians, and others who depend for their living on displays of mannerly civility, are in the habit of suppressing their natural impulses and for this reason are more disease-prone than country folk.

Dr. V., a female Āyurvedic physician with a small practice, enjoyed the variety of life that the Āyurvedic texts regard as existing and good. She said she liked Āyurveda because "each patient is an institution in himself. There are no across-the-board remedies." She was interested in the fact that people with different bodily constitutions (*prakṛti*) showed different kinds of behavior, and that the predominant humor (*dōṣa*) changed as a person's life progressed. Her treatment of a patient, she said, was carried out day by day, by a trial and error method. She also said that she tried to correct sickness with diet, not medicine.[24]

In contrast with Āyurvedic physicians, but in keeping with their own literary tradition, Siddha practitioners often express ideas that are inwardly oriented, magico-mystical, and negative. Whereas the original Āyurvedic texts were composed in Sanskrit in North India, and most Tamil Āyurvedic physicians are Brahmans, Siddha medicine is identified with Tamil and with anti-Brahmanism. The Āyurvedic physician Dr. N. claimed that "Siddha doctors do not study books. They have no literature, only formulas." In the face of such charges, Siddha doctors feel pressed to demonstrate that they do have texts and a systematic philosophy of their own. The fact that they are thus on the defensive may contribute to their apparent negativism. But more important is the fact that they have sought and found their roots in the only other major indigenous science of the body besides Āyurveda: Tantric yoga. In southern India, many Tantric ideas were incorporated into the eclectic philosophical system known as Śaiva Siddhanta. Siddha doctors have adopted this system as their own.

Āyurveda may be characterized as an extroverted medical system. Francis Zimmermann, for instance, has shown that in classical Āyurveda, the body is described not as a more or less sealed container (the way we are prone to see it), but rather as a landscape, an open field with all processes flowing visibly, at or near the surface (Zimmermann 1982). As though in extension of this principle, the Āyurvedic doctors with whom I spoke, such as Dr. M., were quite garrulous and eager to explain what they were doing in their practice and why.

The Siddha tradition by contrast stresses secrecy and concealment. Stories of siddha yogis, as we have seen, have them hiding themselves in all kinds of ways—they become invisible, crawl into caves, lock themselves up in rooms, retreat into trance. The language of the Siddha poetry is notoriously esoteric; modern students of it say it was deliberately made so, in order that Siddha knowledge would not become public. Siddha medicinal recipes are kept secret; some of them involve midnight-graveyard activities. Finally, modern Siddha doctors claim to be able to tell everything about the internal state of a patient just by feeling his pulse, whereas other doctors, they say, can only diagnose a disease on the basis of "outward signs."

The inward orientation of Siddha tradition prompts modern Siddha doctors to search for hidden meanings in their texts—especially hidden correlations between the concepts of Śaiva Siddhanta and those of modern Western science as Siddha doctors understand it. (This attitude, too, has political ramifications, for one of the strategies of the pro-Tamil, anti-Brahman movement in preindependence India was to seek alliance with the British in opposition to the North Indian–controlled Congress Party.) There is a stress upon both mantras and poetry in Siddha medicine, because both have levels of meaning not apparent on the surface. Thus, whereas the Āyurvedic Dr. N. asserts, "Science is not dependent upon language," the prominent Siddha physician Dr. Y. says, "Inner meaning is called science." Reality is hidden. An atom, says Dr. Y., is not visible to the ordinary onlooker, "but the scientist has seen the atom with his electron microscope."

Dr. Y. disagrees with Dr. N. also on the relation between religion and science. The Āyurvedic Dr. N. keeps them separate. Dr. Y. believes that each is the hidden part of the other: "In *Tirumantiram*," he says, "are both science and religion. When you read it as religion, you forget about the science. When you read it as science, you forget about the religion." And whereas the external orientation of Āyurveda led Dr. N. to say that Āyurvedic physicians rarely treat mental disease, the inwardness of Siddha causes another Siddha physician, Dr. A., to say, "unless a drug works in the mind also, it cannot prolong life."

Siddha medicine shares with Āyurveda the theory of the three humors. But Siddha doctors are inclined to interpret the nature of the humors in a strongly antimaterial way. Dr. G., who teaches and practices in a Siddha hospital in Madras, says that the humors are "not substances. They are like feelings, known only by experience." Dr. Y. carries this antimaterialism further. "Matter is impermanent," he says. "There is nothing in *Tirumantiram* about matter. It is all about energy."

Another contrast between the attitudes of Āyurvedic and Siddha practitioners is the antinaturalism of the latter, as compared to the naturalism of the former. Āyurvedic physicians underplay the importance of medicine and stress the importance of food and healing. For Siddha physicians, medicines opposed to the current of life are all-important. Dr. K., a professor at a Siddha medical college, said: "In Siddha, we do not rely upon herbal medicines. We go immediately for the poisonous compounds. Even a second-year undergraduate will freely use them."

For Siddha practitioners, not only medicine but also way of life contributes to sickness or health. But whereas Āyurvedic texts and physicians exhort patients not to suppress their natural urges, Siddha doctors recommend the opposite course. According to the successful Madras physician Dr. A., "There are four ways of lengthening life. First, control hunger. Second, reduce sleep. Third, reduce the amount of fat in the body. And fourth, arouse thirst." Dr. A. explained that Siddhars sought deathlessness, or at least long life, because the cycle of rebirth interrupted the yogi's progress in meditation. Every time he died and was reborn, he had to start over. Dr. A.'s opinion about the means to postpone death reflects the path that the Siddhars themselves were supposed to have followed.

Such expressions of inward orientation and antinaturalism are not limited to educated and successful leaders of the Siddha movement. They reach ordinary practitioners, and affect these practitioners' attitudes toward all of life. One example is Dr. H., a struggling Siddha doctor in southern Madras, who says he did not attend school at all but learned medicine from his father. Dr. H. lives and has his office a half mile down the road from the female Āyurvedic practitioner Dr. V., mentioned above. Dr. V., though her life has not been easy, has an outgoing attitude and seems to enjoy the diversity of the human race. Dr. H. is quite different. When I visit his office he eyes me suspiciously and asks me what I want. I explain that I want to learn a little about Siddha medicine, and am speaking with many doctors. He tells me that he is an uneducated man who has nothing to teach me, but at last he agrees to talk with me for a few minutes.

"Things that happen inside the body cannot be seen," Dr. H. begins. He says that he practices medicine according to the *panchabhuta* (five elements) theory. "Each *bhuta* has a taste, but cannot be seen. Likewise the ten *nadis* (channels), the ten *vayus* (winds) cannot be seen." (The five elements, ten channels, and ten winds are among the ninety-six *tattuvams* or basic components of the human being, listed in Śaiva Siddhanta literature.)

Of the people he sees, Dr. H. says, "Each tribe is different: it has its own customs. Things will never be equalized." He holds his hands when he says this as though they were the pans of an imbalanced scale. "People fight. There is no agreement or harmony (*ottumai*). Change is eternal. The whole world is the same way. The body is the same way. The body cannot be controlled, the senses cannot be controlled. In the same way, society cannot be controlled."

Trance-healing Through the Smallpox Goddess

Siddha poetry and medicine, as I have said, aim at deathlessness through lifelessness. Since life is evolved in the interaction of male and female, and the transformation of one by the other, of one into the other, or one through the other, however exactly it is seen, the avoidance of transformation means a complete isolation of male from female.

There is one other approach to the problem of death, entailing the isolation of female from male from the viewpoint of the female. This approach is expressed in the tradition of goddess-worship and trance-healing in Tamil Nadu.

Like most South Indian deities, especially female ones, the smallpox goddess Māriamman has lived a stormy life, and has strong needs and feelings. Her story is dramatic and impossible, yet in its essence, it is one that many people know they share.

Māriamman begins as Rēnuka Paramēswari, the chaste and perfect wife of her ascetic husband Jamadagni, serving and supporting him, and bearing him a hundred sons. As a perfect woman she has special powers. For instance, she can roll water up in a ball and carry it home without a pot. One day while getting water at the river, she sees the reflection of a beautiful man flying overhead—perhaps the sun, perhaps a celestial spirit, perhaps an airplane pilot (different tellers of the story suggest different beings). Just from looking at this man who is not her husband, she finds that she has lost her magical powers. When she returns home to her husband, he declares that her chastity is lost, and sends her eldest son to kill her. She flees while her son chases her with his sword, and at last she finds refuge in the hut of an untouchable woman, whom she embraces for comfort. The son enters the hut and beheads both women, and returns to his father with bloody evidence of the completed murder. In one version of the story the grateful father grants the son a boon, and the son asks that his mother be revived. In another version, the angry father realizes his mistake, and sends the son to revive the mother. In either case, the son returns, and places the severed heads back on the truncated bodies, but he puts them on wrong. The head of the Brahman woman now has the body of the Untouchable. She returns to her husband, but because her body is untouchable, he sends her away. From that day forth she lives alone, or with her twin in the forest, as a goddess.

When I first heard this story it was told in the first person.[25] I had befriended a woman in Madras who was a medium of Māriamman. She became regularly possessed by the goddess and when she did, the goddess spoke through her and addressed people who came to her with petitions and complaints. When a medium of Māriamman enters a trance, the power of the goddess is strong in her and can both speak and heal.

One day the goddess spoke to me and at my request told me who she was. She told an extended form of the story recounted above. She ended by exhorting me to believe in her and by stressing her identity with the woman whom she possessed—both were married women, both were afflicted with suffering, both were innocent. Women like this medium, because they were like the goddess, would believe in the goddess completely, she said. She told me also, "You must not change your heart. I have truly come here out of earth. But for Tamil women only I am one who will do much good."

The trance-healer and her patients know Māriamman and her story well, for the mythological goddess is regarded as a real person dwelling within the healer (among other places), and her personality, actions, and statements to patients are believed to result from the experiences she has undergone.

From the point of view of this essay, it is important to note that the woman in the story becomes an immortal goddess after she has died, and her powers as goddess of smallpox to heal and to kill seem to stem from this point (the transformation of woman to goddess through the violent death of the woman is not an uncommon theme in southern Indian folklore).

A kind of structure can be worked out for the story of Māriamman, which also seems to underlie the Siddha philosophy. Given that death and nurturance are mutually implicative, denial of one requires denial of both. We have seen how the siddhar cuts himself off in order to be immortal. Māriamman's

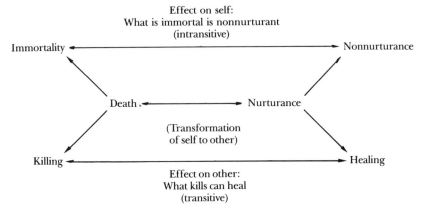

Figure 6.1

immortality, too, comes when she is rather literally cut off, and when she leaves her role as wife and mother. As a state of nurturance is replaced by a state of nonnurturance, a state of subjection to death is replaced by a state of immortality. At the same time, however, a new set of opposites is produced. For death yields not only to immortality as the negation of death, but also to an intensified and transitive version of death, killing. And nurturance yields not only to the negation of nurturance, but also and simultaneously to an intensified and transitive version of nurturance, healing. Death, as a process involving a transformation of self to other, thus breaks into the totally intransitive state of immortality, and the totally transitive act of killing (transitive in that it produces a transformation in the object, the one who is killed, but not in the agent, the killer). Nurturance, also as a process involving transformation of self to other, breaks into the totally intransitive state of nonnurturance, neither taking nor giving, and the totally transitive act of healing (transitive in that it changes the patient, but not the healer). Finally, therefore, as a negation of the single two-sided process, we have four opposites: the state of deathlessness and the act of killing on one side, the state of lifelessness and the act of healing on the other (see fig. 6.1).

Systems built on the negation of some reality are inevitably paradoxical: my description of Siddha medicine gives some idea of its paradoxical quality, and the paradoxes inherent in the image of the smallpox goddess are legendary. As if to restore unity, each of these systems brings together the opposites that it creates, and expresses the idea that what kills can also heal (as in the medicinal poison of the Siddhars, and the dual personality of the goddess), and that what is immortal or deathless is also unnurtured and unnurturing, or lifeless.

A similar structure appears in the mythology of the goddesses Mīnākshi and Kaṇṇaki. The story of Mīnākshi is that she is born three-breasted from a sacrificial fire and becomes a warrior goddess destroying not only demons but everything in sight. Only when she meets her future husband Śiva does her third breast melt away, at which point she becomes a normal, docile female. (In one version of the story, she is just about to kill Śiva when she realizes who he is and her anger disappears.) The story of Kaṇṇaki is that she is a normal, docile wife until her husband is killed, at which point, in her rage, she tears off her breast and destroys by fire the inhabitants of a whole city and finally is apotheosized. In these stories, the normal nurturant form of the woman (two-breastedness) is opposed to a kind of transnurturance (three-breastedness), and a denial of nurturance (one-breastedness), both linked with immortality and with killing.

But the structure of denial of nurturance and death is not confined to mythology. The medium of Māriamman told me that when she was young she had become possessed by the goddess and that the goddess had performed acts of healing through her, but she did not become a professional healer until she fell ill with tuberculosis and came close to death—her kin had in fact already given her up for dead and had begun to mourn her, when the goddess appeared to her in a vision saying that she (the goddess) had been the one to bring on the disease, and she now would end it, which she did. This experience of the medium seems to reflect, in weakened form, the goddess's own death and resurrection—it was, for her, a denial of the power of natural death (and natural healing methods, for she had been to regular doctors, and they had failed to heal her). She had been a good wife and had borne a large number of children, whom she nursed and reared. But as she became a healer the goddess demanded of her that she bear no more children, that she refuse not only to have sex with her husband but even to speak with him, that she make herself sexually unattractive, that she not cook for her family, and that she move away and live separately from them. Her life, therefore, became a life of isolation and one of refusal to nurture. It was a nonnurturant life not only in that she refused to nurture others, but also in that she said that for some time she had felt "no desire," which she explained as no hunger, so that she ate very little, and no desire for human company in general and men in particular.[26] In the stories that she told of her life, the villains and death-dealers all were men, the helpers all women. Most of her clientele were women.[27]

Thus, in many ways she was the reflex of the Siddha yogi, who isolates himself from the world and looks upon women as the source of evil and death.

There are, however, some important differences. The medium, though claiming to desire isolation, in fact lived a very gregarious life. Though the medium was never hungry, the goddess possessing her was often ravenous. Though the medium said she wished to avoid mixing with others, the goddess mixed with them in the most intimate way possible, through spirit possession. Though the Siddha yogi existed in a state of perfect and painless peace, his body and soul united into a single immortal entity, the medium and the goddess each said of themselves that they suffered and that they had no peace. The goddess said she had a form of wind (unstable spirit in search of a body) or of mud (perishable body in need of a spirit), and she said that though she aided others, she could not change her own misery.

This brings us back to the original form of being which these healing systems seek to negate and escape. All the differences between the goddess-medium and the Siddha yogi stem from the fundamental sexual assymmetry of their shared model of life. The Siddha yogi escapes the change that is at the core of natural life by making himself changeless, and isolating himself from the changing female who embodies that life. The goddess and her medium cannot do this, because they *are* female, and so they *are* (in their own eyes as well) the process; they are the change. Thus the name Māriamman, according to the medium, means "the changed mother."

In conclusion, the four systems of thought which have been discussed here can be seen to form a gradient: first, according to how much they embrace the dying-into-another process of life or how much they negate it; and second, according to their high or low evaluation of the feminine ideal. Not surprisingly, the two gradients are one.[28]

At one extreme is modern Śaiva bhakti, which virtually deifies the feminine as the embodiment of love, meltingness, and self-sacrifice, and which takes as its goal the dissolution of the boundaries of the self and the flowing of the self into Śiva as the other. Next is Āyurveda, which accepts the feminine process as necessary for the evolution and liberation of the masculine spiritual entity. Following is the religion of the goddess, which hangs suspended between ideals of isolation and merger, between espousal of the feminine ideal and denial of its validity. Finally comes the Siddha system, which aims to isolate the practitioner totally from all interaction, transform life process into stasis, and radically exclude the feminine from its sphere of being.

It is interesting that the two extremes of this continuum, Siddha medicine and Śaiva bhakti, share many of the same texts, which are voluminous and ambiguous enough to allow widely discrepant interpretations. Also interesting is the fact that the two middle terms in our continuum, Āyurveda and trance healing, are practiced by individuals at opposite ends of the social spectrum.

The dying or ill person in Tamil Nadu who consults a number of healers is likely to receive in some form the message that all these systems share: freedom comes from pain and death is part of life. It is not entirely an optimistic message, nor is it a fair one, for male and female are implicated in the message in different ways. But being expressed so diversely yet consistently through different traditions, that message may at least give the sufferer a sense that his or her experience is not without an overarching meaning.

NOTES

1. Data for this article were collected between January 1975 and August 1976, in Madras and in Kanyakumari District of Tamil Nadu, under a grant from the Social Science Research Council. An earlier version of this article appeared in *Social Science and Medicine* 17 (1983): 935–945.

2. The Āyurvedic texts referred to here are the two earliest known ones, *Śuśruta Saṁhitā* and *Caraka Saṁhitā*, both composed in Sanskrit in northern India and dated sometime between 200 B.C. and A.D. 200.

3. Charles Leslie (1976) refers to this type of healing as "learned magico-religious medicine." The Śaiva gurus are probably the most influential practitioners of this genre in Tamil Nadu.

4. Works by Tirumūlar and Ramalingar actually contain very little in the way of practical medical information, such as descriptions of recipes for medicine, treatments for diseases, body types, and so forth. This kind of information is contained in palm leaf manuscripts that were originally handed down from father to son or from teacher to student, and are now being collected and published by government-subsidized colleges and hospitals. These manuscripts, while rich in practical experiential knowledge, are said by collectors to lack an overall theoretical framework distinct from that of Āyurveda. For such a distinguishing paradigm, present-day Siddha doctors resort to the more famous poetic and philosophical Siddha texts.

5. To the best of my knowledge, the most detailed description in English of yogic philosophy and of the notion of the siddhar is still to be found in Eliade (1969).

6. See, for example, Trawick (1987).

7. See, for example, Zvelebil (1973).

8. A good reference in Tamil is *Cittar Pāḍalkaḷ*, Aru Ramanatan, ed. Madras: Pirema Piracuram, 1968.

9. Material on the cult of Māriamman cited in this paper is drawn from a study by Trawick (Egnor) (1978a, 1982).

10. For examples see Moreno (1982a), Preston (1980, 1982), Beck (1981), and Trawick (1982).

11. Nicholas (1981), Greenough (1980), and Marglin (1987).

12. The necessity of congruence between a medical system and the culture in which it must operate has been stressed by Gould (1965), Marriott (1955), Carstairs (1955), and many others. The nature of this congruence, however, is subtle. It can be a matter of shared unconscious fears, the patient's unspoken worry being confirmed by the doctor's diagnosis (Obeyesekere 1976), of differential development or stress of a given concept in folk and specialist systems of medical knowledge (Nichter 1980), of metaphorical relations between folk categories and specialist categories, or of compromise between folk and specialist categorical systems where incongruities appear (Tabor 1981). Other kinds of congruence between lay and professional conceptual systems can easily be found. A systematic study of the various possibilities would be interesting.

13. Tabor (1981) provides other examples of such processes of mutual adjustment.

14. Leslie (1980).

15. Compare W. T. Jones's point (Jones 1976) that less systematicity in a worldview, that is, less coherence among its various parts, is conducive to greater flexibility.

This is perhaps one of the strongest reasons for maintenance of medical pluralism within a society. A looser medical structure can stretch to accommodate not only the unique needs of particular patients but also whole new medical systems because of the processes of mutual adjustment and gradual incorporation of one another's methods and theories that plural medical systems undergo.

16. Lévi-Strauss (1963*a*). When religion is conceived, as Max Weber conceived it, to be essentially a response to great "problems of meaning," then the boundary between religion (which subsumes myth) and medicine (as a branch of science) begins to fade. Both are built upon the problem of pain. For religion, this problem is framed in terms of theodicy, divine morality ("If God is God, he is not good"), and for medicine, in terms of causation ("The force that through the green fuse drives the flower . . . is my destroyer"). In either case, an insurmountable contradiction is there, like a grain of sand in an oyster, to be continually worked over but never dissolved. Weber himself noted the use of healing metaphors in world religions such as Buddhism and Christianity. In smaller and more tightly knit systems, such as the shamanic one discussed in this paper, the identity between healing and religion is total.

17. Patterned and balanced symbolic relations among competing medical systems, as seen from the layman's point of view, have already been discovered by Gould (1965), Marriott (1955), and Nichter (1980). Gould reports that Rajasthan villagers in the mid-1950s resorted to native medicine for "chronic nonincapacitating dysfunctions . . . conditions manifesting drawn-out periods of suffering" and to Western medicine for "critical incapacitating dysfunctions . . . marked by the opposite inventory of symptoms: that is, maladies involving sudden and often violent onset, and rather complete debilitation." According to Marriott, North Indian villagers saw native medicine as fast and powerful. More recently, Nichter's Kanarese informants described an analogy between Western medicine and temperamental, bloodthirsty local deities on the one hand, and between Āyurveda and the cool-headed, vegetarian Brahmanical deities on the other. The former were seen as hot, fast, powerful, and uncontrolled, while the latter were considered balanced, controlled, nondestructive, and not conducive to "shock" in the patient. This paper considers a similar set of contrasts (see especially the section on Siddha medicine), but among indigenous healing systems rather than between them and exogenous ones.

18. For a more detailed discussion of parallels between Āyurveda and Samkhya, see Trawick (Egnor) (1974).

19. I recorded this interview in 1976 when I was living near the clinic operated by this doctor, Mahadeva Iyer, and studying his practice. For more extensive analysis of the rhetorical structure of this physician's interviews with his patients and with me, see Trawick (1987, 1991).

20. For a more detailed discussion of concepts of the body in Śaiva bhakti, see Trawick (Egnor) (1978).

21. For more on the temple of Murugan at Paṟani, see Moreno (1982*b*).

22. Tabor (1981) has made the same observation.

23. The full text of this discussion is in Trawick (1987).

24. A synopsis of the autobiography of Dr. V., Valliammae, is in Trawick (1980).

25. For full text and commentary see Trawick (Egnor) (1978, 1982).

26. According to personal communication with Gananath Obeyesekere, anorexia is a common complaint of such mediums.

27. Not only in South Asia, but in societies throughout the world, spirit possession occurs as a means for women and others lacking access to the regular channels of power to escape or alleviate oppressive social conditions (Lewis 1971). Frequently spirit possession results in the woman separating herself partly or completely from her family.

28. This association is of course not confined to India. See Beauvoir (1952).

REFERENCES

Amarasingham, Lorna Rhodes
    1980   Movement among healers in Sri Lanka: a case study of a Sinhalese patient. *Culture, Medicine and Psychiatry* 4: 71–92.
Beals, Alan
    1976   Strategies of resort to curers in South Asia. In *Asian Medical Systems*, ed. Charles Leslie, 184–200. Berkeley, Los Angeles, London: University of California Press.
Beauvoir, Simone de
    1952   *The Second Sex*, trans. and ed. H. M. Parshley. New York: Knopf.
Beck, Brenda
    1981   The goddess and the demon: a local South Indian festival and its wider context. *Purusartha* 5: 83–136.
Caraka
    1949   *Caraka Samhita*, ed. and trans. Shree Gulabkunverba Ayurvedic Society. Jamnagar, India.
Carstairs, G. Morris
    1955   Medicine and faith in Rajasthan. In *Health, Culture and Community*, ed. Benjamin Paul. New York: Russell Sage.
Eliade, Mircea
    1969   *Yoga: Immortality and Freedom*. Princeton: Princeton University Press.
Gould, Harold
    1965   Modern medicine and folk cognition in rural India. *Human Organization* 24: 201–208.
Greenough, Paul
    1980   Variolation and vaccination in South Asia, c. 1700–1865: a preliminary note. *Social Science and Medicine* 14D: 345–347.
Jones, W. T.
    1976   World views and Asian medical systems: suggestions for further study. In *Asian Medical Systems*, ed. Charles Leslie. Berkeley, Los Angeles, London: University of California Press.
Leslie, Charles
    1976   The ambiguities of medical revivalism in modern India. In *Asian Medical Systems*, ed. Charles Leslie, 356–367. Berkeley, Los Angeles, London: University of California Press.
    1980   Medical pluralism in world perspective. *Social Science and Medicine* 14B: 191–196.

Lévi-Strauss, Claude
1963a   The structural study of myth. In *Structural Anthropology*, 206–231. New York: Basic Books.
1963b   The sorcerer and his magic. In *Structural Anthropology*, 167–185. New York: Basic Books.

Lewis, I. M.
1971   *Ecstatic Religion*. New York: Penguin.

Marglin, Frederique Apffel
1987   Smallpox in two systems of knowledge. Manuscript, Smith College.

Marriott, McKim
1955   Western medicine in a village of North India. In *Health, Culture and Community*, ed. Benjamin Paul. New York: Russell Sage Foundation.

Moreno, Manuel
1982a   The appropriation of order in a Hindu festival. Manuscript.
1982b   The god of healing poisons: thermic complementarity and exchanges in two South Indian pilgrimages. Manuscript.

Nicholas, Ralph
1981   The goddess Sitala and epidemic smallpox in Bengal. *Journal of Asian Studies* 41(1): 21–44.

Nichter, Mark
1980   The layperson's perception of medicine as perspective into the utilization of multiple therapy systems in the Indian context. *Social Science and Medicine* 14B: 225–234.

Obeyesekere, Gananath
1976   The impact of Ayurvedic ideas on culture and the individual in Sri Lanka. In *Asian Medical Systems*, ed. Charles Leslie, 201–226. Berkeley, Los Angeles, London: University of California Press.
1977   Psychocultural exegesis of a case of spirit possession in Sri Lanka. In *Case Studies in Spirit Possession*, ed. Vincent Crapanzano, 235–294. New York: Wiley.

Preston, James
1980   *Cult of the Goddess: Social and Religious Change in a Hindu Temple*. New Delhi: Vikas.
1982   The goddess Chandi as an agent of change. In *Mother Worship*, ed. James Preston, 210–226. Chapel Hill: University of North Carolina Press.

Śuśruta
1907   *Śuśruta Saṁhitā*, ed. and trans. K. K. L. Bhishagratna. Calcutta, India.

Tabor, Daniel
1981   Ripe and unripe concepts of health and sickness in Ayurvedic medicine. *Social Science and Medicine* 15B: 439–455.

Trawick (Egnor), Margaret
1974   Principles of continuity in three Indian sciences. Master's thesis, University of Chicago.
1978a   The sacred spell and other conceptions of life in Tamil culture. Ph.D. Diss., University of Chicago.
1978b   A Tamil priestess. Manuscript. Western Washington University. Bellingham, Wa.

1980   On the meaning of sákti to women in Tamil Nadu. In *The Powers of Tamil Women*, ed. Susan Wadley. Syracuse: Maxwell School of Citizenship and Public Affairs.

1982   The changed mother, or, what the smallpox goddess did when there was no more smallpox. *Contributions to Asian Studies* 18: 24–45.

1987   The Ayurvedic physician as scientist. *Social Science and Medicine* 24 (12): 1031–1050.

1990   *Notes on Love in a Tamil Family*. Berkeley, Los Angeles, Oxford: University of California Press.

1991   An Ayurvedic theory of cancer. *Medical Anthropology* 13: 121–136.

Weber, Max

1964   *The Sociology of Religion*. Boston: Beacon Press.

Zimmermann, Francis

1982   *La Jungle et le Fumet des Viandes: un theme ecologique dans la medicine hindoue*. Paris: Gallimard-le Seuil.

Zvelebil, Kamil

1973   *Poets of the Powers*. London: Rider.

SEVEN

Science, Experimentation, and Clinical Practice in Āyurveda

Gananath Obeyesekere

Though medicine, in most cultures, extends beyond the realm of disease into larger problems of existence, it must at minimum attempt to cure disease or ameliorate it. But no matter what the mode of therapy used—magical, physical medicine, or whatever—success and failure are built into systems of medicine. The individual curer must justify his therapy in terms of practical criteria of efficiency, since it would be hard to defend a therapy that does not work consistently. The afflicted person must also feel that his affliction is "cured," or he must know that his condition is incurable or a difficult one that can only be ameliorated at best. Medicine is also part of the public domain and, however esoteric the medical theory, physician, patient, and community are linked together in an intersubjective network defining the nature of symptoms as well as types of medicine and their relative efficacy. The efficacy of a cure raises the following questions: Does the medicine work? What are the signs of its success or how do we know it works? When it does not work, what explanations can we give? In other words, the essentially pragmatic function of medicine forces public discussion of issues pertaining to the effectiveness of a therapy and the form of medicine it enshrines; truth or falseness of a therapy depends on the practical criteria pertaining to efficacy.

Medicine is rarely focused on therapy alone, or given exclusively to medical prescription. It often must justify the therapy in terms of some rational scheme. The theoretical rationale for therapy is only part of the public domain, for most of medicine is knowledge held by specialists. But specialists, even if they belong to esoteric schools or confraternities, must justify to themselves and to rivals that beyond the efficacy of the therapy is its validity. I am not suggesting that this form of intersubjective validation is universal, but that it is widespread in medical practice cross-culturally. Medical specialists are forced into debate among themselves or others, not only regarding therapy, but also regarding the rationale or the theory for the therapy. This is not always readily apparent. A shaman may say that the efficacy of his therapy depends on his "power." But power, like faith, is not an abstract force; it is locked into a cosmology, into a pantheon of supernaturals and, ultimately, into beliefs about the derivation and maintenance of that power.

What has the preceding argument to do with "science"? In order to open up for discussion the *idea* of science, I shall formulate its parameters as follows: (1) the formulation of one's knowledge of the world in abstract and conceptual form; and (2) empirical verification and intersubjective validation of that knowledge. The question now arises whether medicine is an appropriate arena for dealing with science in the manner defined above. It seems clear, at least in terms of the foregoing discussion, that the second criterion of empiricism exists in medical practice with sufficient frequency for it to be used in our analysis.

Empiricism is everywhere grounded in experience, even if it deals with the experience of supernatural beings or entities, but empiricism alone is not science according to our definition. It must be associated with the second criterion that requires a theoretical, metatheoretical, or conceptual rationale. Yet one must make a distinction between *any* "rationale" for explaining the therapy and the specific one pertaining to conceptual formulation highlighted here. For example, many medical systems have rational explanations for illness and therapy in terms of gods, demons, spirits, and other personalized entities. I reject Horton's thesis that these explanations are strictly parallel to that of modern science;[1] in my definition they are not. I agree with Horton that these supernatural beliefs might be systematically and rationally formulated, but, though they are systems of thought, they are not systems of science. As systems of thought they deal not only with medicine but, more fundamentally, with broader issues of human existence and being and sometimes even salvation. This would hardly do for a definition of science. But the fact that therapeutic efficacy could be rationally defended in terms of a larger belief system implies that, in some instances, the rationale may develop from such personalized explanations as found in religion, to more impersonal explanations couched in abstract and conceptual form.

Understanding the conditions that foster such a development, or the parallel existence of at least two forms of rationality, is one of the long-term goals of my research. However, insofar as medical practice entails both empirical validation and a rationale for illness causation, therapy, and practice, we argue further that in a very basic sense science is based on two experiential values. First, it is "ontological," insofar as it is based on our species experience; second, it is founded in practice. Though the ontological ground of science is in the human propensity to give rational meaning to what we do, conceptual thought is a further development and is not synonymous with all forms of rationality, including the religious.

How, then, shall we approach this problem of the development of conceptual thought from the larger problem of rational thought? For present purposes I would like to deal with it definitionally, as Max Weber did. Though Weber's idea of practical rationality of the sort embodied in the Protestant Ethic is well known, he had a lesser known but, in my view, a more interesting view of rationality as "the kind of rationalization that the systematic thinker performs on the image of the world: an increasing mastery of reality by means of increasingly precise and abstract concepts."[2]

I label this definition theoretical, metatheoretical, or conceptual rationality insofar as it is a systematization of thought through the use of abstract terms or concepts. It is clear that conceptual rationality can exist without empirical verification. Philosophical beliefs, such as abstract religious doctrines like Buddhism or commentaries on religious doctrines by thinkers, all can produce highly systematized abstract thought without being grounded in systematic empiricism.

But when the two combine, we have the beginnings of science. When medicine, for whatever reasons, postulates explanations in abstract form, it must produce a "science of medicine" since the second criterion of empirical verification is intrinsic to most, if not all, forms of medicine. The existence of a science of medicine, in turn, may help us answer questions pertaining to the nature of science—its development or evolution, its goals, its ontological interests, its conceptions of truth, and so forth, though perhaps not, as Popper cautions us, the prediction of its future.[3]

This is where Āyurveda comes in. We all know that Āyurveda possesses a highly abstract metatheoretical framework for explaining diseases, similar in form to theories in the social sciences and psychoanalysis. Like the latter, the highly abstract metatheoretical framework, unlike philosophical and religious speculations, does not exist without empirical verification, but is grounded in well-recognized procedures of validation and experimentation. But, though Āyurveda is a science in our sense of the term, there are no professional scientists of Āyurveda, that is, those whose main role is the generation of scientific knowledge through research. Āyurveda practitioners are physicians and their science emerges out of their medical practice. But it is also obvious that some are more interested than others in the practice of science in the course of their practice of medicine, and it is these "out-of-the-ordinary" individuals whom we sought to interview in our research. We selected a small number of physicians from a variety of backgrounds, including Dr. W. A. Fernando, whose practice I describe below. He comes from a family tradition of Āyurvedic physicians in Sri Lanka; he knows Sanskrit well and can quote freely from classic Sanskrit texts. His office is a room in the side of his house and one wall is lined with old and frayed printed texts in Sanskrit and Sinhala. Dr. Fernando is not familiar with English and his knowledge of Western medicine and physiology is minimal, coming from newspapers, Sinhala texts, and dialogue with fellow physicians. He can occasionally give English equivalents for Āyurvedic terms, but this knowledge is widespread among contemporary Āyurvedic physicians. Some of it is incorporated into Āyurvedic texts written during this century. Our strategy for research was a very simple one. We watched Dr. Fernando treat patients in his consulting room. We tape-recorded sessions that we thought might turn out to be interesting. In Āyurveda there is virtually no physical examination: the patient lists his symptoms while the doctor probes him with further questions. Then the doctor prescribes a medication with instructions on regimen. We interfere at this point, and often in the presence of the patient we ask him to explain or elaborate on the features of symptomatology and the medication that did not seem clear to us. A more detailed discussion of select cases takes place after office hours. In the following account we use a mere fraction of the data collected.

The Man Who Couldn't Pass Wind

This case is typical of the patients that consult Āyurvedic physicians, for most go to Western doctors and government hospitals for acute illnesses. Our patient is a thirty-two-year-old man who complains of a pain on the left side of his stomach. He feels a revulsion for food and has no appetite. He also often experiences nausea, and complains that his stomach is constantly puffed up (*pippila*). He had gone to a Western physician who gave him some medicines but these unfortunately produced hives (*palu*). His boss asked him to consult Dr. Fernando, who gave him several decoctions (*kasāya*) over a three-month period. He says that he feels very much better now. This is his fourth visit.

He tells the doctor that his stools are hard and he finds it difficult to pass them.

Doctor: But do you pass stools at least once a day?
Patient: Yes, because I have trained myself to "go out" in the mornings.
   [This is a typical Sinhala (and South Asian) practice where people have trained themselves to pass stools first thing in the morning. If this routine is upset or if the passage of stools is difficult people get quite anxious.]
Doctor: So you don't feel fully comfortable, and you feel that your stools should pass more easefully.
Patient: Yes, sometimes I feel as if I want to let out air (*vāta*), but none comes out. With difficulty a little escapes, but with real difficulty.
Doctor: [for my benefit] There is another disease (*leda*) which has been linked to your (previous) disease—that is *arśas* (hemorrhoids and related diseases).
   [With deliberate good humor, the doctor adds:] Western doctors have only one type of *arśas*, but we are the proud possessors of several. Western doctors say there is *arśas* only if there is blood and hemorrhoids, but we have several. Here's a *kalka* (paste), mix it (generally with honey or

sugar) and eat a quarter of the portion I have given you daily. Also take the following decoction, *kasāya*.

The doctor writes out the prescription in Sinhala on a narrow sheet of paper. The patient gives him a twenty-rupee note. The doctor changes the money and gives it back. The patient then gives him a few rupees. This is the accepted convention. There is no standard fee, each patient gives what he can afford. Generally the doctor charges a fixed fee only for medicines that he himself has prepared. The convention is for the patient to present a sheaf of betel leaves with money placed in it as he enters the doctor's office. If the patient is poor the doctor invariably returns the money.

The dialogue continues, stimulated by my presence.

> *Doctor:* There is a possibility that your disease may end up as *arśas*. [To me] Diseases of the bowels are of four chief types, these being: *arśas*, hemorrhoids; *atisāra*, dysentery, which could arise anywhere in the intestines; *ajīrna*, indigestion occurring in the upper part of the intestines; *grahani*, diarrhea which arises at the point where the big and the small intestines join (*grahanisthāna*).

He now quotes a Sanskrit couplet (*śloka*) that he translates for me. It says that *arśas, grahani, atisāra,* and *ajīrna* have *sāmanya hētu*, similar causes or antecedent conditions; they arise from different parts of the intestines. Thus, all four types have the same source of *duśya* ("disruption"), and therefore the same *hētu* ("cause"). He says that this patient's disease started from the top part of the intestines but now it is confined to the area below.

> *Doctor:* Isn't it a great relief if you can pass air without discomfort?
> *Patient:* Yes.
> *Doctor:* It is a big trouble (*loku karadarayak*) if the *vāta* does not go out in the right manner.
> [Now the doctor further explains to us what he meant by the last statement.]
> In medicine one important *nīti* has to do with *anuloma-pratiloma* (literally, "in the direction of the hair"; "against the direction of the hair"). When *anuloma guna* ("the property of *anuloma*") is realized troubles will go away.

I will now consider the prescription for the decoction given by Dr. Fernando containing, among other items, the following ingredients: roots of *tippili* (*Piper longum*); *aralu* (*Terminia chebala*); roots of *dēvadāra* (*Cedrus deodara*); roots of *sivi* (*Piper chawya*); *iṅguru* (ginger); *ratnitul* (*Plumbago rosea*).

The effect or *vipāka* of this prescription is to develop an appetite or *bada ginna* (literally, "belly heat"), not in excess, but a modulated heat or appetite (*sādhārana ginna*). The combination of these items is known as *behet yōgaya*. The major property or *guna* of these medicines is *ūṣna vīriya* ("the strength of *ūṣna* or heat"); some items also produce *grahi gunaya* ("the property of absorbency"). Consider some of the terms employed. In ordinary language use in Sinhala, *baḍa ginna* means "hunger" or "appetite," and one of the problems of the patient was just this. The term *baḍa ginña*, literally means "belly heat" and is derived from the technical language of Āyurveda according to which the food that one ingests is initially cooked in the stomach. The main humor that is responsible for cooking the food is *ūṣna*, or "heat." The Sinhala *gini* is derived from the Sanskrit word *agni*, the element of heat. Since the patient's problem is the lack of heat or fire to cook the food, he suffers from a loss of appetite. Thus, the prescription must correct this and produce a combination of ingredients or *behet yōga*, that will have the *guna* ("property") to increase the strength or *viriya* of heat. However, loss of appetite is not the only problem of the patient: his stools are hard and he cannot pass wind. This is due to the *pratiloma* (against the hair or "contrary flow") of the humors (*doṣa*), essences (*dhātu*), and waste products (*mala*) of the body. If the *guna* or property of *anuloma* ("normal flow") is present in the body and works in the right manner, there will be no accretions or accumulations (*bäñḍīma*) of waste and the bodily substances will flow in the right direction. Thus, *anuloma-pratiloma* is a key principle or law or *nīti* that must be considered in this case and in every case. *Nīti* refers to a fundamental principle that is applicable in a wide range of cases. In this patient's case it refers to the impeded flow of bodily waste or *mala*, but the principle could as easily apply to the flow of *doṣa* ("humors") and *dhātu* ("bodily essences"). The doctor gave an example of a person who has had an impeded blood flow—the effect of *pratiloma* on the *dhātu* or essence of blood. Blood flows through our *nalana-hara* ("nerves and channels"), propelled by the element air or *vāta*. *Vāta* is the force that sends the blood coursing through the channels and nerves of the body. Now, owing to a variety of immediate causes or *hētu*, the element air (*vāta*) and the bodily essence, blood, can move in different directions. This is *pratiloma*, a contrary flow that might produce the illness known as *vāta-rakta* ("air-blood").

Now we can go back to the decoction prescribed by Dr. Fernando for the man who could not pass wind. The doctor's strategy in the prescription is to provide medicines that will help cook the food in the body, and also ensure *anuloma guna* ("the right flow"):

tippili (*Piper longum*): has the property (*guna*) of cooking or ripening (*dīpana*) and also has *anuloma guna*, and consequently can assist the normal flow of bodily wastes. It reduces the swelling in the stomach and bowels by getting the liquid out of the swellings. *Tippili* can scratch or irritate the inside of the swelling in order to get the liquid out.

aralu (*Terminalia chebala or gallnut*): has two *gunas*. Primarily *anuloma guna*, that is, it sends the waste in the normal direction by its emetic properties. It also helps to cook the food.

sivi roots (*Piper chawla*): it destroys *sema* (*sleśma*, "phlegm"), evens out any excess *vāta* ("air"), and increases the quantity of heat manifest as *pitta* or bile. The latter is necessary since the patient has a loss of appetite owing to the absence of heat that cooks the food in the stomach.

ratnitul (*Plumbago rosea*): is good for stomach disorders and is also, according to Dr. Fernando, a germ killer. It is also recommended for *arśas* ("hemorrhoids").

inguru (ginger): increases the property of heat. All three of the above ingredients have *dīpana guna*, which cooks the food in the stomach by their heating properties. They also have *grahi guna*, helping to solidify the waste matter that has been loosened by the emetic properties of *aralu* (gallnut), and helps eject such waste.

dēvadāra roots (*Cedrus deodara*): this ingredient helps *samana* ("even out") the *doṣa* ("humors"). Since the prescription contains a large amount of heat-increasing ingredients, *dēvadāra* will help "even out" or cut down excess heat or *ūṣna* that might build up in the body.

In examining this prescription one can see the clear relationship between the Āyurvedic theory and practice. The properties of ingredients are well known and they are combined to suit the particular case. This combination of ingredients (or the *guna* or properties of ingredients) is known as *behet yōga*, or *samyōga*. In the above case we have presented only a segment of a prescription; in addition, the doctor prescribed another *pēyāva* or "herbal tea" to be taken twice daily in the morning and evening. This tea repeats some of the ingredients of the other prescription (for example, *aralu, tippili*) but adds new ones, such as *kalāñduru ala* (*Cyperus rotundus*), which creates *ruccā* or the taste for food, and also possesses the property of "cooking" (*dīpana*).

Most of Dr. Fernando's prescriptions are standard in the sense that they are found in either Sanskrit texts or Sinhala texts or handed down from his family tradition or that of his teachers. But, though standard, they are never rigidly adhered to. Variations on the standard prescription can take the following forms:

(a) Combination of two prescriptions. Depending on the individual case, Āyurvedic physicians often combine two prescriptions together;

(b) Deletions from the standard prescription. For example, both the prescriptions (the decoction and the tea) given to the patient contained *aralu* or gall nut. Since this might be excessive it could be removed from one prescription. Deletions constantly occur in Āyurvedic clinical medicine and are based on the recognition that the standard prescription may not fit the individual patient. Thus, a deletion may be followed by a substitution or addition. One can, for example, delete *aralu* (gall nut) from the prescription and add *vī pori* (puffed rice), which will help bind the stools (the rice is boiled with the other ingredients and strained);

(c) Additions to standard prescriptions are very common in Āyurveda and are again based on the individual case. For example, there are many other ingredients that have the *guna* appropriate for the case of the man who couldn't pass wind. *Magul Karaṅda* (*Pongamia glabra*) has high *dīpana guna* and can help the cooking of the food in the belly, while the various parts of the tamarind tree (leaves, stems, bark, roots) have the *pāsavana guna*, that is, help the conversion of food into the next stage of *rasa* ("chyle"), and so on to the other stages. Or, to state it differently, this ingredient (tamarind) helps convert food into the *dhatu*s or essences of the body. If there occur several new additions and deletions to a prescription, one is effectively on the way to inventing a new prescription. For example, Dr. Fernando was treating an old lady who was paralyzed from a stroke. He used a standard Sanskrit prescription containing eleven ingredients. But he deleted one of these and added three more: *kaluduru* (black cumin), *tippili* (*Piper longum*), and black pepper. The rationale was clear. The ingredient was dropped from the prescription because it was unknown in Sri Lanka. The three added ingredients suited the complications of this particular patient whose channels and nerves were blocked by phlegm that had hardened. These three substances help loosen the phlegm; they also have *anuloma* properties that then send the deranged humor on the normal path.

It should be clear, then, that combinations of prescriptions, additions to them, and deletions and substitutions may produce a complicated balancing of ingredients, based on the Āyurvedic humoral theory. Since not all prescriptions are standard, the way is open for clinical experimentation to meet the demands of the individual case. In an earlier article I have labeled this mode of experimentation "*samyogic* experimentation."[4] *Samyogic* experimentation is the manipulation of ingredients to produce a new prescription very much in the manner of a chemist combining elements to produce a new compound, but it occurs entirely in a clinical setting. It is through this form of experimentation that Āyurvedic physicians invent new medical prescriptions, either for well-known diseases from the classical Sanskrit or indigenous Sinhala traditions, or when confronted with new diseases. I have cases of *samyogic* experimentation to create new medical prescriptions from several physicians I have interviewed, but none from Dr. Fernando. However, Dr. Fernando, like most other skillful physicians, uses this form of clinical experimentation to constantly delete and add new ingredients to well-known textbook prescriptions, and then the new prescription may end up by becoming a standard one—at least for his family tradition. This is especially relevant when a prescription from a Sanskrit text contains medical ingredients that are unknown in Sri Lanka. Then the doctor, or the tradition from which he comes, would substitute a known ingredient for the unknown one. But the substitution is not made on the basis of guesswork or trying to approximate the Sanskrit ingredient. Quite the contrary; it is based on a theoretical understanding of the disease, and consequently one may end up with a substitute ingredient that is functionally equivalent, but substantively different from, the original.

Principles and Causes

Since the patient suffered from *ajīrna*, which was caused, in his case, by food becoming noxious, it was absolutely essential that his daily diet be carefully controlled. He should avoid "cold" foods as much as possible, such as milk, bananas, buffalo curd, cold water, melons, and so forth. In other words, the regimen or *pattiyama* (Sanskrit, *patya*) is an absolutely essential part of the cure. The doctor gives advice on *pattiyama* or regimen for practically every patient who consults him. Most often *pattiyama* pertains to diet, but this is not all, and in some instances it could extend to everyday living. For example, the *pattiyama* for a patient suffering from catarrh would entail avoidance of contact with dew, going about in the heat of the sun, and keeping up late at night. In some instances *pattiyama* may include restrictions on one's sex life; in others it might extend to prayers and meditation.

The importance of *pattiyama*, or regimen, is expressed in what Dr. Fernando calls *nīti*, literally meaning "law," but perhaps better translated as "principle" or even "rule." As usual, he quotes *śloka*s (couplets) from later Sanskrit works (*saṃgraha*), such as *Bhaisaja Ratnavāliya* or *Sri Yoga Ratnakāraya*:

> *vinā tu bhiṣajair vyādih pathyād eva vilīyate na tu pathyavihīnasya bheṣajānām śatair api*
> [A disease is cured without medicines by regimen alone. But not by even hundreds of medicines if one lacks regimen.]

This, of course, is a general principle; there could be more specific principles derived from or related to the above. Thus:

> *vīryādhikaṃ bhavati bheṣajam annahīnaṃ hanyā(t) tadâ mayam asaṃśayam āśucaiva tad*
> *bāla-vrddho yavati mrdavo nipīya glāniṃ parāṃ nayati câsubhalakṣayaṃ ca*
> [A medicine without food becomes stronger, then it can kill a disease very fast, no doubt.
> If children, old people, young women, and feeble people take that course, it takes them to extreme malaise and innumerable calamities.]

There are two principles here that are applicable to patients. First, there is the more basic principle that states that the *vīriya*, or strength, of a medicine is greater if given with a low diet. Patients who take Āyurvedic medicines are urged to go on a low diet, so that the medicine can be well absorbed by the body. Nevertheless, this principle cannot be applied in all cases; thus, there is another *nīti* or principle that provides an exception, or a way out of this rule. For example, if the above principle is applied to the very young, the old, and the weak, they will get weaker still, body strength deteriorates, and the disease will get worse. Dr. Fernando then quotes yet another *nīti* ("principle") which, rendered into English, goes as follows:

> If the patient has signs of deteriorating strength (that is, weakening of *dhātus*), then you can give him suitable food; strength will be restored because of the food; and owing to the patient's strength the opportunity exists to cure the disease.

"If we rigidly stick to a regimen (*pattiyama*) the patient will die. You must preserve the patient's life to cure his disease," Dr. Fernando laughed. "But remember, even for a weak person we cannot discard *pattiyama* totally. We must try to devise minor regimes suitable for the specific condition."

Principles or *nīti* are then very often applied in Āyurvedic clinical practice. This is not readily apparent when a physician prescribes medications or a regimen, but underlying them is a principle. Sanskrit texts are full of rules or principles, but they are not always clinically relevant for Āyurvedic practitioners. The relevance of the rule is based on clinical applicability, itself based on the efficacy of the rule in treatment. The rule is not only related to practice but, as with experimentation, it is rooted in the general theory of Āyurveda. But it must be reiterated that the mere fact that a rule or principle is theoretically relevant does not mean that it is used; use or practice depends on the clinical efficacy of the rule.

Principles or rules must be differentiated from causes, or *hētu*. Dr. Fernando's criticism of popular Sinhala texts is that they contain one stanza that deals with the symptoms of the disease and another that prescribes a medication. The texts, he said, echoing Kuhn without having read him, are useful for "ordinary physicians" who can identify a disease on the basis of symptoms (*rōga lakaṣaṇa*) and prescribe a cure, but they do not give one an understanding of the disease. Such understanding must deal with causes, and causes in turn make sense only in terms of the larger theory of Āyurveda: that of constituent elements of the universe (*bhūta*), the humors (*doṣa*), and the essences of the body (or *dhātu*).[5] In any one disease many causes may be operative; therefore, one has to consider the root cause (*mūla hētu*) of a disease. But, once again, the root cause is not fixed: it changes with the problem under consideration. Thus, one can say that the root cause of the *ajīrna* in our patient who couldn't pass wind is food that went noxious; but one can shift ground and make a more general point that the root cause of several *other* diseases could be *ajīrna*. One cause can be rooted in another cause. Furthermore, the root cause and the root location (*mūla sthāna*) of the disease may be connected, and both must be known in order to prescribe the proper medication. For example, the root causes of the *ajīrna* of our patient are the foods that became noxious, but the root location of the disease may be in some specific part of the intestines.

Innovation and Bricolage

Principle or rule, experimentation, innovation, cause—these ideas are found in Āyurveda. They do not exist in an *ad hoc* manner in clinical practice but are grounded in the highly abstract theory of Āyurveda.

I shall now discuss situations in which the theoretical grounding of medical ideas fail, and result in nontheoretical understanding or *bricolage* (in Lévi-Strauss's usage). In several interviews with doctors, I have come across *bricolage* when they have had to confront diseases they were not familiar with, especially diseases given well-known Western labels such as syphillis, polio, cancer, and so forth. I am not making a general proposition that whenever an Āyurvedic physician treats a patient with a disease from the Western repertoire with no parallel in the Āyurvedic tradition, he must inevitably end in *bricolage*. This would be false, since I can document cases in which the new disease has been creatively incorporated into Āyurvedic theory. Nevertheless, it is his confrontation with new and relatively unknown diseases that forces the physician into *bricolage*. I shall document this form of thinking from one of Dr. Fernando's cases.

The case is that of a female patient (age thirty-six) who had been diagnosed by Western doctors as suffering from a terminal cancer that had spread from the intestines to the pancreas. She was given two to three months to live. The patient's family came to see Dr. Fernando as a last resort, a not untypical action in Sri Lanka. They did not tell the patient about the nature of the disease in order not to discourage her. The doctor told the patient's family that all he could do was to try his best, but they should not hold out much hope. He felt absolved from any responsibility if she were to die. "Āyurveda says that you should treat any patient who comes to seek your help." This is simply an affirmation of *his* view of Āyurveda, for many classic texts are not that explicit about the ethics of treating terminal cases.

Dr. Fernando gave her a *behet yoga* (combination of medical ingredients) that contained, among other things, three crucial items: *karañda* (*Pongamia glabra*), papaya, and *kudumirissa* (*Toddalia aculeata*). Dr. Fernando justified the use of these ingredients with the following reasons:

> *Karañda* (*Pongamia glabra*):
> The cancer was located in the intestines. One of the most serious diseases of the intestines is *arśas* (hemorrhoids) and sometimes a serious case of *arśas* can present symptoms very similar to cancer. *Karañda* is excellent for *arśas* as well as for a variety of wounds and abscesses in the stomach and the duodenum (*grahani*). It is also used for curing any kind of wound in general and sometimes for *ajīrna*. Consequently, it appears in many "medical combinations" (*behet yoga*). Hence, he decided to use the five parts or *pancañga* of the *karañda* tree: roots, bark, flowers, leaves, fruit.
> *Papaya*:
> The papaya is never mentioned in classic sources, since it is not indigenous

to Sri Lanka. It is, however, well known to many indigenous (*desīya*) traditions as especially effective for liver (*ākmāva*) conditions, internal wounds
(*visarpa*), and *granti dosa* ("glandular troubles"). He initially prescribed ripe
papayas, but later included the "five parts" of the tree boiled, strained, and
then consumed.

Kuḍumirissa:
This is a thorny vine referred to in Sinhala texts. These texts refer to *kuḍumirissa* as especially effective for *pilikā* ("growths"). Dr. Fernando said that,
though the word *pilikā* is used for cancer nowadays, in traditional Āyurveda
it was used for certain kinds of external wounds only. "So I used the indigenous tradition of medicines from the repertoire known as *geḍi-vana-pilikā*
("boils-wounds-growths"), and selectively combined them into my prescriptions for this patient. I did all this on the basis of my previous experience as a
physician." The patient's most conspicuous symptoms were pain, inability
to eat, distended stomach, bad bowel movements, and sleeplessness. Gradually, these symptoms diminished and she passed the deadline of the three
months given to her by Western physicians. "Consequently, both the patient
and I were encouraged. The family of the patient who had given up hope
now became enthusiastically supportive of her. After a course of treatment
which took about nine months, she was cured. This was fifteen years ago and
she still comes to me for minor illnesses."

Consider what has occurred here. Dr. Fernando is confronted with a disease, "cancer," from the Western repertoire. Diseases are not an entity but a
conception, and the conception of cancer is well known in contemporary Sri
Lanka. Posed with this "new" disease, Dr. Fernando uses his experience to
invent several prescriptions from a variety of ingredients that are known to
be efficacious for the presenting symptoms. He has not understood cancer
theoretically, that is, he has not been able to explain the disease in terms of
Āyurvedic theory and develop a prescription on a theoretical base. Rather,
he is putting together things in a manner of a *bricoleur*. It is ad hoc experimentation, not the kind of *samyogic* experimentation that I spoke of earlier. It
is not different in principle, I think, from the Western treatment of cancer
(until very recently) where therapy was at best peripherally related to a
theoretical understanding of the disease, since such an understanding barely
existed.

It is instructive to get back to Dr. Fernando's successful treatment of the
cancer patient, and its aftermath, to highlight other features of both *bricolage*
and Āyurveda. The limitation of *bricolage* is precisely the absence of theoretical understanding, for without theory it is difficult to construct a prescription
to suit the wide range of symptoms represented by cancer. If all patients who
came to see the doctor suffered from the identical form of cancer, then he
could replicate his previously successful treatment irrespective of a theoretical knowledge of the disease. But each time a patient comes with a cancer, Dr.
Fernando would have to put together a *behet yōga*, or "combination of medical

ingredients," from the existing repertoire to deal with the presenting symptoms of each case. It is true that some of the ingredients such as *karaṅḍa* (*Pongamia glabra*) would remain constant, but others must surely be invented to meet the variations in symptoms in each case—an extremely difficult task.

This is *our* criticism of *bricolage*. Dr. Fernando did not quite see it in this way, though he says his treatment of the patient was done "without much knowledge." His view of the course of treatment for cancer illustrates a further important feature of Āyurvedic medicine, though not of *bricolage*. Three others who heard of his successful treatment of cancer came to him for help. They took treatment from him, but they gave up after some time. It was clear, said Dr. Fernando, that his treatment was not successful in these other cases. Therefore, he felt that he should abandon treating cancer patients. He knew that people get well all the time, with or without medication, and that cancer patients were no exception. He felt that his success in the first case may have been fortuitous, since there were three failures subsequently. Moreover, he was fully aware that his treatment was not based on much knowledge, by which he meant theoretical knowledge. What we have here is a feature of Āyurvedic medicine applicable to innovations either on the level of *bricolage* or of *samyogic* experimentation, namely "clinical falsification." Falsification is built into clinical practice in Āyurveda: if a prescription does not work, it is abandoned. It is immaterial whether the prescription is from a hallowed Sanskrit text, or one invented by a physician—the ultimate test is its efficacy in a clinical situation. The situation here is quite different from what occurs in magical medicine or ritual curing, where falsification need not result in the revision or abandonment of the cure. Rather, failure itself could be attributed to a variety of causes such as taboo violation, incorrect performance of ritual, and so forth. In ritual curing, a client may seek another curer because he is dissatisfied with the prescription or cure. The specialist, however, does not abandon his procedure that easily, even if there is "clinical falsification," since his repertoire of actual cures is strictly limited. By contrast, in Āyurveda the uses of theory in conjunction with *samyogic* experimentation have produced, and continue to produce, a huge repertoire of prescriptions. To put it differently, the generation of new medical prescriptions is possible because Āyurveda is a science of medicine. And, like its Western counterpart, the development of a scientific attitude in Āyurveda presupposes either a demystification of magic, or its methodological isolation from clinical practice.

A Charter for Clinical Practice in Āyurveda

I now present the gist of a talk given by Dr. Fernando at a congress on Āyurveda sponsored recently by a Sri Lankan newspaper. His thesis is stated below:

When mankind arose on the earth, from whatever reasons, they contracted various diseases. To cope with these, people learned basic medical techniques and cures largely through observation and trial-and-error learning. Dr. Fernando stated that even animals consume various plants when they have discomforts. For example, when they want to vomit, dogs will eat grass, and in that sense vomiting is a natural medicine. Sometimes, they will eat leaves to cure an indigestion (*ajīrna*).[6]

Mankind developed in various ways but still there was no science of medicine. Then after some time infectious diseases began to spread. The sages (*rsis*) who had cultivated their intellects and practiced *samādhi* and *vratas* ("contemplation and vows of devotion to God") in order to live long could no longer do so, and there was also a decline in their life spans. Now, these people got together and had discussions about what they should do. The classic works do not state that they discovered the medical system out of their own intellects, but rather that they obtained it from Sakra (Indra). But we cannot accept this, argued Dr. Fernando. We must infer that these discoveries were made through constant discussions among themselves. But even this kind of thinking may fail and a person may withdraw into the forest and make new discoveries through the cultivation of his mind.

He illustrated this with an example of a Sanskrit grammarian, Ācārya Anubhūtisvarūpa, who was searching for an elusive law of grammar that would help him complete his project.[7] He thought he grasped it intuitively, but he could not formulate it. His colleagues were also aware of this, and since he could not complete his grammar (owing to the absence of this one law) he fell into a deep shame. He withdrew from society and went into the forest in order to give up his life there. Now this grammarian was a person who observed *vratas* (vows) and also possessed *dhyāna* ("trancelike") powers. Sakra (Indra) saw this unusual person with his divine eye. He came to the earth in the guise of an *udākki* drummer, and beat a stanza on the drum. Our grammarian and sage wrote it down and soon realized that this was the elusive law that he was looking for. But this story (as stated traditionally) is not correct, says Dr. Fernando; in reality the sage himself discovered the law through contemplation in the forest. But this is not what he told the public. He said that he managed to complete his grammar through Sakra's (Indra's) aid. He did this to express his *bhakti* (devotion) to god before society. In truth he himself discovered the law.

Dr. Fernando then proceded to summarize the origin myths of Āyurveda found in Suśruta and Caraka. In both these texts, knowledge of medicine was transmitted from Brahma or Indra, and through them to a human being (Dhanvantari or Bharadvaja) who ultimately proclaimed the divine truths to the world. Dr. Fernando says that, as a Buddhist, he cannot accept the idea that Brahma created everything. "We accept Buddhist views and, consequently, we find the theories on origin in the old texts unacceptable." He reiterated his views on natural cures, and the importance of trial-and-error learning in the origins of Āyurveda. He then quoted another example:

> Say, for instance, someone had fever. It was observed that his body temperature was high and that he had no desire for food. It could then be inferred that food was not good for this condition and he had to go on a low diet. But this, of course, wasn't enough, and it was evident that further treatment was necessary. So certain medicines were given: some of these succeeded and others did not. But this is not what the book says. According to the book [that is, classic texts], Brahma knew that diseases would befall humans and therefore he created the Āyurvedic system. [He laughed.] Really, can anyone seriously believe a story like that?

It is evident that Dr. Fernando has a critique and an interpretation of the classic Sanskrit origin myths of Āyurveda. However, his own interpretation is also a pragmatic (or scientific) myth-charter for the kind of Āyurveda he advocates. He is, on the one hand, thoroughly familiar with a wide range of Sanskrit texts and constantly quotes couplets from classic sources like Suśruta and Caraka. Yet, on the other hand, he does not accept the tradition uncritically; the validity of a medication is in its clinical efficacy. The Āyurvedic theory of the humors, no matter how abstract, is still a theory relevant to clinical practice. Some elements of that theory he does not accept, as he does not accept classic prescriptions that do not work. *Ojas*,[8] for example, is an important concept in classic Āyurveda, but it is of little clinical use, and neither he nor other Āyurvedic physicians in Sri Lanka find it useful. "You cannot treat problems pertaining to *ojas*," he said. So it is with any prescription. The prescription is a carefully constructed work, based on the theory. These doctors keep no files. The patient brings with him the previous prescriptions, and by looking at these prescriptions physicians can recollect or reconstruct the nature of the patient's disease. If one changes physicians one brings the old prescriptions along and the new doctor can once again fathom the interpretation of the disease and its devolution. The prescription then is a scientific document that provides a language of intersubjectivity among the community of physicians.

Dr. Fernando's origin myth is a charter for the special kind of Āyurvedic practice that, I believe, took root in Sri Lanka among its more sophisticated physicians and the traditions they represented. This is a concern with an experimental method that I have called *samyogic* experimentation. It is at base a development of simple trial-and-error knowing, as Dr. Fernando states in his origin myth, but it is not synonymous with it, since it has evolved a long way from trial-and-error learning. For according to the origin myth, further developments occurred through public argumentation and debate among learned practitioners. But neither empiricism that lies at the base of *samyogic* experimentation nor discussion and debate are the exclusive sources of knowledge. Theoretical knowledge and laws could also be derived from inward contemplation. But it is also clear that knowledge cannot and did not come from God; that would violate the tenets of Buddhism as it violates the special kind of empiricism that underlies much of Āyurveda, whether Sanskritic or Sri Lankan. The tradition that Dr. Fernando subscribes to carries to a logical conclusion this form of empiricism, which must invariably lead to a denial of divine origin. Dr. Fernando attributes the dethroning of God to his Buddhist inheritance. This must at least be partially true, since Buddhism explicitly dethrones Brahma, and popular texts lampoon his omniscience. Along with the dethronement of God, the complicated metaphysical ideas based on *puruṣa* and *prakṛti* that link the Sanskrit tradition of Āyurveda with the Sāṃkya philosophy of Hinduism lose much of their significance.[9] Buddhism helps create a tradition of Āyurveda without God, and without a complicated metaphysical framework.[10]

NOTES

1. Robin Horton, "African traditional thought and Western science," in *Rationality*, ed. Bryan Wilson (Oxford: Basil Blackwell, 1979), 131–171.

2. Max Weber, "Social psychology of the world religions," in *From Max Weber*, ed. Hans Gerth and C. Wright Mills (New York: Oxford University Press, 1946), 293.

3. Karl Popper, *The Poverty of Historicism* (London: Routledge Kegan Paul, 1960).

4. G. Obeyesekere, "Science and psychological medicine in the Āyurvedic tradition," in *Cultural Conceptions of Mental Health and Therapy*, ed. A. J. Marsella and G. M. White (Dordrecht, Holland: D. Reidel Publishing Company, 1982), 235–250.

5. In an earlier article I briefly summarized this larger theory of Āyurveda.

The fundamental principles (*mūla dharma*) of Āyurveda include the doctrine of the five *bhūtas* or basic elements (atoms) of the universe, the *tridoṣa*, or three humours, and the seven *dhātus*, or components of the body. The five elements are ether (*ākāśa*), wind (*vāyu*), water (*ap*), earth (*pṛthvi*), and fire (*agni* or *tejas*). These elements are constituents of all life and as such also make up the three humours and the seven physical components of the body. As the five elements contained in food are "cooked" by fires in the body, they are converted into a fine portion (*āhara-prasāda*) and refuse (*kitta* or *mala*). The body elements are produced by successive transformation of the refined food substance into chyle (*rasa*), blood (*rakta*), flesh (*māmsa*), fat (*medas*), bone (*asthi*), marrow (*majja*) and semen (*śukra*). Semen is said to be the most highly refined element in this body, the "vital juice" that tones the whole organism. (Filliozat 1964: 27)

Physical health is maintained when the three humours are in harmonic balance, but when they are upset they become *doṣas*, or "troubles" of the organism. The universal element (*bhūta*) of wind appears in the body as a humour, also called wind (*vāyu*); fire appears as bile (*pitta*); and water as phlegm (*kapha* or *sleśman*). Illness is due to upsetting the homeostatic condition of these humours (*tridoṣa*). The more serious condition is one in which all three humours are upset (*sannipāta*). When a *doṣa* is "angry" or excited it increases in proportion to the other humours. The aim of medication is to reduce or control this excess. The excited *doṣa* may also damage one or more *dhātu* (blood, flesh, fat, etc.) so that treatment must aim to restore the affected body substance. (Reproduced from Obeyesekere, "Science and psychological medicine," p. 237)

6. In another interview Dr. Fernando referred to the observational basis for the discovery of "lizard oil" (*kaṭusutel*) in local traditions of Āyurvedic toxicology. When a cat eats a lizard (*kaṭussa*) it gets thin, and if it continues to eat lizards it will die. Thus, we can say from observation that lizard meat has the property, or *guna*, of causing bodily weakness (*kṣaya*). One can then make "lizard oil" and try out its capacity to cause weakness or *kṣaya*.

7. I have not been able to locate this personage in Sanskrit linguistics. Dr. Fernando says that he got this example from a commentary on Panini's grammar.

8. Monier-Williams's *Sanskrit-English Dictionary* translates *ojas* as "vitality that infuses the body."

9. For an account of the relationship between Sāṃkya philosophy and Āyurveda, see G. Obeyesekere, "The theory and practice of psychological medicine in the Āyurvedic tradition," *Culture, Medicine, and Psychiatry*, vol. 1, no. 2, 155–181.

10. Research for this study was made possible by a grant BNS-8213698 from the National Science Foundation for a project entitled, "Science Experimentation in Non-Western Medicine."

EIGHT

Interpretations of Illness: Syncretism in Modern Āyurveda

Charles Leslie

Cultural Continuities and Historical Discontinuities

Anthropologists who first wrote about curing practices in rural India in the 1950s emphasized the familiarity of laymen with Āyurvedic concepts. Humoral ideas were used in food preparation, personal hygiene, and domestic rituals, and villagers commonly interpreted their own illnesses by using concepts of humoral pathology. The anthropologists reasoned that since these ideas were continuous with those of Āyurvedic physicians, consultations with them were fully understood by laymen, who in turn complied with their recommendations. In contrast, encounters with "Doctor medicine" were said to be incomprehensible. Injections, surgical procedures, and diagnostic instruments were symbols of power to villagers, who wanted access to them for serious trauma or illness. But on the whole they thought that government doctors were avaricious, and that the people in charge at primary health centers were neglectful, dishonest, and insulting. Even though government workers might occasionally treat them with respect and provide inexpensive care, villagers often considered them to be a last resort.

Indigenous medical practitioners were observed to use stethoscopes and antibiotics in the 1950s, and since the anthropologists who recorded these observations wanted to introduce more cosmopolitan medicine to rural communities, one would have expected them to favor this development. Instead, they assumed the perspective of allopathic physicians who asserted that these elements of medical syncretism signified quackery. This was perhaps inevitable since the anthropologists were acting as consultants to doctors in government health services who encountered a massive problem of noncompliance and underutilization in rural areas. The anthropologists accepted the doctors' definition of the situation in trying to explain their problem. Assuming that to understand someone was to agree with him, the anthropologists argued that villagers understood indigenous practitioners and thus complied with their advice, while they failed to understand the doctors. A more skeptical approach would have considered compliance problematic in either case, and a more evenhanded approach would have judged the syncretism of village practitioners to be a normative cultural practice rather than an aberration.

However one dates the emergence and historical development of cosmopolitan medicine, vaidyas and hakims were in contact with its practitioners from its beginning. Indian physicians in eighteenth-century Calcutta and Bombay adopted "English medicine," which they proudly combined with indigenous practices, and during the first quarter of the nineteenth century the East India Company sponsored a program to train "native doctors" that integrated European anatomy and medicine with instruction in Āyurveda and Yunāni tibbia. This program, taught in vernacular languages, was terminated in 1835 when a new policy was adopted to teach European knowledge in English medium schools. The debate at that time was whether the Indian and Western civiliations were historically continuous with each other, and whether modern science was historically discontinuous with ancient science.

Sir William Jones had shown that Indian languages were related to those of Europe, establishing the continuity of Indo-European civilizations. The Orientalists in the nineteenth century were his heirs in disputes about how to introduce Western science to India. They maintained that modern science had originated in ancient Greece, and that the middle ages were a discontinuity in this tradition only in the sense that they constituted an interval of stagnation, though a rather long one, in its progressive development. In their view an enlightened antiquity related to Greece had existed in India, and had suffered a similar medieval decline. A renaissance of Indian civilization would reassert continuity with its past, just as the Italian Renaissance had reasserted European continuity with classical Greece and Rome. The East India Company should encourage this enterprise by helping to revive and strengthen indigenous medical institutions. The method would be to translate and teach new scientific knowledge in vernacular languages, thus facilitating its assimilation to the local culture and reawakening the native spirit of scientific inquiry among vaidyas and hakims. The Orientalists joined the idea of progress to a heroic conception of civilization. Creative work in science and the arts, and an economy and government that fostered these things, were the measure of a civilized society. Material progress and scientific discoveries were signs of spiritual continuity with the past. The life of a civilization was not sustained by repetition and holding on, but by inv   )n, adventure, and progressive change.

Whether modern science and medicine were grounded in Greek tradition or a break from it made little difference to those who opposed the Orientalists, for in either case they maintained that contemporary Indian civilization was inferior to the West. Although the Orientalists lost the debate on educational policy in British India, the point is that they provided the ideological platform for an indigenous movement that has transformed traditional medical learning in modern South Asia. The leaders of this movement adopted technology, ideas, and institutional forms from the evolving cosmopolitan system to found pharmaceutical companies, colleges, and professional associations, and to reinterpret traditional knowledge. They translated Sanskrit classics into English and vernacular languages, wrote manuals and modern textbooks for students, and published journals and popular tracts. They lobbied to create state and central government agencies that would support indigenous medicine. In short, the syncretism between Āyurveda and cosmopolitan medicine which anthropologists first noted in rural India in the 1950s was a far-reaching and long-standing aspect of Indian society, and it has greatly affected the ways that people interpret illness. In South Asia today syncretic practitioners of Āyurveda and Yunāni medicine far outnumber physicians with degrees from cosmopolitan medical colleges.

My first research in South Asia was a survey of indigenous medical schools during the summers of 1961 and 1962. In retrospect the 1960s appear to be the closing decade of more than a century of medical revivalism inspired by the Orientalist rhetoric. By the end of the nineteenth century its advocates held common cause with the independence movement, and during the 1920s and 1930s they trained a generation of practitioners who imagined a comprehensive national medical system that would be inspired by Āyurveda and that would assimilate cosmopolitan medicine to indigenous culture. Āyurveda dominated the effort because Hindus outnumbered Muslims, and with the exception of men like Hakim Ajmal Khan in Delhi, they were its most vigorous leaders. Nevertheless, the same rhetoric served both Hindu and Muslim revivalists, who were joined by a shared nationalism and need to confront the advances of modern science.

The Political Context: Pandit Shiv Sharma in Sri Lanka

The structures of meaning in diagnoses of illnesses are not limited to the technical meanings of medical concepts, but are situated in and draw significance from other cultural domains. They are not confined to dyadic doctor-patient relationships, but are negotiated by many actors in complex social settings. Since medical systems and health cultures are pluralistic, a single episode of illness may be diagnosed in different ways, and the ways in which it is diagnosed symbolize many more things than biological malfunction. The political symbolism of Āyurvedic medicine was unmistakable when I visited Sri Lanka in 1962, the year that a Buddhist priest was executed for having assassinated Prime Minister Bandaranaike.

As a Minister of Local Administration in 1937, Bandaranaike had been

Chairman of the Board of Indigenous Medicine, a position he held until 1944. In the early 1950s he led the opposition to politicians who had inherited power at independence. Identifying them with the colonial past, Bandaranaike appealed to Singhalese sentiments about language, religion, and history. Āyurvedic practitioners played a prominent role in his election. They were divided, however, between those who wanted to elevate the status of Āyurveda by assimilating modern diagnostic technology, medicine, and surgery, and the advocates of "pure Āyurveda," who thought that this would degrade their tradition. The man who assassinated Bandaranaike in 1959 was an advocate of purity. Six people were arrested at the time, including the Minister of Health and a faculty member of the Government College of Indigenous Medicine.

The Minister had been embroiled in a highly publicized dispute with the Principal of the College, Dr. R. B. Lenora. The Minister opposed his efforts to add x-ray and laboratory facilities to the teaching hospital, to improve instruction in anatomy and surgery, and to raise the standards of examinations. Her tactic was to appoint her supporters to the Board of Indigenous Medicine to which Dr. Lenora was responsible. According to Dr. Lenora, one of the men she appointed had failed his examinations at the college five times.

Another tactic of the Minister of Health was to use the Colombo Plan for mutual aid between South Asian countries to invite Pandit Shiv Sharma, the leading advocate of "pure Āyurveda" in India, to recommend policy to the Government of Ceylon. The invitation was made with the understanding that his report would reverse an earlier committee report that had recommended an integrated program of indigenous and cosmopolitan medicine. That committee had been chaired by a well-known physician and educator from Calcutta who was trained in both medical systems, but Shiv Sharma's credentials were also impressive. He was trained in Sanskrit and medicine by his father, who was the Rāj Vaidya to the court of the Māhārāja of Patiala. In this setting Shiv Sharma had also acquired an aristocratic manner and a perfect command of the English language. When Māhātma Gandhi's dying wife requested an Āyurvedic physician, he had been summoned, and he had been repeatedly elected President of the All India Āyurveda Congress.

In contrast, Dr. Lenora belonged to the generation of college-trained physicians who had imagined a national medical system inspired by indigenous tradition but incorporating modern science and technology. He had earned a scholarship from the Oriental Medicine Society in Ceylon to attend the Jamini Bhushan Āstānga Āyurveda College in Calcutta, a school founded by a vaidya who was also trained in cosmopolitan medicine, and famous for its integrated curriculum. Lenora later studied medicine in Edinburgh and Glasgow, and by the time of independence was a prominent physician in Colombo. He was Principal of the College of Indigenous Medicine in 1954 when it celebrated its twenty-fifth anniversary. He contributed an article, "Progress of Āyurveda," to the commemorative volume. The following abstract, composed of direct quotations from that article, indicates the substance and manner of the integrationist argument.

> Āyurveda is a science which had its origin over three thousand years back and had been gradually developed . . . into a complete science capable of dealing with any type of ailment of the human body, including major surgery and ear, nose and throat diseases. But the advent of Foreign invasion . . . terminated the further development on Āyurveda lines. . . . No science, including medicine, could ever be permanent. . . . The trend of modern medicine is to discard what is found to be wanting in treatment and diagnosis, and adopt new and better methods. . . . The researches done in the field of Bacteriology, and modern mechanical aids in diagnosis, such as Cardiac Catheterisation, Bronchoscopy, Air Encephalography, Arteriography, Thoracoscopy, etc., and the research in the field of Antibiotics, Chemotherapeutic drugs and Radioactive isotopes have completely revolutionized the concept of medicine of the present day. . . . But unfortunately the events where Āyurveda is concerned have been quite the opposite . . . hardly anything has been added to Āyurveda by its followers in spite of Āyurveda being poor in analgesic drugs, and drugs that can be used in medical emergencies. . . . The worst possible harm has been done by some political leaders by giving undue praise to the Āyurvedic Physician and keeping him satisfied and ignorant. . . . Criticism is leveled at me for pointing out defects in Āyurveda, and praising the foreign science and yet being the head of an Āyurvedic Institution. Criticism can be constructive or destructive. There can be no progress in any science unless one sees and analyzes the defects and puts these defects in order. . . . The institution of which the Silver Jubilee is celebrated today has been in existence for the last 25 years. Yet, as yet, there are no facilities for X-rays, Pathological Work, Post-Mortem Examinations, etc., in spite of the Post-Mortem room being the place where over jubilant medical man comes down to earth on many occasions. . . . Āyurveda has had a glorious day, and in spite of being over 3000 years old is still holding its own. . . . I would like to appeal to my allopathic colleagues to be more tolerant and understanding of their Āyurvedic Colleagues and help them to give up their erroneous ideas and help the development of a science of which we all are bound to be proud. . . . I would also like to appeal to my Āyurvedic Colleagues to seek more light and not to accept blindly everything infallible because a Rishi has proclaimed a method or a medicine. . . . Research, more Research, and reliable research can and will give results of which we can some day be proud.[1]

Dr. Lenora lost the dispute with the Minister of Health and resigned from the College in 1956. The Minister was supported by physicians and bureaucrats with the main responsibility for running governmental institutions and for regulating private practice throughout the island. They did not want to enhance the claims of Āyurvedic practitioners to equal status with allopathic doctors. Despite the fact that Dr. Lenora proposed to raise standards at the college, they interpreted his program as one that would lower standards by increasing the legitimacy of physicians trained outside of "regular medicine." Pandit Shiv Sharma was a perfect ally for the Minister of Health and her supporters because he recommended that the teaching hospitals at indigenous medical colleges eliminate whatever uses they had made of modern diagnostic technology, chemotherapy, and surgery, and that the curriculum in the first years of training be limited entirely to concepts and practices from ancient and medieval texts. Students at the college in Colombo went on strike when the new policy was adopted, and Dr. Lenora raised money for 115 of them to complete their education at integrated colleges in India.

In these kinds of conflicts the criticism of their own institutions by integrationists like Dr. Lenora was used against them by opponents. In working to improve the colleges they too asserted that the graduates were poorly trained. The fact that they were better equipped to help patients than they would be with less instruction or none at all in cosmopolitan medicine was ignored by Pandit Shiv Sharma and by the Minister of Health on the principle that a little learning was a dangerous thing because it encouraged practitioners to exceed their limitations. A sore point for graduates of the Āyurvedic colleges was that they were largely excluded from government posts equivalent to their training, and a sore point for "qualified doctors" was that the college-trained Āyurvedic physicians competed with them in the fee-for-service market.

Self-instructed in the use of modern diagnostic technology, Pandit Shiv Sharma himself ordered laboratory tests and x-rays for his patients, and his only son became an allopathic doctor. The irony of these facts was widely known by protagonists in the conflict over policies affecting Āyurveda but Shiv Sharma was protected from their use against him by his reputation as a polemicist. Furthermore, he symbolized a rare and desirable conciliation of identities for many upper- and middle-class Indians. He was a Pandit who won golf tournaments at his club, an Āyurvedic physician with cosmopolitan manners, a Brahmin, vegetarian, and sophisticate who quoted Sanskrit ślokas and joked in English. He was acquainted with powerful people, from his youth in Patiala to the patients whom he attracted even as a young practitioner. Finally, his advocacy of pure Āyurveda flattered an Aryan sense of continuity and self-sufficiency while accommodating policymakers who also wanted the whole imported package of professional medicine from Europe and America.

Altogether these things earned more political clout for Pandit Shiv Sharma than any other spokesman for Āyurveda in the postindependence period. In 1938, at the age of thirty-one, he had become the youngest president in the history of the All India Āyurveda Congress. He was given the office by Congress leaders who respected his father and thought that his ability as a speaker would be useful to their cause, but once in office he seized control of the

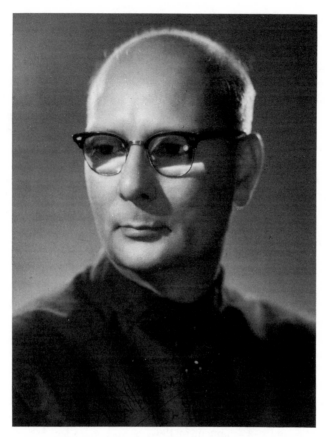

Fig. 8.1. Pandit Shiv Sharma (1906–1982).

organization. He moved its headquarters to Lahore, where he lived and could appoint his followers to staff positions, and he recruited new members by appealing to vaidyas without institutional training who were threatened by college-educated practitioners who demanded a separate and higher status in the regulations for registering practitioners. He also expanded membership in the Āyurvedic Congress by recruiting people who would be loyal to him. During the next seventeen years he used the Congress as a platform to gain national attention, serving as its president seven times and engaging in factional disputes with other leaders, some of whom were far more accomplished than himself. For example, he quarreled with Pandit Yadavji Tricumjee Acharya from Bombay, who was also an advocate of "pure Āyurveda," and with Kaviraj Gananath Sen from Calcutta, who was perhaps the best-known advocate during the 1920s and 1930s of an integrated medical system.

By the time that the Minister of Health invited Shiv Sharma to Sri Lanka his reputation as a critic of the Āyurvedic and Yunani colleges had been disseminated in English language and vernacular newspapers. He announced what all middle-class urban people already knew, that the students in these colleges used them as "backdoors to the practice of allopathy," but he went on to call the colleges "refugee camps for incompetent practitioners," a disgrace to the nation and a scandalous plot by allopathic doctors to destroy the integrity of Āyurveda. He cared less about Yunāni tibbia, maintaining that it was derived from Āyurveda and kept alive by Muslim communal sentiments in India long after it had disappeared from its homeland. Condemning vaidyas and hakims who used antibiotics, he projected the image of a future in which a pure Āyurveda would thrive in an independent manner alongside the technically impressive but iatrogenic system of cosmopolitan medicine, eventually absorbing it into its own comprehensive and philosophically grounded being.

The twain would meet, but not now, and not until circumstances would prevent Āyurveda from being overwhelmed. In the meanwhile, Pandit Shiv Sharma proposed an Asian Health Organization on the pattern of the World Health Organization, except that it would be devoted to Āyurveda. The Ministry of Health published a plan in 1960, and according to Shiv Sharma, the government of Sri Lanka inquired whether the People's Republic of China would join a project of this kind that would also include Chinese medicine. The Chinese did not respond, and shortly thereafter the thought of further effort was abandoned when China invaded India.

Following his success in Sri Lanka, Shiv Sharma helped to persuade state after state in India to reduce cosmopolitan medical training in their Āyurvedic colleges. Elected to Parliament in 1967, he sponsored legislation to reorganize the support for Āyurveda by the central government, and he approved the officer to manage these affairs in the Ministry of Health. He had himself appointed Chairman of the Ministry's Central Council for Research on Indigenous Medicine, and very largely dominated national policy through the 1970s. By the time that he died in 1982 (he was born in 1906), the extensive system for professional education, research, and practice had been brought under central government control. By then, too, the Orientalist rhetoric that he employed had lost its power to influence policy as the Chinese model for using indigenous resources in a state system of health services, and the World Health Organization rhetoric of "Health for all by the year 2000" passed Shiv Sharma by. Borrowing the new language of primary health care, a major program to train Community Health Workers was launched and gave token recognition to indigenous medicine while ignoring its professional institutions. Despite Shiv Sharma's political successes, these institutions are still committed to medical syncretism. The *Shuddha*, or pure, policy has been implemented by people who feel that they have to prove the value of Āyurveda by using the language of modern science. Shiv Sharma, like Dr. Lenora, recommended research and more research toward this end. Both purists and integrationists have always rejected chemical studies of plants which are as likely as not to show that they do not possess qualities attributed to them. They call instead for research "on the lines of Āyurveda." In practice this means the study of texts, ethnobotany, and clinical hospital research using traditional medicine. But the diagnoses of illnesses in this work employ modern techniques along with those of Āyurveda, and the traditional nosology is translated into cosmopolitan medical categories. Double blind methods are often said to be used, and the results are presented in statistical form employing measures from modern biology. Having discussed this work over many years with knowledgeable people, including researchers themselves, I am convinced that no one really expects anything new to come from it. It is, after all, directed toward verifying longstanding practices, and the results are uniformly positive. Meanwhile, most registered practitioners, and particularly those trained in colleges, are convinced that for the good of their patients, and to support themselves in practice, they cannot give up vitamin and antibiotic injections, or symbols of medical expertise such as the stethoscope.

Dr. C. Dwarkanath, Captain Srinivasa Murti, and the Orientalist Tradition

I want to analyze the syncretic system of Āyurveda by recounting the career and ideas of one of its most accomplished and articulate representatives. Dr. C. Dwarkanath was Advisor on Indian Systems of Medicine in the Ministry of Health from 1959 to 1967. He was Pandit Shiv Sharma's main opponent in New Delhi during this period. They were the same age, but in contrast to Shiv Sharma's aristocratic background, Dwarkanath was middle class. His father was a bank auditor in Madras, and though several cousins became physicians, he was the only member of the family to study Āyurveda, entering the government School of Indian Medicine in Madras when it opened in 1925.

The Principal of the new school, Captain Srinivasa Murti, decided that Dwarkanath was the most talented student in the class, became his patron, and inspired his career. Born in 1887, Srinivasa Murti had earned medical and law degrees from the University of Madras. He served as a medical officer during the first World War, and continued to use his military title after leaving the service in 1921. In that year he was appointed secretary to a Committee on Indigenous Systems of Medicine for the Government of Madras. The Committee was the first of its kind, and created a stir among hopeful revivalists throughout India. Srinivasa Murti wrote a report published in 1923, including a ninety-eight-page monograph, *The Science and the Art of Indian Medicine*, which was one of its appendices. In 1924 he was made Principal of the school that was created to be the first step in a program outlined by the Committee to build a national system of medicine.

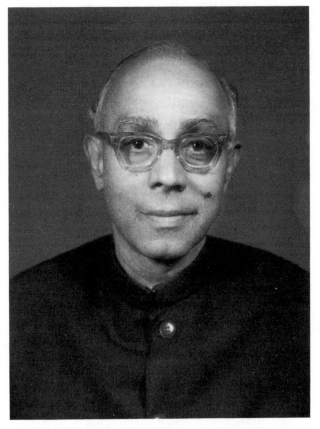

Fig. 8.2. Dr. Chandragiri Dwarkanath (1906–1976).

Twenty-six years later Dr. Dwarkanath became the secretary for a similar committee, which this time was created by the newly independent Government of India. The report that he wrote was essentially an updated version of the earlier one, and in it he reprinted Srinivasa Murti's monograph. This work defined the intellectual direction of Dwarkanath's career. Its argument was practically an outline of the three-volume study, *Fundamental Principles of Āyurveda*, which he published while serving as the Principal of the Government Āyurvedic and Unani College in Mysore. Having said this, we must say at once that Srinivasa Murti drew his ideas from Bengali intellectuals who in the Orientalist tradition set out to document the accomplishments of ancient Indian science, and to reestablish its continuity with the modern world.

These Bengali scholars were a living presence in India during the early part of Dr. Dwarkanath's career. Two of the grand figures were Jagadis Chandra Bose (1848–1937) and Prafulla Chandra Roy (1861–1944), professors of physics and of chemistry at Presidency College, the most prestigious school in India. Bose gained international recognition in the 1890s for research on electromagnetic waves, and then began experiments to show that living and nonliving things responded similarly to changes in their environment. From 1903 on he studied plant physiology to prove that plants experienced emotions—for example, in responding to music—and that they enacted a moral life. He founded the Bose Research Institute in 1917, with modern laboratories in a building that resembled a Hindu temple. Ostensibly Bose remained entirely within the sphere of modern experimental science, but his vitalism and his proofs for an organic model of physical phenomena seemed to validate Hindu philosophy, and to contribute a distinctively Indian perspective to world science.[2]

P. C. Roy was more pragmatic and humble in his scientific work than Bose, but equally famous and revered. He earned a doctorate in chemistry at the University of Edinburgh, and was offended when he returned to Calcutta in 1888 to be offered a teaching post below the rank of less qualified Englishmen. Nevertheless, he attracted ambitious students, and he wrote an influential two-volume *History of Hindu Chemistry* based mainly on the texts of Āyurveda. Inspired by the Swadeshi movement to promote Indian enterprise, he founded the Bengal Chemical and Pharmaceutical Works. Gaining wealth, he contributed to charities, assisted other business entrepreneurs, and encouraged scholars such as B. N. Seal, who wrote *The Positive Sciences of the Ancient Hindus*, and G. N. Mukhopadhyaya, who wrote a three-volume *History of Indian Medicine*. Other Bengali authors published English translations of classic Āyurveda texts between 1900 and the first World War, and Kaviraj Gananath Sen composed his famous Sanskrit textbooks incorporating modern anatomy and physiology. Over ninety scholars and political leaders met in Calcutta in 1905 to plan a national university that opened the following year, and included in its general science courses "truths embodied in Oriental learning, and in medical education specially of such scientific truths as are to be found in the Āyurvedic and Hakim systems."[3]

These efforts were the source of Srinivasa Murti's ideas about medical reform, along with his membership in the Theosophical Society, which, with its headquarters in Madras, was a center for Hindu revivalism. After Dr. Dwarkanath graduated from medical school, Srinivasa Murti encouraged him to continue studying, and helped him to win a scholarship in 1934 to spend a year at the University of Hamburg medical school.

A 1948 reprint of Srinivasa Murti's monograph opened with a quotation from the Congress politician, Rajagopalachari, recommending that Āyurvedic colleges include instruction in cosmopolitan medicine, and that vaidyas

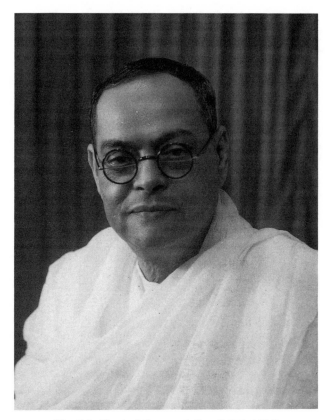

Fig. 8.3. Kaviraj Gananath Sen (1877–1944).

cooperate with doctors in research on the principle that "Truth and Science are one. There can be no competition between truth and truth, but only between truth and error."[4]

The first section of the monograph argued that the Indian traditions were as scientific as those of the West, and since truths could not contradict each other, religious and scientific truths were compatible. This at least was the case in Hinduism, which Srinivasa Murti asserted to be undogmatic because it maintained different interpretations of scriptural authority. The differences within Hinduism were said to be comparable to different theories and hypotheses in Western science.

Just as alternative geometries were used in Newtonian physics and relativity theory, Āyurveda used an alternative set of postulates to those of cosmopolitan medicine. Among the *Ṣaḍdarśana*, or six traditional systems of Hindu philosophy, the *Nyāya, Vaiśeṣika*, and *Sāṅkhya* systems were to Āyurveda what modern chemistry, physics, and biology were to cosmopolitan medicine.

Thus, volume one of Dwarkanath's *Fundamental Principles of Ayurveda* was devoted to epistemology and the atomic theory in *Nyāya Vaiśeṣika* tradition. Volume two, "Outlines of Samkhya Patanjala System," set forth the twenty-five *tattva* that compose and evolve in the universe—matter, intelligence, self-consciousness, the five subtle and five material elements, the five organs of sense, the five actions, and mind and soul. This system also includes the three qualities, or *guṇa*, that predominate in things as they evolve, and are important organizing ideas in many spheres of Indian life: *sattva, rajas,* and *tamas,* which Dwarkanath translated as essence or intelligence, energy in motion, and mass or inertia.

Dwarkanath quoted the Bengali Orientalist, Brajendra Nath Seal, and Western authors—Alexis Carrel's *Man the Unknown,* James Jeans's *The New Background of Science,* and so on—the point being that Western science confirmed the Hindu *Darśana.* Yet his and Srinivasa Murti's argument was ambivalent. Their conception of science was that it dealt with eternal truth. This conflicted with the power in modern science to discover new truths that make former ideas obsolete. The very faculty that brings fame to modern scientists reveals the theoretical imperfection of the whole enterprise, for Srinivasa Murti and Dwarkanath argued that as modern science eliminated the errors of its past it moved toward the unchanging, complete, and perfect truths of Hindu theory. For example, the *Mahāpañcabhūta,* or five elements—ether, air, fire, water, and earth—correspond with hearing, touch, sight, taste, and smell, and because these senses are the only ways that we can perceive the world, the concept of five elements "provides the advantage and satisfaction of having a complete theory valid for all time."[5]

When advocates of "modern Western medicine" demanded that Āyurveda be explained "in terms of Western Science," and in a manner "clear to persons of ordinary intelligence not proficient in or acquainted with even the elements of the Darshanas,"[6] they were as arrogant and foolish as vaidyas would be if they asserted that the validity of cosmopolitan medicine depended on the ability of doctors to explain its theories to people with no understanding of modern science. Dwarkanath objected to using the term humor to translate *doṣa,* as P. C. Roy had done, following common practice by calling *kapha,* phlegm; *pitta,* bile; and *vāta,* wind. Instead, Dwarkanath wrote that they described functions of the body, with *vāta* designating "processes of the central, vegetative and autonomous nervous system," *pitta* denoted functions of the nutritional system, including "the thermogenetic" and "activities of glandular structures, especially enzymes and hormones, whose functions . . . [are] tissue building and metabolism," and *kapha* referred to what "Western physiologists include under . . . the skeletal and anabolic systems."[7]

Srinivasa Murti had written that the three humors could not be defined, but only their effects observed, like electricity in modern science.[8] Yet neither he nor any other Indian writer to my knowledge ever advanced a position as extreme and consistent as the one that Manfred Porkert has used to interpret Chinese medicine, insisting that a complete epistemological break exists between Chinese and cosmopolitan medicine, the one dealing with "functions" and the other with "substrata," so that a technical European vocabulary must be invented to translate and describe Chinese humoralism.[9] A similar position would maintain that Āyurveda cannot be translated by using concepts from modern science because it deals with an entirely different aspect of reality.

In contrast, Indian translators and writers of both purist and integrationist persuasions have used the language of cosmopolitan medicine. Srinivasa Murti wrote that "for a proper appreciation of the treasures of Āyurveda by the present generation of intellectuals in India and the world at large, it is necessary to present them, wherever possible, in the language of modern science."[10] He and Dwarkanath described Hindu atomic theory as "strikingly modern," with concepts that anticipated quantum mechanics, and different combinations of "proton-electron bricks" composing the five elements. To describe the *rasa, vīrya, vipāka,* and *prabhāva* conceptions of the way medicine and food juices are digested and assimilated, Dwarkanath wrote:

> Endless debates on and discussions of these concepts have been going on. . . . There is, however, sufficient evidence in the authoritative classics . . . to justify a proper evaluation of them now, in the light of facts of the modern science. . . . The obvious method for resolving these problems is to make a fresh approach to them . . . in the words of Albert Einstein: "To raise new questions, new possibilities, *to regard old problems from a new angle* requires creative imagination and marks a real advance in science." The elucidation of the old concepts of virya and vipaka now offered is the outcome of an approach, not only *"to regard old problems from a new angle"* but also to regard new facts of modern science from an old angle.[11]

The motive force of Dwarkanath's career was this effort to translate between Āyurveda and cosmopolitan medicine, to prove thereby that Hindu theories were more inclusive and valid than the limited and changeable truth of modern science. His ambivalence grew from a conflicted belief in the superiority of Āyurveda, and the wound of its inferior status in India and abroad.

Dr. Dwarkanath was appalled as a student by the inability of vaidyas to demonstrate their diagnostic procedures in the college hospital, and by the disparity between their practices and the texts they quoted. They obviously did not do what the texts prescribed, though they referred to them as scripture. In contrast, allopathic physicians demonstrated concepts and facts exactly as they appeared in the textbooks, showing more exact and objective diagnostic techniques than the vaidyas possessed. They also demonstrated effective interventions, such as surgery and chemotherapy, for problems that left the vaidyas standing by helplessly.[12]

Dwarkanath said that he had to learn Āyurveda independently because the vaidyas who were instructors at his college were incompetent teachers. Modern Āyurveda, he declared, was a ruin, a vestige of its past. Of the eight branches that had composed a comprehensive medical system in antiquity, only *kāyachikitsā*, or internal medicine, remained in practice. Yet vaidyas continued to memorize and quote texts that they neither understood nor used for the other seven branches. Even at Jamnagar, where he was Professor of *Kāyachikitsā* at the Post-Graduate Training Center from 1956 to 1959, he ran into "orthodoxy" when the Principal, Vaidya B. V. Gokhale, objected to experiments that involved animal sacrifice. Also, the Director of the institutions at Jamnagar played politics to keep the purists and integrationists divided. Endless time was spent in factional scheming rather than constructive work.

The fallen state of Āyurveda, with its ignorant, incompetent, and mendacious practitioners was a bitter theme for Dr. Dwarkanath. He would hold his fingers in the shape of a lotus blossom, which is the form of the heart in Āyurveda. The heart is the organ of consciousness; it opens and closes in wakefulness and sleep. He would quote the appropriate Sanskrit verse, opening his lotus-formed hand, and declare that this was not a poetic metaphor to the traditionalists, who piously believed this nonsensical anatomy. He would throw it out, because he loved Āyurveda, along with whatever else failed to stand up under rigorous scientific scrutiny.

Dr. Dwarkanath was known for these opinions, but I would have misunderstood them if I had not read his books. In the volume where he took Einstein's advice to regard old problems from a new angle, he outlined the doctrine of the six rasa, or taste: sweet, sour, saline, pungent, bitter, and astringent. He described their differing qualities (*guṇas*), and eight potencies (*vīrya*): light or heavy, cold or hot, unctuous or not, and dull or sharp. He related their *vipāka*, or changing taste as digestion transforms food and medicinal juices, and finally, the *prabhāva*, or specific action that may differ from the one indicated by other qualities. Along the way he related these ideas to the chemistry of carbohydrates, glucose, amino acids, and so on, and summarized the whole scheme in figure 8.4.

Dr. Dwarkanath took this kind of analysis further in his most ambitious book, *Introduction to Kāyachikitsā*, published in 1959. This work exhibited greater acquaintance with British and American medical books and journals than his earlier textbooks. For example, in describing *śleṣmaka ojas*, phlegm semen, the most refined and vital body substance, Dr. Dwarkanath reasoned that it was "for the most part" produced in the liver, and that it circulated in the blood as "a very stable compound consisting of (lipo-) proteins of high molecular weight."[13] He then reviewed current research in the United

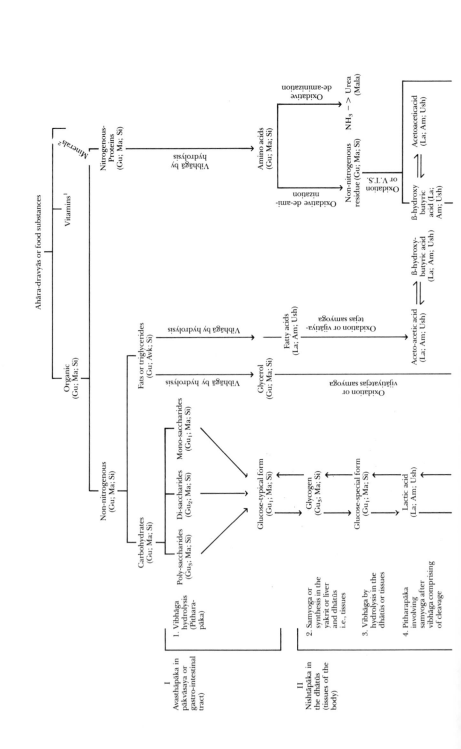

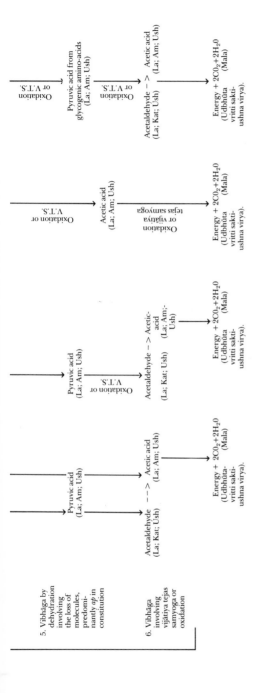

5. Vibhāga by dehydration involving the loss of molecules, predominantly *ap* in constitution

6. Vibhāga involving vijātiya tejas samyoga or oxidation

Pyruvic acid (La; Am; Ush)

Acetaldehyde (La; Kat; Ush)

Energy + 2CO₂+2H₂0 (Udbhūta-vritti sakti-ushna virya).   (Mala)

Oxidation or V.T.S.

Pyruvic acid (La; Am; Ush)

Acetaldehyde – > Acetic-acid (La; Kat; Ush)   (La; Am;-Ush)

Energy + 2CO₂+2H₂0 (Udbhūta vritti sakti-ushna virya).   (Mala)

V.T.S. or Oxidation

Acetic acid (La; Am; Ush)

Oxidation or vijñūya tejas samyoga

Energy + 2CO₂+2H₂0 (Udbhūta vritti sakti-ushna virya).   (Mala)

Oxidation or V.T.S.

Pyruvic acid from glycogenic amino-acids (La; Am; Ush)

Oxidation or V.T.S.

Acetaldehyde – > Acetic acid (La; Kat; Ush)   (La; Am; Ush)

Energy + 2CO₂+2H₂0 (Udbhūta vritti sakti-ushna virya).   (Mala)

K E Y

Gu₁ = Guru of first degree
Gu₂ = Guru of second degree
Gu₃ = Guru of third degree
La = Laghu
Ma = Madhura

Am = Amla
Katu = Katu
Avk = Ayaktarasa
Si = Sita virya
Ush = Ushna virya

Note: This schema represents the reconciliation of the views of Charaka and Vāgbhaṭa of three vipākas viz., madhura, amla, and katu and the two vipākas of Susruta viz., madhura and katu. According to this reconciled view, all food substances when subjected to energy releasing reactions alternately undergo madhura –> amla < – katu vipākās.

(1) Vitamins which are defined as organic compounds do not appear to undergo transformation similar to those to which carbohydrates, fats and proteins are subjected to. They are required (a) for the promotion of normal growth and maintenance of animal life; (b) they are effective in small quantities; (c) they do not furnish energy and are not utilized to form part of animal structure; (d) they are essential for the transformation of energy and regulation of metabolism, and (e) as parts of the enzyme system, they catalyze the reactions within the organism, and therefore operate within a narrow range of temperature and pH.

(2) Minerals as a rule are ushna in virya in view of their electrically charged ions which represent kinetic energy. They are sita in virya when their ions are not dissociated and ushna when dissociation of their ions from the molecules has taken place.

Figure 8.4   A schematic representation of the transformation of food substances or āhāra dravyās in the course of digestive and metabolic processes, furnishing general details of the biochemical steps as per facts of modern physiology *vis à vis* the Āyurvedic concepts of Rasa, Guna, Virya, and Vipākā.

States on the role of serum properdin in natural resistance to infections, and, comparing properdin to *śleṣmaka ojas*, he concluded:

> As stated by James B. Conant, "We can put it down as one of the principles learned from the history of science that a theory is only overthrown by a better theory, never merely by contradictory facts." Proceeding on these lines, it may be said that modern researches . . . are not contradictory to the existing Āyurvedic conceptual scheme of *śhleishmika ōjas* . . . [but] appear to amplify the latter theory. . . . While it is not . . . claimed that serum protein, properdin, is *śhleishmika ōjas*, the resemblance they bear to each other . . . is striking. . . . Together they form part of the still larger scheme of *kapha* (or shleshma) organization of the body.[14]

I offended Dr. Dwarkanath by questioning his conflation of Sanskritic and modern biological concepts. Srinivasa Murti had written, "We should not torture Āyurvedic texts to read into them modern allopathic teachings through forced comparisons and fanciful interpretations."[15] Dwarkanath was convinced that his own and Srinivasa Murti's interpretations avoided this error. But self-deception is not the most interesting issue for us in considering his work.

Though Dwarkanath was a college-educated physician who used the title of doctor and wanted to improve cosmopolitan medicine in the Āyurvedic curriculum, and Shiv Sharma was a Pandit who opposed this policy, claiming that college-educated practitioners had never attained the "stature which the products of the *Guru Shishya Parampara* achieved,"[16] I believe that Dr. Dwarkanath was the more traditional and perhaps the more religious intellectual. Shiv Sharma could trim his sails to suit the company in a way that Dwarkanath could not. He was witty and at ease with powerful politicians and businessmen. He traveled and lectured abroad with successes Dwarkanath would not have managed. Yet when one allows for inconsistencies in the publications and speeches from different parts of his career, it is clear that Shiv Sharma's ideas resembled those of people he opposed. Indeed, he borrowed material from Srinivasa Murti, Dwarkanath, and other integrationists. Except for his polemical skills, none of his interpretations of Āyurveda was original. A less polished and energetic man would not have had Pandit Shiv Sharma's political success. Yet, he was successful because he was on the winning side. The policy he worked for was the one advocated by most of the people in power. With few exceptions, political leaders felt that doctors should determine health policies and the interest of the organized profession was to keep as much control as it could over new technology and the market for medical services. The "pure" curriculum curtailed training in modern diagnostic and therapeutic techniques for students in the indigenous medical colleges. Middle-class people who were sensitive to foreign conceptions of India, and whose children might become doctors, did not want their government to get out of step with the world system by integrating Āyurveda with cosmopolitan medicine.

Meanwhile, people of all social classes use indigenous medicine, so that a substantial market has existed for this system. The demand for Āyurveda supported practitioners and companies that manufactured indigenous medicines, and they developed professional institutions to improve their lot competitively with the expanding system of cosmopolitan medicine. The Orientalist rhetoric provided a definition of their situation, and a moral platform for dealing with it. Dr. Dwarkanath worked in that tradition. The interesting question about his work concerns its relationship to the whole tradition of South Asian humoralism. Was the Orientalist effort an epistemological break, a genuine historical discontinuity?

The Orientalists asserted that Buddhist objections to dissection and the conquests by Muslim and British invaders·who patronized rival systems caused the moral decline of vaidyas who retreated to dogmatism and secrecy. But this was mythology. Āyurvedic practices in the eighteenth and nineteenth centuries were different from those described by the classic texts, but this did not mean that Āyurveda was a ruin and vestige of its past. Physicians probably did not practice medicine at the time the texts were written in exactly the ways they prescribe. They are normative works, and what books say that people should do is always problematic in relation to their actual behavior.

Cosmopolitan medicine has undoubtedly broken with humoral traditions, and one might think that a self-declared modernist like Dr. Dwarkanath was on the other side of that epistemological chasm trying to build a bridge for other practitioners to cross over. In some moods this is probably how he imagined himself, but if one reads his books the structure of his thought is clearly that of the classic theories. He stood on the humoral side of the chasm trying to find a way across with traditional concepts, using odds and ends from biomedicine to give the appearance that the sides were joined. But an operative science requires a consensus, a community of workers, and no modern medical scientist will find colleagues to cross this makeshift structure.

Diagnostic Practices in Modern Textbooks, among Physicians in a Teaching Hospital, and by a Renowned Rural Practitioner

The first problem in describing how patients are diagnosed and treated in modern Āyurveda is to indicate the range of practitioners. Pandit Shiv Sharma's patients had the same kind of dyadic, fee-for-service relationship with him that they had with allopathic doctors, except that he emphasized humoral balance and the simplicity and mildness of his prescriptions, in contrast to surgery and the side-effects of chemotherapy. Consultations with him by politicians like Moraji Desai and G. L. Nanda had religious and nationalistic connotations that would be unusual when ordinary people consult vaidyas. Also, Shiv Sharma offered an "alternative therapy" with pastoral connotations for some of his patients who had read about "holistic health" in domestic or foreign magazines. He was in this sense an unusually stylish vaidya. He even arranged for his son to study acupuncture in Japan and Hong Kong. Although Shiv Sharma did not use the symbolism of the stethoscope, I spent some time with him in New York looking unsuccessfully in medical supply houses for a gadget that would not cost too much, and would fit into his suitcase. He wanted it for his office, where it would intrigue patients and serve as a conversation piece.

In contrast, most vaidyas have plain-looking clinics open to the street in a market area, and consultations with them are brief. The patient or an accompanying person will recount symptoms, and the physical examination will be limited to a glance at the tongue or a momentary reading of the pulse. The prescription may be an injection, along with an Āyurvedic medicine to take orally, and some instruction about food. The vaidya's reasoning will not be discussed unless the patient takes the initiative. The notion that patients normally consult vaidyas at length and have the diagnosis and treatment carefully explained to them is not true, at least as far as I have observed. Consultations in the outpatient clinics of Āyurvedic hospitals often last a minute or two, so that even in teaching institutions practices do not always follow textbook instructions for diagnosing patients. Finally, I have sat with Pandit Shiv Sharma and his secretary while he dictated letters to patients who had consulted him by mail. In Delhi, hakims meet every week to answer patients who have written to the clinic of Hamdard, one of India's largest pharmaceutical companies for indigenous medicine.

We have discussed the syncretism of Āyurveda and cosmopolitan medicine, but Āyurveda and Yunāni tibbia also borrow from each other, homeopathic medicine is used by many vaidyas, and, in another direction entirely, some practitioners combine Āyurveda with tantric ritual. Confronted with the pluralism for which South Asia is famous, I will describe two studies that illustrate patterns of diagnosis and treatment.

Daniel Tabor studied with vaidyas in the hospital of the H. O. Nazar Āyurveda College in Surat, and with the retired principal of the college, Sri Bāpālāl G. Vaidya (1897–1983). Our material is from an article that he published on the use of *āma* (unripe) and *pakva* (ripe) categories to interpret illnesses. These Sanskrit terms are related to the vernacular categories, *pakkā* (perfect) and *kaccā* (imperfect), which are used for all sorts of things: *pakkā* food is fried in clarified butter, *pakkā* housing is built of stone or brick with a tile roof, and *pakkā* roads are paved, while *kaccā* food is boiled, *kaccā* houses are built of mud and straw, and *kaccā* roads are unpaved.

Following Francis Zimmermann, Tabor pointed out that the *āma-pakva* concepts belonged to the ecological concern in Āyurveda with the flow of juices in the landscape and within the body, their physiological transformations and management. Now that Zimmermann has published a major book,[17] it would be interesting to take this further, but rather than consider Āyurveda from the perspective of critical historical scholarship, I want to relate Tabor's description of practices in Surat to ideas in Dr. Dwarkanath's book on *kāyachikitsā* and to other syncretic textbooks, such as M. Visweswara Sastry's *Rugniviścaya: Clinical Methods in Āyurveda*,[18] or Bhagwan Dash's *Fundamentals of Āyurvedic Medicine*.[19] They outline the following concepts of illness and diagnostic procedures for students of Āyurveda.

A person is an organization of ether, air, fire, water, and earth in living exchange with similarly organized elements in the world around him. Illnesses are classified as *nija* or *āgantuja* according to whether they originate in the internal or external environment, but even when the origin is external, for example, from events causing fright or anger, the disorder upsets the internal ecology that leads to illness.

The governing forces maintaining internal order are the three humors (*tridoṣa*): phlegm (*kapha*), which has lubricating and cooling functions; bile (*pitta*), which digests and transforms substances; and wind (*vāyu*), which circulates nutritive substances and eliminates wastes. The humors move throughout the body, but phlegm centers in the upper part, bile in the middle region, and wind in the lower part of the trunk. Diagnoses identify which humor or combination of humors has become vitiated (*dosa dusti*), or has increased and become aggravated (*doṣa vrddhi*).

Food juices enter the body and are transformed by digestive fire (*jāṭharāgni*, or *kāyāgni*), and as they circulate they undergo further transformations by fires within the elements (*bhūtas*) and tissues (*dhātūs*) that compose the body. Exchanges also occur and may become disordered between the five sense organs (*indriyas*) and their objects, with each sense dominated by one of the five elements and reacting to its counterpart element in external objects (*arthās*). Sinful actions in this or previous lives, and supernatural interventions cause disorder, but, along with variation of food intake, the most common external sources of illness are ecological changes of season (*ṛtu*). Seasonal changes encourage the accumulation of one or another *doṣa*, its spread through the body, and its return to normality.

How individuals respond to all these variables depends on their temperament, age, sex, caste, occupation, personal habits, and so on. It also depends on astrological circumstances, which these textbooks neglect, though they are a central concern to almost everyone in South Asia at critical junctions in their lives. For the most part, however, vaidyas defer to professional astrologers in using this and other forms of divination.[20]

The *āma* (unripe) that Daniel Tabor wrote about is caused by inadequate digestive fire that leaves a residue of uncooked or unripe food juice. This matter spoils and circulates through the body to clog channels and accumu-

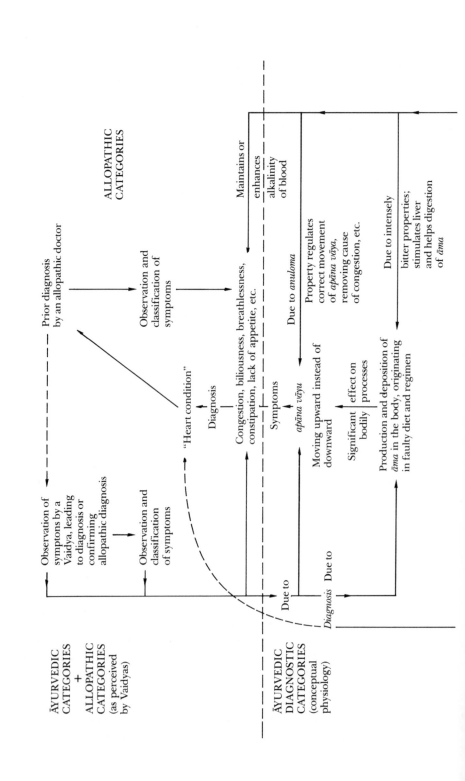

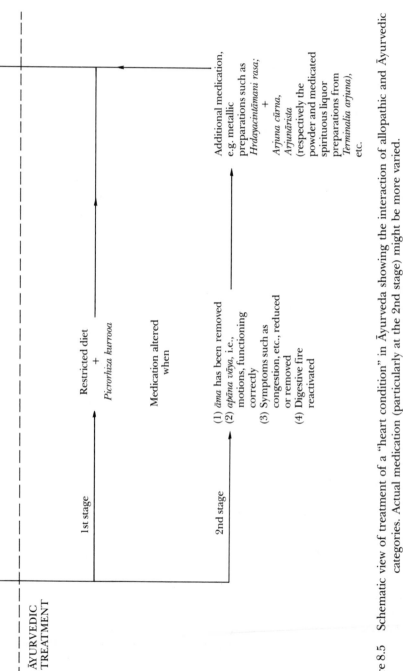

Figure 8.5 Schematic view of treatment of a "heart condition" in Āyurveda showing the interaction of allopathic and Āyurvedic categories. Actual medication (particularly at the 2nd stage) might be more varied.

late in congested places where it impairs the fires that sustain surrounding tissues. Eventually a *sāma* state may be reached in which spoiled matter causes malfunctions in all seven body substances (*dhātu*). Diarrhea, fevers, rheumatism, and other maladies are caused by *āmā* and *sāma* conditions. "In fact," Dr. Dwarkanath wrote, "most of the diseases included under *kāyachi-kitsā* may be stated to be the outcome of *āma* and *sāma*."[21] Bhagwan Dash agrees, writing that "the *āma* and aggravated *doṣas* are present along with the vitiated *srotas* (channels) which include the *dhātus* (tissue elements) in all the endogenous type of diseases."[22] And Bāpālāl Vaidya, Tabor's teacher, "concluded that *all* diseases were due to unripe food-juice."[23]

Tabor described various illnesses that involved *āma*, and for heart conditions he diagrammed diagnoses and treatments to show how Āyurveda and cosmopolitan medicine were combined (fig. 8.5). He wrote that "the diagnosis of a heart condition, usually, though not always, originated from an allopathic doctor," and "was often retained, along with whatever additional Āyurvedic diagnosis might be made."[24] Vaidyas at the teaching hospitals where Tabor studied described the initial symptoms as congestion, breathlessness, biliousness, anorexia, and constipation, but they attributed these symptoms "to the *apāna vāyu* (the downward wind) going up instead of down."[25] The reversal of the wind that normally facilitates evacuation was caused by *āma* having accumulated over a long period.

The preliminary treatment for heart conditions was to put the patient on a light diet (*laghu*, or light in the humoral sense, as well as small in amount), along with a bitter herbal medicine to enhance digestion. This regimen would stop the accumulation of *āma* and restore the movement of wind downward to remove the remaining spoiled juice from the body. Sri Bāpālāl Vaidya also believed that these patients had acidic blood and the herb would restore its normal alkaline quality. In the second stage of treatment, complex medicines were used to restore the heart itself.

Referring to the conception of the heart in Āyurveda, which Dr. Dwarkanath ridiculed as the vessel of *ojas* (semen) and the lotus-shaped seat consciousness, Tabor wrote:

Among the practitioners in Surat . . . the allopathic description of the structure and function of the heart was accepted as correct, though in other contexts some of the Āyurvedic functions would be retained (e.g. the heart as the repository of "vital essence"). The category of "heart disease" . . . was therefore somewhat ambiguous; but this very ambiguity allowed the assimilation of modern anatomy and physiology to the more general categories of Āyurveda. The problems involved in making equivalences or identifications between the two realms of discourse . . . are considerable; but in the clinical situation these identifications were made or assumed as necessity dictated. The diagnosis of a "heart condition," if originating from an allopathic doctor, could therefore be accepted and treated on lines largely dictated by the conceptual physiology of Āyurveda.[26]

Āyurvedic textbooks say that a diagnosis should consider the regional ecology, the season of the year, current weather conditions, and how compatible these things are with the patient's constitutional disposition. The vaidya should consider how the illness began and its stage of development, the patient's caste and whether the messenger sent to fetch him belongs to a lower caste, or is dirty, or arrives at an inconvenient time. His investigation should determine: (1) the primary cause of the illness (*nidāna*); (2) the prodromes (*pūrvarūpa*); (3) the fully expressed symptoms (*rūpa*); (4) the response to trial therapy (*supaśaya*); and (5) the mature form of the illness (*samprāpti*, literally, the onset), including the *doṣa* involved, its nosology, and so on. These categories were used in the classic *Mādhavanidāna*,[27] but the procedures for applying them must be inferred from lists of diseases and their symptoms, or of medications and their uses. Bhagwan Dash and Lalitesh Kashyap have translated a sixteenth-century work of this kind.[28] Visweswara Sastry's *Rugviniścaya* is a manual prepared for students at the College of Integrated Medicine in Madras which simply lists 326 pages of symptoms and diseases— seven kinds of *gulma* (stomach upset), thirty-five kinds of *kuṣṭha* (skin disease, including leprosy), seventeen kinds of *unmāda* (madness), and so on.

According to the textbooks, diagnoses are based on the knowledge of the authorities, the patient's narrative and response to questions, and the vaidya's observation of physical signs. These observations are said to constitute an eightfold physical examination: the pulse, which is complex and revealing; the moisture, color, and texture of the tongue; body heat; luster and skin color; and conditions of the voice, eyes, urine, and feces. Actually, high-caste practitioners may refrain from touching their patients, and it is hard to believe that a direct examination of stools was ever a normal diagnostic practice. Vaidyas commonly ask about the color, odor, and consistency of stools, and patients may anticipate such questions by volunteering information.

The Āyurvedic textbooks do not describe how to apply diagnostic concepts, and the classic texts lack case material that would clothe their theories with empirical flesh. Of course, diagnostic skills are learned by observation and imitation even when the technology of cosmopolitan medicine is at hand, but despite the rationally ordered nosology and etiological concepts in Āyurveda, the skill of using them depends entirely on tacit knowledge.

Ethnological studies are essential to learn how vaidyas diagnose their patients. I have indicated the social and political background of modern Āyurveda, and Tabor's material illustrates this tradition in a teaching hospital, but we have still not described the clinical construction of a diagnosis. When we examine the stories of people in trouble which compose such material, the inescapable fact comes forward that medical practice is always a moral enterprise. A dilemma of the textbooks is that they want to present Āyurveda as an analytic technology, but the concepts resist this treatment because they are an iconic dramaturgy for enacting, reconciling, and undoing conflicts.[29]

Our case material, drawn from an article by Mark Nichter,[30] describes the traditional practice of a hereditary vaidya and Pandit in a South Indian village. Pandit Ganapathy learned Āyurveda from an older brother. Their father was a practitioner, as are three other brothers. Pandit Ganapathy's wife's father was a vaidya, and she assists Ganapathy, who has a reputation for special skills in dealing with women's complaints. His village is off the main road, and difficult to reach for over half his patients who come from towns or a major city fifty miles away. The trip to consult him is a pilgrimage for patients who come after having consulted other vaidyas, doctors, compounders, and ritual specialists. His fees are high, and though patients may be discouraged or anxious, the family members who accompany them are hopeful that the malady can be explained and treated. Thus, consultations are longer and more deliberate than for accessible and less renowned vaidyas.

Ganapathy and a prominent astrologer refer clients to each other, and Nichter compares the ways they negotiate interpretations of illness. Both receive difficult cases, and their clients initially volunteer little information, relying on the specialist's power of observation and intuition to grasp the issues and to direct the enquiry. From the appearance, name, and the relationships to the patient of the accompanying person or persons, the vaidya and the astrologer anticipate particular family problems. The manner of their initial presentation of the illness, and their responses to questions help to confirm or modify these impressions. The astrologer uses several techniques of divination to draw out the patient and to orient his enquiry. Nichter writes, "A consultation alters a client's everyday conception of self as he is made more aware of influences from beyond the sphere of normal comprehension; influences that are accepted as real but about which little is actually known."[31] Through palm reading, the toss of cowrie shells, and astrological calculations, "a client gains a degree of freedom from the responsibility of his own acts; he is able to talk about these acts no longer having to bear full responsibility for them."[32] This allows the astrologer to pursue the consultation in a way that resembles psychological counseling in other societies.

Nichter describes a mother whose son had run away from home after failure in examinations that would have qualified him for a prized job, and after refusing to marry a girl who would bring a substantial dowry that his family expected to use in arranging a marriage for his sister. When the astrologer attributed these events to Saturn, and defined the period for its negative effect on the boy's life, the visibly relieved mother poured out stories of his illnesses, fights at home and school, and other troubles, revealing that his father feared that the family's misfortunes were due to sorcery. Comparing the astrologer's procedure to consultations with vaidyas like Pandit Ganapathy, Nichter writes:

> Vaidyas subtly discuss with their patients sensitive issues relating to family interrelationships and personal problems by referring to humoral imbalances much the same way as astrologers refer to stars and planets. As in the case of the astrologer, an important part of the vaidya's therapy is making explicit hidden emotions and displacing responsibility . . . instead of stars and planets, reference to body constitution, humors, states of hot/cold, diet, season, etc., serve as the vaidya's critical points of reference.[33]

Nichter describes how Pandit Ganapathy questioned a young unmarried woman who was accompanied by her mother, and who had been previously treated by another vaidya, an allopathic doctor, and an exorcist. She suffered from back pain, weakness, poor sleep, malaise, and anorexia. In the course of the consultation, and in a private discussion with Ganapathy's wife who examined the color of her urine, other symptoms emerged that were embarrassing to the patient, and led to a diagnosis of *dhātu* loss (the *dhātu* referred to is semen). Ganapathy prescribed a medicine to increase the patient's weight, another to restore and increase her semen, a blood purifier, a cooling oil for the forehead to induce sleep, and a special diet. During the consultation the Pandit ventilated problems that had caused the family to postpone the patient's marriage because they needed the money she earned in a cottage industry, while at the same time he legitimatized the somatic complaints and circumscribed the further postponement of a search for a suitable groom by defining the goal of restoring the patient's vitality and weight as preparation for marriage.

Indians commonly assume that illnesses arise from a concatenation of events, so that it is reasonable to consult different specialists for the same illness if it seems intractable. They expect different interpretations under these circumstances, and to pursue different remedies concurrently or in sequence. This may look inconsistent to an outside observer, and cosmopolitan medical practitioners disapprove of this "shopping around" because it ignores their claim to exclusive authority to diagnose and treat illnesses. The more pluralistic medical systems are, the greater autonomy laypeople have to interpret their own illnesses and to make choices about how to combine the ideas and advice of different specialists. South Asian anthropologists have illustrated these points in many articles, but among them the ethnography in Nichter's work is particularly rich.[34] We will close this section with an example from the essay we have already discussed.

A type of illness patients bring to Pandit Ganapathy is called *gulma*. Visweswara Sastry's textbook listed seven types of *gulma*. He gave the symptoms for the first type as weakness (*daurbalya*), benign tumor (*mūdhagranthi*), *sūla*, anorexia (*annādvēsa* and *aruci*), restlessness (*arati*), diarrhea (*atisāra*), languor (*tandrā*), vomiting (*chardi*), burning sensation in the throat and stomach (*dāha*), fever, (*jwara*), fatigue (*klama*), and ulcers (*arumṣi*).[35] Ganapathy related *gulma* to duodendal ulcer, and said that this malady had a high rate in South India. He considered it an *āma* disorder, caused by poor digestion, and Nichter comments on the central role of shared food in Indian households, so that conflicts in maintaining extended family units and in their division into separate hearths is symbolized by the shared digestive cycle of household members and its disruption.

But just as the symptoms of *gulma* and duodendal ulcer resemble each other, they also resemble *kai visha* (hand poison), a form of sorcery involving food that causes "indigestion an hour or so after eating a meal, burning sensation, and a feeling that there is a ball in the stomach."[36] The same malady may therefore be diagnosed and treated in different ways. Pandit Ganapathy treated such a patient with medicines to digest the *āma*, and to correct the *doṣa* imbalance caused by *gulma*, but he also referred him to an astrologer, and this specialist "tossed cowrie shells . . . and decreed the patient suffering from *kai visha*."[37] In Indian society Āyurveda thus lives side by side in complementary relationships with ritual curing and cosmopolitan medicine, as well as in the competitive and conflicted relationships we described earlier in this essay.

Conclusion

The following concepts are replicated in many domains of knowledge: the five elements (*pañchabhūta*); the hot-cold, light-heavy, subtle-gross, and other qualities of things (*guṇas*); the flavors (*rasa*), bitter, sweet, sour, and so on, and the transformation of flavors (*vipāka*); the potency (*vīrya*) and specific action (*prabhāva*) of foods; and the body substances (*dhātu*) and constitutional types (*sattva, rajas,* and *tamas*) that correspond to one or another dominant humor (*dosa*). Humoral language describes the elaborate Indian cuisine, and the musical forms appropriate to different seasons of the year and times of day. It encodes the colors, substances, and arrangement of offerings to the gods, dance, and forms of art other than music or dance. Peasant farmers use it to combine the humoral qualities of soils with those of seeds, water sources, and kinds of fertilizers, attempting to harmonize their properties to insure good crops. Humoral language defines personal characteristics, kinship, and relationships between castes. No wonder, then, that modern science can be unsettling when educated Indians realize that it is grounded in a different conception of knowledge than the one that in ritual and daily life forms their sense of reality and truth. And no wonder that Āyurvedic physicians (and allopathic doctors, though this has not yet been studied) reconcile humoral concepts with biomedical knowledge. Dr. Dwarkanath and many other

Āyurvedic scholars I have known have felt deeply that a way of life is at stake in their interpretation of illnesses, and not just a set of medical practices. Our narrative of Dr. Lenora, Pandit Shiv Sharma, Dr. Dwarkanath, Sri Bāpālāl Vaidya, and Pandit Ganapathy moved from political controversy about how Āyurveda should be taught to an analysis of the conceptual structure of modern Āyurvedic thought in textbooks, in clinical teaching, and in private practice. I have illustrated related styles of professional Āyurvedic medicine in the practices of Shiv Sharma, physicians at an Āyurvedic college, and of an educated village healer. Physicians of this kind define the Āyurvedic tradition in publications and teaching, and their practices are exemplary for laypeople as well as for other vaidyas. In the public's eye (insofar as publics are created in India by the mass media popular culture) professional Āyurvedic institutions cannot compete with biomedical institutions in creating striking new diagnostic and therapeutic technology. The physicians we have described are sometimes painfully aware that cosmopolitan medicine dominates the Indian medical system, yet a substantial market exists for commercial Āyurvedic products and for consultations with practitioners. The structural reasons that medical pluralism is a prominant feature of health care throughout the world are that biomedicine, like Āyurveda and every other therapeutic system, fails to help many patients. Every system generates discontent with its limitations and a search for alternative therapies. Similarly, moral conflicts dispose people to different interpretations of illnesses. Āyurveda, biomedicine, and other traditions provide different rhetorics of responsibility and different meanings for suffering. I have shown how large-scale historical changes frame the interpretations of illnesses employed by Āyurvedic physicians, and at the same time help define the character in this century of Indian civilization, for I believe that Āyurvedic scholars are correct in feeling that more is at stake in the interpretation of illness than a set of medical practices.

NOTES

1. R. B. Lenora, "Progress of Āyurveda," in the *Silver Jubilee Souvenir* (Colombo: Government College of Indigenous Medicine, English language section, 1954), 4–6.

2. See Ashis Nandy, *Alternative Sciences: Creativity and Authenticity in Two Indian Scientists* (New Delhi: Allied Publishers Private Limited, 1980), 17–91.

3. Haridas Mukherjee and Uma Mukherjee, *A Phase of the Swadeshi Movement: National Education, 1905–1910* (Calcutta: Chuckerverty, Chatterjee and Co., 1953), 47.

4. G. Srinivasa Murti, *The Science and the Art of Indian Medicine* (Adyar, Madras: The Theosophical Publishing House, 1948).

5. Ibid., 55.

6. Ibid., 57.

7. C. Dwarkanath, *The Fundamental Principles of Ayurveda, Part III, Ayushkamiya and*

Dravyadi Vignana (including Rasabhediya) of Ashtanga Hridaya (Mysore: The Hindusthan Press, 1954), 17–18.

8. Srinivasa Murti, *Science and Art*, 59–60.

9. Manfred Porkert, *The Theoretical Foundations of Chinese Medicine: Systems of Correspondence* (Cambridge: MIT Press, 1974). See also, Manfred Porkert, *The Essentials of Chinese Diagnostics* (Zurich: Chinese Medicine Publications Ltd., 1983).

10. Srinivasa Murti, *Science and Art*, 80–81.

11. Dwarkanath, *Fundamental Principles*, 143–144.

12. The same experience was reported to me by former students of other schools, including Dr. K. N. Udupa, who studied Āyurveda at Banaras Hindu University and later became the Director of the Institute of Medical Sciences at that university, and Vaidya B. V. Gokhale, who was trained at the Āyurveda Mahavidyala at Poona, and became the first Principal of the Post-Graduate Training Centre in Āyurveda at Jamnagar. In other interviews during the 1960s and 1970s, faculty members and students at various colleges told me that students ridiculed teachers who quoted slokas and pontificated to disguise their inability in hospital wards and outpatient clinics to apply the concepts of Āyurveda in a convincing manner, and that the most effectively taught courses at their schools were the ones that dealt with cosmopolitan medicine. However, Dr. Udupa and Vaidya Gokhale maintained that cosmopolitan medicine failed in many cases where Āyurveda succeeded, and, like Dr. Dwarkanath, they wanted to improve its institutions.

13. C. Dwarkanath, *Introduction to Kāyachikitsā* (Bombay: Popular Book Depot, 1959), 266.

14. Ibid., 289–291.

15. Srinivasa Murti, *Science and Art*, 85. Dwarkanath wrote, "Much of text-torturing and forced interpretations have been resorted to, to prove that every modern discovery had either already existed in the old doctrines or were anticipated by them. It will, therefore, be our purpose to make a critical, dispassionate and scientific study of the doctrines basic to Āyurveda, so that they may be understood in a proper perspective" ("Introductory and outlines of *Nyāya-Viaśeshika* system of natural philosophy," in *Fundamental Principles of Āyurveda* [Mysore: The Banglalore Press Branch, 1952], 4). Even so, his method resembled that of Kaviraj Gananath Sen, who asserted that although ancient Hindu anatomy was comparable to that of modern biology, all of the original texts had been lost so that only fragments survive in passages of the remaining texts. These passages "bristle. . . with omissions, interpolations and inaccuracies" introduced by later writers who "in their ignorance of the true meaning of ancient texts, have only burdened the literature with what may be called 'Fanciful Anatomy'" (introduction to the first 1911 edition of *Pratyksha Sariram*, 3d edition, 1921, 7).

16. Shiv Sharma, "Presidential address at a special session of the All India Āyurvedic Congress held at Ghaziabad, Delhi, on 11th and 12th August, 1951" (pamphlet), 3.

17. Francis Zimmermann, *The Jungle and the Aroma of Meats: An Ecological Theme in Hindu Medicine* (Berkeley, Los Angeles, London: University of California Press, 1987).

18. M. Visweswara Sastry, *Rugviniścaya: Clinical Methods in Āyurveda* (Madras: College of Integrated Medicine, 1956).

19. Vaidya Bhagwan Dash, *Fundamentals of Āyurvedic Medicine* (Delhi: Bansal & Co., 1978).

20. Dr. Chandrasekhar G. Thakkur, a vaidya and astrologer who has made several lecture tours of the United States, is the author of *Introduction to Āyurveda: Basic Indian Medicine*, 2d ed. (Jamnagar: Shri Gulabkunverba Āyurvedic Society, 1975) and of *Medical Astrology* (Bombay: Ancient Wisdom Publications, 1976). Another reason that the modern Āyurvedic textbooks neglect astrology is that it is the specialization of practitioners other than vaidyas. Finally, these texts are striving to make Āyurveda a science equivalent to cosmopolitan medicine, and this makes astrology along with other forms of divination and ritual curing inappropriate.

21. Dwarkanath, *Introduction to Kāyachikitsā*, 69.

22. Dash, *Fundamentals of Āyurvedic Medicine*, 101.

23. Daniel C. Tabor, "Ripe and unripe: concepts of health and sickness in Āyurvedic medicine," *Social Science and Medicine* 15B (1981): 442.

24. Ibid., 448.

25. Ibid.

26. Ibid., 449.

27. See the splendid translation of the first ten chapters of this work with later commentaries and modern analysis by G. J. Meulenbeld, *The Madhavanidana and Its Chief Commentary* (Leiden: E. J. Brill, 1974).

28. Vaidya Bhagwan Dash and Vaidya Lalitesh Kashyap, *Diagnosis and Treatment of Diseases in Āyurveda Based on Āyurveda Saukhyam of Todarananda*, Part 2 (New Delhi: Concept Publishing Company, 1982). This is the fourth volume in the series. Vol. 1 was on materia medica, vol. 2 on principles, and vol. 3 was part 1 of five projected volumes on diagnosis and treatment. Vols. 8 and 9 will be on specialized therapies and iatrochemistry.

29. Henry R. Zimmer describes the classic tradition from this perspective, saying that "Hindu physiology unfolds like a spectular romance of the three humors, with their quarrels and appeasements, aggressions and defeats." He illustrates the tradition by summarizing a seventeenth-century didactic play about a struggle between the king of disease and the ruler of the body. See H. R. Zimmer, *Hindu Medicine* (Baltimore: The Johns Hopkins Press, 1948), 61ff and 138.

30. Mark Nichter, "Negotiation of the illness experience: Āyurvedic therapy and the psychosocial dimension of illness," *Culture, Medicine and Psychiatry* 5 (1981): 5–24.

31. Ibid., 9.

32. Ibid.

33. Ibid., 10. Judy Pugh has analyzed the work of astrologers in Banaras in this manner, using extensive case material and comparing differences between the Hindu and Muslim communities. See Judy Pugh, "Astrological counseling in contemporary India," *Culture, Medicine and Psychiatry* 7, no. 3 (1983): 279–299.

34. Some of Mark Nichter's publications are: "Health ideologies and medical cultures in the south karana areca nut belt," Ph.D. diss., 2 vols., University of Edinburgh, 1977; "Patterns of curative resort and their significance for health planning in South Asia," *Medical Anthropology* 2 (1978); "The layperson's perception of medicine as perspective into the utilization of multiple therapy systems in the Indian context," *Social Science and Medicine* 14B (1980): 225–233; "The ethnophysiology and folk diete-

tics of pregnancy: a case study from South India," *Human Organization* 42, no. 3 (1983): 235–246; and "Modes of food classification and the diet-health contingency: a South Indian case study," in *Modes of Food Classification in South Asia*, ed. R. Khare and K. Ishvaran. In press.

35. Sastry, *Rugviniścaya*, 280.
36. Nichter, "Negotiation of the illness," 20.
37. Ibid.

NINE

Gentle Purge: The Flower Power of Āyurveda

Francis Zimmermann

Contemporary advocates of Āyurvedic medicine in Western countries associate it with one of the most attractive values of our time, a value we borrowed from the classical Hindu tradition—that of nonviolence. The more Āyurvedic doctors criticize modern scientific medicine for its harmful side effects, the more they stress the nonviolent, nonoperative character of their own system. Humoral balance, the proper nourishment of the tissues by soothing drugs and massages, and the integration with the environment are said to offer an alternative to the harshness of biomedicine. This modern version of Āyurveda appeals to an ideal also shared by environmentalists in which the soft, the gentle, the harmless, the cool, the refreshing, and the natural are qualities rooted in the soil, in the cycle of the seasons (which is praised as manifesting spiritual values that elude an economic calculus), and inscribed in the fabric of life itself, that is, in the vital fluids of humoral physiology. Nonviolence is thus akin to humoralism. Far from being obsolete, the humoral concept of temperamental fluid is revived in our modern partiality for environmentalism and holistic medicine.

In the classic texts two kinds of medications prevailed: calming drugs and baths were used to modify the body's internal tension and temperature, and these were distinguished from purges and emetics to eliminate the peccant humors and other pathogenic excreta. According to the classic texts, oil baths, sudorifics, and massages are merely preliminaries to the more drastic action of evacuants. Herbalized oil embrocations, warm baths and poultices, and massages with and against the hair soften and liquefy humors in the body channels. They bring the vitiated organic fluids back into the central system (*koṣṭha*), the alimentary tract. Here they are cooked by evacuant medications before they are expelled. Oily, tepid, and gentle massages temper the violence of purges and emetics. This is what is taught in the classic

texts. However, in contemporary practice in South Asia, as well as in Āyurvedic therapies exported to the West, practitioners avoid using emetics or
drastic purgatives. All violence has disappeared from medications aiming to
cleanse the patient's humoral system. Neither red (the red of bloodletting),
nor black (the black of chemical oxides), but green—the green of herbs fresh-
ly gathered, a symbol of nonviolence: this is the new motto of Āyurveda's
flower children.

The modern emphasis on gentle elements in Āyurveda changes the tradition significantly. For example, in a treatment that draws patients from
many parts of India to the southern state of Kerala, practitioners have substituted the ambiguous concept of five actions (*pañcakarma*) for the more basic
concept of catharsis, purification and evacuation (*śodhana*), and they have
reduced the actual practice of the five actions to nonoperative therapeutic
methods by scoring out vomition and by focusing on massages. This treatment has been exported to other parts of India, where it is taught in Āyurvedic colleges, and to Europe and America. We concern ourselves here with
these recent alterations of the classical doctrine, in order to reveal the significance of catharsis—both purification and purgation—in historic Āyurveda.
We do not hesitate to cite Sanskrit texts. A hitherto unknown literary piece of
evidence will be presented, which illuminates the division of the ancient
medical profession into (1) physicians who act by means of the scalpel, forceps, and evacuants; (2) those who act by means of baths, poultices, massages, and soothing drugs; and (3) those who prescribe regimen and diet.
Parallel Latin texts show that Āyurveda and Hippocratic medicine belong to
the same Indo-European tradition. According to this tripartite division,
catharsis belongs to the category of *extractive* methods. Since these methods
are intrinsically violent, they require soft and gentle correctives selected from
the category of *calming* methods. Therefore, catharsis and nonviolence are
complementary to each other within a dialectical system. Gentle medications
are historically understood only in relation to violent, extractive methods.
The subject of this paper is the dialectic of purity and violence, catharsis and
nonviolence, strong evacuants and gentle massages.

CATHARSIS AND THE VALUES OF NONVIOLENCE

I am addressing the ideological discourse in which the practice of evacuant
therapies is wrapped up. Quoting from advertising material, colored booklets
on glossy paper published by some fashionable health centers, and cata-
logues of medicines offered for sale by leading Āyurvedic companies, I will
try to relate what they say to what is said in the classic texts, to reveal distortions, biased translations from Sanskrit into English, and a general trend
toward turning the ancient wisdom, the ancient Art of Catharsis, into a set of
commodities.

The equivalent of Greek *katharsis* existed in the Sanskrit *śuddhi* and *śodhana*, "purification, evacuant therapy." The purifications of Āyurveda require confinement to bed. In ancient times they were inseparable from religion and ritual, but today they are administered in India by registered practitioners in government hospitals and private-sector nursing homes, and they have become commodities that compete with other kinds of paramedical techniques in the health-care market. The herbalized oils used in these treatments have become an article of export. In mentioning only oils, I am simplifying a most complicated Galenic pharmacy, which offers also herbal teas, powders, butters, and so on. Oils are the most typical Āyurvedic remedies because they exemplify the prevalence of unctuous substances (*sneha*) and illustrate the principle of polypragmatic use: as potions when recooked 101 times, as enemas, inunctions, and so on. They are medicated with spices through a process of cooking and straining that continues over a period of at least five days and nights. An ambiguity in their being either taken internally or applied externally corresponds to the ambiguity of catharsis itself. Catharsis combines inside and outside, potions and baths, enemas and massages, aiming to invade the patient's body from all sides and through all apertures. Stereotyped formulations exist of the principle of polypragmatic use. For example, *catuṣprayoga*, "the four modes of administering (a dose of medicine)," involves potions, errhines, unctions, and baths.[1] The image of the body is of a network of innumerable channels open to attacks by evacuant medicines so that the body can be soaked through and drained off. Catharsis is a *dehavyāpti*, "a pervasion of the body";[2] the medicines pervade the channels and soak up the vitiated humors before being discharged. Sesamum oil is a good vehicle for active medicinal ingredients because it is exquisitely pervasive or *vyavāyin*, "insinuative." "*Insinuative* means: ready to pervade the body. A drug is insinuative, which, as soon as it is consumed during a meal, pervades the body all over before it is subjected to coction."[3] Coction means more than simply digestion, it is also the ripening of morbific matter before elimination from the body. In the course of Āyurvedic evacuant therapies, the herbalized oils bring the vitiated humors back into the alimentary tract, where they are cooked. Defecation and vomition are the results of such humoral coction.

In humoralist physiology, disease is internalized and liquefied as vitiated humors run astray, hidden in the depths of body channels. No strict demarcation exists between fluids and tissues. The medicated fluids of pharmacy and the vitiated fluids of physiology are two sides of the same nexus. We shall avoid the details of pharmacy here, but the ideological distortions of bodily techniques which I will describe could be richly documented also in pharmacy. For example, decoctions, the most familiar medicines, were formerly made in principle from fresh plants. The crushed leaves, stems, or roots that were not soluble in water were eliminated by filtering the decoction. The remedy was a liquid into which the active principles of medicinal plants had passed. Nowadays in manufacturing tablets, however, the vegetable materials are pulverized and may be incorporated into tablets without any cooking. The liquid phase may thus be entirely eliminated. To make tablets digestible, modernizers reason that the choice of ingredients should be more restrictive than the original recipe. The ideas of fluidity, solubility, and water conceived of as a vehicle and medium for humoral control are devaluated, and the spirit of Āyurvedic pharmacy is lost.

A similar ideological distortion can be observed in therapeutics. The classic techniques of oleation and sudation stressed the skin and tissues, but the bony framework and articulations have now become the focus of attention. A misunderstanding occurs in using the term *massage* to refer to Āyurvedic baths, inunctions, and embrocations. The underlying idea is that the skin is a path through which remedies are absorbed and humors exuded. The concept of classic Āyurvedic massages is of a fluid metabolism through the skin, not of mechanical pressure exerted on the muscles. Only recently, under the influence of Western anatomical thinking, the Hindu fluid conception of the human person which pervades Āyurveda gave way to a Western concept of physical therapy in which the solid parts of the body play the title role.

The first part of this essay is based on the assumption that, willingly or not, the discourse of contemporary practitioners on catharsis betrays its classical sources and needs to be deciphered in the light of the learned tradition. To illustrate the theme of nonviolence, I will cite an advertisement for the Maharishi Āyurveda Prevention Centers™ in North America.[4] The keynote for all their cures is rejuvenation. This is in accordance with one feature of the classical system: rejuvenation is the archetype of hospitalization. Hospitalization in Āyurveda is not only a confinement to bed, a special diet, an abstention from work, but also a way of ritualizing the cure. Accordingly, the rejuvenation programs offered to wealthy patrons in modern Āyurvedic sanatoria, although they are cast in the prosaic mold of massages and evacuant therapies, are tinged with the spiritualizing flavor of ancient mystery cults. The Maharishi's advertisement reads:

> *Rejuvenation program (Panchakarma)* . . . an individualized purification and rejuvenation treatment supervised by a specially trained physician. The recommended program requires two hours per day over a period of seven consecutive days. While the . . . Panchakarma Program varies for each person, there are common features. These include Āyurvedic massage with specific herbalized oils, heat treatments, and internal purification procedures. The rejuvenation program is gentle, natural and extremely relaxing. It eliminates imbalance in the physiology and effectively promotes ideal health. Thousands of people have already participated in this program and have experienced its rejuvenating and revitalizing effects. Additional programs are available for weight loss and weight gain, stress management, and other special health concerns. (Maharishi, 10)

In referring to the Sanskrit texts and notions alluded to in this document I do not advocate a scriptural fundamentalism. I want to acknowledge that Āyurvedic practices described in the Maharishi's brochure are genuine while at the same time exposing their bias toward gentleness and showing that they involve an ideological confusion of Āyurvedic categories.

This rejuvenation program overlooks the rituals described in the classic texts and equates "rejuvenation" (rasāyana) with the "five actions" (pañcakarma). It further confuses the classic tradition by associating rejuvenation with internal "purification" (śodhana). Strictly speaking, the pañcakarma are not the same as the five śodhana.[5] The śodhana are the evacuants proper: vomition, purgation, evacuative enemas, evacuative errhines, and bloodletting. While the pañcakarma include vomition, purgation, evacuative enemas, and errhines, they omit bloodletting and include instead calming and repletive oily enemas that differ from evacuative enemas. The relatively minor medication with repletive errhines is neglected in the traditional lists, but it belongs to the pañcakarma group. All procedures may be classified according to whether they are evacuant (śodhana) or calming (śamana), depletive (laṅghana) or repletive (bṛmhaṇa). The realm of therapeutics divides in the cosmic duality of the unctuous or repletive and the dry or depletive. Furthermore, the dry group divides again into the evacuant and the calming.[6] Purification, in the strict sense of the word, designates the śodhana treatments and if need be the laṅghana, or the methods of fasting and reducing one's weight, a fixed list of which is indicated in table 9.1.

Among the pañcakarma, the boundary between the first four evacuative actions and the fifth unctuous action should be emphasized, because an ideological shift along the diagonal from upper left to bottom right on table 9.1 has occurred among Āyurvedic practitioners who drop the harshest and driest medications and favor the gentlest and most unctuous. Thus, the violence of catharsis has been erased.

VIOLENCE OF THINGS, VIOLENCE OF BEINGS

There is a violence inherent in medical operations. Within the classical tradition of Āyurvedic medicine, this violence was acknowledged and provided for. However, among the more orthodox Brahminic circles, violence came to be defined as a kind of pollution inherent in beings. Consequently, the medical concept of catharsis was subjected to a dramatic shift of meaning. In order to be "pure," it had to be "gentle." We are facing here the same semantic drifts as those affecting purity and auspiciousness. T. N. Madan has shown that śuddha, "pure," is not generally used to refer to events.[7] An important distinction should be made between objects and persons, on the one hand, and events and performances on the other.[8] One will say "a pure mind," referring to a person, but "a violent purge," referring to an event. When the

TABLE 9.1.   The Main Divisions of Therapeutics

		Evacuant (śodhana)		Calming (śamana)
Depletive (laṅghana)	Bloodletting	Five actions (pañcakarma): 1. vomition 2. purgation 3. evacuative enemas 4. errhines		A fixed list of seven: 1. [dissolving] digestive (pācana) 2. [stimulating] digestive (dīpana) 3. hunger 4. thirst 5. gymnastics 6. heat 7. wind
Repletive (bṛmhaṇa)			5. oily enemas	Diets (meat-soup, etc.) and body techniques (oil-bath, etc.) Calming the humor wind or the conjunction of bile and wind

SOURCE: After Vāhaṭa, Aṣṭāṅgahṛdaya, sūtrasthāna 14, 1–7.

distinction is blurred, that is, when you say "a pure purge" or "a nonviolent practitioner," as in the flower power discourse, ethics merges into physics, or the world of actions into the world of things.

Let us come back to the Maharishi's advertisement. It does not distort classic Āyurveda when it claims that rejuvenation therapy should be individualized, with the sequence of prescriptions varied to account for each person's constitution. The concern for gaining or losing weight and the theme of stress management resonate with modern Western culture, but also occur in the classic texts in the dialectic of increase (vṛddhi) and decrease (kṣaya) of all saps and humors, and in the principle of "clarity, purity, serenity [of mind]" (sattva) which is destroyed by illness, but restored through the wisdom of Āyurvedic regimen. These classical ideas can be read between the lines in the Maharishi's advertisement. Yet new accretions have been introduced to fit the modern division of labor in the medical field. The same brochure goes on to describe the so-called Panchakarma Program, after the physician has evaluated the patient's needs. The first phase is that of home preparation. A special diet to prepare the body tissues is recommended several days prior to hospitalization. The rejuvenation procedures in the hospital begin with unctions (abhyaṅga), herbalized oils. Massages, oil baths, or inunctions correspond to the oleation (*snehana*) phase in the classical scheme. Then come the sudation procedures, for which the technical names given in the Maharishi's brochure are quite significant:

Heat treatments (*Swedana, Pizichilli, Pindaswedana*, etc.)
These treatments vary from special herbalized steam to oil treatments or herbal packs. They are specified by the doctor based upon your individualized rejuvenation program. (Maharishi, 11)

"Sudation" (Sanskrit *svedana*) in the classic tradition is only a preliminary to the evacuants that will come afterward, but here becomes a full-fledged set of techniques. These techniques are special treatments practiced in Kerala. The Pizichilli (Malayalam *piḷiccil*) is a massage with a medicated oil squeezed out (*piḷiccu*) of a piece of muslin used as a sponge. The Pindaswedana (Sanskrit *piṇḍasveda*) is a massage and sudation (*sveda*) by means of boluses (*piṇḍa*) of rice soaked in an herbal tea (a decoction of the roots of the Indian mallow, *Sida rhombifolia*) kept warm on the fire. A color plate in the booklet illustrates the technique of *śirodhārā*, in which a stream (*dhārā*) of medicated oil is directed on the patient's head (*śiras*). The oil flows from a vessel with a hole at the bottom which hangs above the brow of the patient, who lies on his back. The last treatment mentioned in the Panchakarma Program is that of internal cleansing by means of evacuants: purges, enemas, errhines. I wonder whether catharsis occurs here as a third phase in a sequence, from oleation to sudation to evacuation, or simply is an alternative to massages and heat treatments.

In any case, instead of a fixed sequence, from oil to heat to catharsis, culminating in the final process of discharging unwanted excreta—which is the traditional method of *pañcakarma*—we now have a panoply of alternative actions: massages, heat treatments, and/or internal cleansing. I would like to suggest that catharsis has changed imperceptibly into a kind of physical therapy. However, while Western physiotherapists are dealing with the solid parts of the patient's body, their South Asian competitors aim to tackle the internal movement of bodily fluids.

The conclusion can be warranted by further readings through the superabundant literature of modern Āyurvedic advertising. I shall limit myself to another document, the *Medicine Catalogue* of Vaidyaratnam P. S. Varier's Arya Vaidya Sala, a well-known Āyurvedic trust based at Kottakal in South India:

Special Treatments . . . for Rejuvenation and Cure. . . . The principle underlying these methods of treatment is one of detoxication of the subject. Application of warmth (*svedana*) and oily massage (*snehana*) to the body promotes better circulation of blood in the system and free diaphoresis. The daily laxative usually given during the course of the treatment ensures satisfactory evacuation of the bowels and better cleansing of the alimentary tract. The fat contents and medicinal factors in the unguents are absorbed by the skin, resulting in the toning up of the subject. The soft oil massage itself has a marked soothing effect on the nervous system as a whole. . . . These measures give nature the fullest chance; there is no forcing of a tired system to work, no whipping up of a fallen horse.

That massage of all kinds plays an important role in every system of science of healing is evident from its popularity as an inevitable adjunct in Physiotherapy. What is achieved by artificial means such as Electrotherapy, Occupational therapy, etc., is achieved in Kerala by the scientific system of massaging. Modern types of massages known as Effleurage, Petrissage and Tapotement, etc., cannot yield as much good results as the Kerala massages. Pressure is applied not only by the palms but also by the soles of the feet as necessitated by circumstances. (Vaidyaratnam 1976, 58–59)

The second paragraph clearly turns tradition around to suit a modern division of labor in which physical therapy is made a specialty of Āyurveda. To one who knows the tradition this is particularly evident when the doctors pretend to be resorting occasionally to massages "by the soles of the feet." This is not an Āyurvedic procedure, although it is alluded to in the classic texts;[9] this is a technique evolved by fencing-masters in the gymnasiums (Rosu 1981; Rosu and Jobard 1987; Zarrilli 1984, 1989). To conclude on this particular point, the so-called Āyurvedic system of massaging is a modern, syncretic addition grafted onto the classical tradition.

The first paragraph I have quoted from this catalogue of medicines produced by the Arya Vaidya Sala is plagiarized verbatim from a handbook written by Vayaskara Mooss, *Special Treatments of Kerala.*[10] It offers an admirable blending of the three basic ideological themes underlying the modern practice: detoxication to cleanse the body channels, oleation to tone up the tissues, and *vis naturae medicatrix*, when nature is given the fullest chance. Yes indeed, a purge may be prescribed to evacuate the humors, but it should be an unctuous purge to nourish the tissues, a gentle purge to assist natural healing. The violence of catharsis is transformed with the nonviolence of oil bath.

What remains unsaid in this modern presentation of Āyurveda is that catharsis itself is violent and dangerous. An internal tension exists in the classic sequence of therapeutic procedures. Unctuous and warm medications are given to temper the violence of catharsis and keep it under control. Yet oleation and sudation can also result in violent effects when dosage is wrong or when they are not properly prepared for. Fasting must precede oleation especially with an obese, phlegmatic patient. The undigested food and overflowing phlegm should be drained and dried out by fasting lest oleation result in retch and nausea. Humoral catharsis fundamentally is a two-phase process, in which each of the two phases presents violent aspects. Oleation and sudation are meant to agitate, liquefy, and mobilize the vitiated humors that are lying stagnant and sticky in the channels and tissues, in order to bring them back into the alimentary tract. This agitation (*utkleśa*) is a first violence, although it is a necessary phase in catharsis.[11] Then, when the humors are back in the alimentary tract, the second phase, that of humoral coction (*doṣa-pāka*) proper, may begin. Evacuative medications will cook, ripen, and eliminate the humors. This coction is a second violence, resulting in vomition or diarrhea. One possible method of keeping the whole process under control is to institute a dialectic of agitation and coction, the unctuous and the purgative. This is made perfectly clear by the therapeutic programs laid down in the classic texts. According to these texts, all the procedures we are discussing require the patient to be hospitalized for seven, fourteen, or twenty-one days, during which the violence of evacuants is systematically tempered by their alternating with oil baths. Oleation is an inescapable requisite. Should the patient be subjected to more than one type of evacuant, the sequence of operations would be, for instance: oleation, sudation, purgation, oleation, sudation, oily enemas, evacuative enemas, oleation. Actually, most therapeutic programs prescribed nowadays involve only one type of evacuant, but in any case one may not omit the oleation and sudation procedures required before every evacuation, or the final oleation.[12]

Whenever catharsis is achieved by enemas, the program is devised for bringing about a soft progression from oily enemas through the more drastic evacuative ones. Oily enemas are alternated with purgative ones on the following patterns:

> *Karma* program of enemas: this is a sequence of 30 enemas, that is, an oily one [hereafter coded as O] to begin with, then 12 purgative ones [P] alternated with 12 oily, and 5 oily at the end—that is, schematically, the pattern OOPO-POP. . . OPOOOOO.
> *Kāla* program: a sequence of 15 enemas on the pattern OOPOPOPOPO-POOOO.
> *Yoga* program: a sequence of 8 enemas OPOPOPOO.
> One should not indulge in oily enemas nor in purgative ones taken separately. When taken alone, the oily enema produces *utkleśa* [that is, both an agitation of the humors and nausea which is the perceptible symptom of the hidden agitation], and it destroys the digestive fire. When taken alone, the purgative enema may provoke wind disorders. Therefore, one should always balance the purgative enemas with oily ones, and the oily enemas with purgative ones.
> Enemas are curative to all the three humors precisely because this method is based on a reasoned combination (*yukti*) of the unctuous and the cathartic.[13]

In the classical presentation of catharsis, nonviolence results from the reasoned adjustment (*yukti*) of two potentially violent phases to each other, namely, agitation and expulsion. Precisely this internal balance of the whole process is overlooked in the recent descriptions.

When stressing the soft and gentle quality of Āyurvedic treatments, the ideological discourse of modern advertising visualizes gentleness in the properties of oils and in conspicuous gestures of massage. The unctuous quality of oils and the fluid gestures of massage provide images of nonviolence. Instead of being the harmonious result of careful adjustments, this nonviolence is the property of a commodity. You buy this nonviolence in commercially produced oils and massages.

OPERATIVE MEDICINE IN THE INDO-EUROPEAN TRIAD

The old Hippocratic method of *expectation*, the method of waiting upon the efforts of nature in the treatment of disease, prefigures the current quest for gentleness in the competitive marketplace of alternative medical care. However, expectation should be understood as a counterbalance to the method of *operations*. Furthermore, expectation and operation are only part of a more comprehensive system of therapeutics that prevailed in classical India and the Western ancient world. Therapeutics was divided into three categories: manipulations, medicaments, and diets. A well-known formulation of this trifunctional division is found in Celsus (A.D. first century):

> During the same times [that is, the Hellenistic period of late Antiquity] the Art of Medicine was divided into three parts: one being that which cures through diet, another through medicaments, and the third by the hand. The Greeks termed the first *Diaitetike*, the second *Pharmaceutike*, the third *Cheirourgia*.[14]

Medical historians have debated whether these sentences distinguished three distinct professions or alluded instead to a purely theoretical division within one and the same practice. On the one hand, other Latin sources indicate that in Celsus's time, surgery began to split off from the other parts of medicine and to provide for its own "professores" like Philoxenes in Alexandria, who wrote specific treatises of surgery.[15] On the other hand, Celsus was looking at therapeutics from the point of view of a full-fledged physician, and in the context of an ideal synthesis of medical knowledge, in which dietetics, pharmaceutics, and surgery represented three therapeutical methods for one and the same art.[16] This is no news to medical historians in the West. What has remained unnoticed, however, is that the very same division appears in Āyurvedic Sanskrit texts. The trifunctional division of medicine is common to both Greece and India.

The encounter is significant enough to justify our quoting the Sanskrit phrases. The division can be traced first in the *Carakasaṃhitā*, where it appears incidentally, applied against worms and parasites:

> The extraction (*apakarṣaṇa*) of all worms is to be done first, then the dissolution of the basic factor (*prakṛtivighāta*), and thereafter the abstinence from things that are said to be triggering off infestation (*nidānoktānāṃ bhāvānām anupasevana*).
> Extraction is removal effected by hands, after duly considering [whether it

will be] with the help of a [surgical] instrument of without any instrument. The extraction of worms should be done logically (*nyāyatas*), by the medication corresponding to the place where the worms have gone in the body; there are four such medications: head-purgation (*śirovirecana*) [by errhines], vomition (*vamana*), purgation (*virecana*), and purgative enema (*āsthāpana*). This is the method of extraction.

The dissolution of the basic factor producing these worms is the prescription of pungent, bitter, astringent, alkaline and hot drugs, and whatever else is antagonistic to [and will dissolve] phlegm and stools. This is dissolution of the basic factor.

Thereafter, abstinence from things that are said to be triggering off infestation is the avoidance of whatever is mentioned in the list of drugs that trigger off infestation and others of the kind.

Such is therapeutics according to its characteristics (*iti lakṣaṇataś cikitsitam*).[17]

My rendering of the terminology is at variance with other translations because I want to highlight the trifunctional division of etiology and therapeutics into (1) the *localization* of a given disease and its extraction; (2) *humoral causes* and the pharmaceuticals counterbalancing them; and (3) *circumstances* and the rules of diet to check them. The three main Sanskrit terms are: (1) *sthāna*, the affected places in the body; (2) *prakṛti*, the basic factors of humoral pathology; and (3) *nidāna*, the occasions, or better, the *accidents* in the medical sense of the occurrences or circumstances that trigger a disease. The question of causality should be addressed, and especially the distinction between *humoral causes* and *accidents*—between *prakṛti* and *nidāna* in Sanskrit—since it has parallels in the Hippocratic tradition.

The foregoing division in Caraka dates from the beginning of our era and is elaborated further in the A.D. seventh century in the *Aṣṭāṅgasaṅgraha*:

But again, [therapeutics] is divided into three parts: extraction, dissolution of the basic factor, and avoidance of what triggers off the disease (*apakarṣaṇam prakṛtivighāto nidānatyāgaś ca*), each one being further subdivided into external and internal.

External extraction (*bāhyam apakarṣaṇam*): in case of nodules, tumors, sties, parasites, arrowheads, etc., with the help of knives, hands, forceps, etc. Internal extraction (*ābhyantaram punar*); by means of vomition, purgation, etc. (*vamanavirecanādibhiḥ*).

Dissolution of the basic factor: calming [medications] (*prakṛtivighātaḥ saṃśamanam*). External: inunctions, sudation, poultices, affusions, massages, etc. Internal: what is absorbed and calms the humors without agitating them (*ābhyantaram yad antaram amupraviśyāvikṣobhayad doṣāñ chamayati*).

Avoidance of what triggers off the disease: according to the state of humors (*yathādoṣam*), the avoidance of either hot or cold foods, physical exercise, etc., and the nonconsumption of either unctuous or dry things, etc.[18]

This scheme, in which the internal extraction of catharsis belongs with the external extraction of surgery, is summarized in table 9.2.

TABLE 9.2.   The Trifunctional Division of Therapeutics

	External applications	Internal medications
Operative medicine to extract peccant matter	Surgery manipulations like: lancing, incising, bursting	Evacuants, or catharsis (Sk. *śodhana*): vomition, purgation
Calming medications (Sk. *śamana*)	Oleation, sudation Special treatments like: oil-baths, massaging, *piṇḍasveda*	Galenic compositions, pharmaceuticals to be taken internally: digestives
Regimen and diet	Hygiene Rules of conduct Physical exercise Shifting habits, from sun to shade, or vice versa	Dietetics Nourishment Shifting diets, from unctuous to dry, or vice versa

SOURCE: After Vāhaṭa, *Aṣṭāṅgasaṅgraha, sūtrasthāna* 12, 3–4.

Following a seminal article by Emile Benveniste forty years ago, Georges Dumézil, in a recent review of the extant evidence on medicine and the Three Functions, has shown that ancient India, Iran, and Greece shared a common division of the art of healing into charms, surgery, and vegetable drugs.[19] This medical scheme corresponded to the trifunctional division of society in the overall Indo-European ideology, charms being there for sacredness and decision, surgery for violence and action, and drugs for productiveness and fertility. To Dumézil, it was an example of the trifunctional ideology's ability to reproduce, so to say, within itself: while medicine globally belonged under the Third Function, it was again subdivided into three functions. When compared to the documents cited by Benveniste and Dumézil, the foregoing quotations from Āyurvedic treatises seem to confirm the Indo-Europeanists' findings, although they introduce an important change of meaning in the division. Extraction corresponds to surgery, the battlefield, and violence, that is, the Second Function. Calming medications correspond to vegetable drugs and the Third Function. But the remaining category, regimen and diet, is a secularized version of the First Function, that of decision and sovereignty. Charms and rituals, the magical and religious dimensions of medicine, have been replaced by counseling and hygienics.

In any case, vomition and purgation are clearly defined as extractions. Contrary to modern practitioners' claims that *pañcakarma* is nonoperative,[20] a structural approach to the whole system shows that the modern avatars of ancient catharsis involve violence.

CONCLUSION

Let us come back to the complex system of therapeutic methods offered nowadays by Āyurvedic doctors in the form of rejuvenating cures. What this paper has attempted to demonstrate is that, in accordance with the classical tradition, these methods combine violence, gentleness, and counseling; they combine extraction, unctuous massages, and dietetics; they combine what after Dumézil we have come to call the Three Functions; and violence is one of these functional categories of traditional thought in India as well as in Europe. Within that scheme, nonviolence does not mean violence *erased* but violence *managed*. Beneath the lenient discourse of flower power and alternative medicine, and all attempts to establish gentleness as the motto of a radical break-up with the evils of modern medicine, medical history and structural anthropology are able to trace and to unearth a true line of continuity— continuity in the management of violence.

ACKNOWLEDGMENTS

I would like to thank Charles Leslie for his devoted and inspiring comments on a previous draft of this essay, and for his indefectible support as teacher, friend, and trusted guide in this field of studies. Thanks also go to Lee Mullett for her assistance in editing the text.

NOTES

A few standard abbreviations are used for references in the following notes, namely, Ah. for *Aṣṭāṅgahṛdayasaṃhitā*, As. for *Aṣṭāṅgasaṅgraha*, and Ca. for *Carakasaṃhitā*.

1. See, for example, Indu on Ah. *Cikitsā* XXII, 44c (*Aṣṭāṅgahṛdayasaṃhitā* 1939, 731b, n. 6): *catusprayogaṃ—pananasyābhyañjanasekaprayogam*. Errhine: a medicine to be snuffed up the nose.

2. As. *Sūtra* XXVIII, 43 (*Aṣṭāṅgasaṅgraha* 1980, 213a): *nirūhavīryeṇa dehavyāptaye tanmanās tiṣṭhet* [the patient] "should lie on his back, concentrating his mind on the process, to obtain the pervasion of his body by the energy of the purgative enema."

3. Parameśvara on Ah. *Sūtra* V, 55b (*Aṣṭāṅgahṛdayasaṃhitā* 1950, 88 under verse 59b): *vyavāyi vyāptiśīlam. yad dravyam abhyavaharaṇasamanantaraṃ dehe sarvatra vyāpya punaḥ pākaṃ prayāti tad vyavāyi*. Cakra on Ca. *Sūtra* XIII, 98d (*Carakasaṃhitā* 1941, 87b): *vyavāyi akhiladehavyāptipūrvakapākagāmi* "insinuative: that which pervades the whole body before being subjected to coction."

4. These centers are recent innovations of the religious movement called Transcendental Meditation. The Maharishi gained many followers in America and Europe in the 1960s, particularly after the highly publicized pilgrimage of the Beatles to his Ashram at Rishikesh. One wonders whether the abbreviation "TM" printed in exponent to all their titles means "Trade Mark" or "Transcendental Meditation"; probably both, thus illustrating a typically Hindu rhetorical device, that of "double meaning" (*śleṣa*).

5. See, for example, Ca. *Sūtra* II, 14d (def. *pañcakarma*), Ca. *Sūtra* XXII, 18 (*śodha-na* excluding oily enemas); Ca. *Sūtra* XXVI, 10 (def. *pañcakarma*); Ca. *Siddhi* II (complete study of *pañcakarma*); Ah. *Sūtra* XIV, 1–7; Ah. *Sūtra* XXVII, 8 (bloodletting opposed to *pañcakarma*); Ah. *Cikitsā* VII, 108ab ("*pañcakarma* and bloodletting").

6. Ah. *Sūtra* XIV, 4a (*Aṣṭāṅgahṛdayasaṃhitā* 1939, 223a): *bhūtānāṃ tad api dvaidhyād* "due to the duality in creatures. . ." that of "unctuousness" (*snehana*) and "dryness" (*rūkṣaṇa*).

7. "The word *śuddha* [pure], in contrast to *śubha* [auspicious], is not generally used in everyday speech to refer to events" (Madan 1985, 17).

8. T. N. Madan (1985, 23) borrowed the distinction from British philosophers of language and pragmatics like Austin. Good old continental existentialists have taught the same distinction between "essence" (which can be said to be pure) and "existence" (which can be said to be happy).

9. Ah. *Sūtra* III, 10d: *pādāghāta* "massages by the feet."

10. Precisely, from the introduction to that book (Mooss 1983, vii–ix) written by L. A. Ravi Varma in 1944 for the first edition.

11. Ah. *Sūtra* XVIII, 58cd–59ab: *malo hi dehād utkl/(Aṣṭāṅgahṛdayasaṃhitā* 1963, 121): *ūṣādibhir yathotkl]eśya hriyate vāsaso malaḥ/snehasvedais tathotkliṣṭaḥ śodhyate śodhanair malaḥ* "just as stains are removed from cloths by agitating them with the help of lye, so the humors are removed from the body by agitating them with the help of oleation and sudation, before their being evacuated with the help of evacuants."

12. Ah. *Sūtra* XVIII, 57cd–58ab.

13. Ah. *Sūtra* XIX, 63ab–67ab.

14. Celsus, *De Medicina*, Prooemium, 9 (Trans. Spencer, Loeb Classical Library).

15. The best discussion to date is that of Mudry (1982, 17 and 67); also Mudry (1985).

16. As Charles Daremberg argued convincingly (Daremberg 1865, 450; Daremberg 1870, I, 196).

17. Ca. *Vimāna* VII, 14–15.

18. As. *Sūtra* XII, 3–4 (*Aṣṭāṅgasaṅgraha* 1980, 109).

19. Published a few months before his death (Dumézil 1986).

20. G. D. Singhal has published the *pañcakarma* section of the *Suśrutasaṃhitā* (Singhal 1979) under a most significant title: "Non-Operative Considerations in Ancient Indian Surgery." He should have said, "Operative but Nonsurgical."

REFERENCES

Acarya, Jadavaji Trikamji, ed.
1941   *Carakasaṃhitā*, 3d ed. Bombay: Nirnaya Sagar.
Aṣṭāṅgahṛdayasamhitā. See Kunte, Navre, and Harisastri 1939; Mooss 1950–1963.
Aṣṭāṅgasaṅgraha. See Athavale 1980.
Athavale, A. D., ed.
1980   *Aṣṭāṅgasaṅgraha*. Pune: Athavale.
Carakasaṃhitā. See Acarya 1941.
Celsus
1935   *De Medicina*, ed. and trans. W. G. Spencer, vol. I. Cambridge: Harvard University Press.

Daremberg, Charles
1865   *La Médecine, Histoire et Doctrines*, 2d ed. Paris: J.-B. Ballière.
1870   *Histoire des Sciences Médicales*, 2 vols. Paris: J.-B. Ballière.
Dumézil, Georges
1986   La médecine et les trois fonctions. *Magazine Littéraire* 229 (April 1986):
        36–39.
Kunte, A., K. Navre, and P. Harisastri, eds.
1939   *Aṣṭāṅgahṛdayasamhitā*. Bombay: Nirnaya Sagar.
Madan, T. N.
1985   Concerning the categories *śubha* and *śuddha* in Hindu culture, an explora-
        tory essay. In *Purity and Auspiciousness in Indian Society*, ed. J. B. Carman
        and F. A. Marglin, 11–29. Leiden, Holland: E. J. Brill.
Maharishi
1985   *Maharishi Āyurveda Prevention Center*.™ Brochure published by the Maha-
        rishi Ayurveda Corporation of America.
Mooss, Vayaskara N. S.
1950–   *Aṣṭāṅgahṛdayasamhitā*. 2 vols., with Paramesvara's commentary *Vākyapra-*
1963   *dīpikā*. Kottayam: Vaidya Sarathy.
1983   *Āyurvedic Treatments of Kerala*, 3d ed. [1st ed., 1944 under the title *Special
        Treatments. . . .*] Kottayam: Vaidya Sarathy.
Mudry, Philippe
1982   *La Préface du De Medicina de Celse*. Rome: Institut Suisse de Rome.
1985   Médecins et spécialistes. Le problème de l'unité de la médecine à Rome
        au Ier siècle après J.–C. *Gesnerus* 42 (1985): 329–336.
Rosu, Arion
1981   Les *marman* et les arts martiaux indiens. *Journal Asiatique* 269 (1981): 417–
        451.
Rosu, Arion, and Myriam Jobard
1987   Arts de santé et techniques de massage en Inde. *Annales de Kinésithérapie*
        14 (1987): 87–91.
Singhal, G. D., et al.
1979   *Non-Operative Considerations in Ancient Indian Surgery*. (Based on *Suśruta-
        saṃhitā, Cikitsāsthāna* 24 to 40.) Varanasi: Institute of Medical Sciences at
        the Banaras Hindu University.
Vaidyaratnam
1976   *Medicine Catalogue 1976*. Kottakal: Vaidyaratnam P. S. Varier's Arya
        Vaidya Sala.
Zarrilli, Phillip
1984   *The Kathakali Complex, Actor, Performance and Structure*. New Delhi:
        Abhinav.
1989   The three bodies of practice (Āyurvedic and Yogic dimensions of a tradi-
        tional South Indian martial art: Kalarippayattu of Kerala.) *Social Science
        and Medicine* 28 (12): 1289–1309.

TEN

Of Ticks, Kings, Spirits, and the Promise of Vaccines

Mark Nichter

The environment is not just pretty trees and tigers.

Agârwal 1985

Kyasanur forest disease (KFD) is an arbovirus infection found only in south-west peninsular India. Resembling influenza, at onset KFD is marked by sudden chills, fever, frontal headaches, stiffness of the neck, and body pain. Diarrhea and vomiting often follow on the third day. High fever is continuous for five to fifteen days, during which time a variety of additional symptoms may manifest themselves, including gastrointestinal bleeding, persistent cough with blood-tinged sputum, and bleeding gums. In more serious cases, the infection progresses to bronchial pneumonia, meningitis, paralysis, encephalitis, and hemorrhage. After an afebrile period of one to two weeks, fever may once again return for two to twelve days, accompanied by central nervous system abnormalities (Banerjee and Bhat 1984).

    KFD was first identified in March 1957 in the forest areas adjoining Shimoga District, Karnataka State.[1] Relatively few deaths were attributed to the illness until the early 1970s, a time of extensive deforestation in Shimoga preparatory to intensive plantation agriculture. Suddenly in December 1982, an epidemic of a then-unidentified disease swept through four villages of Beltangady Taluk, South Kanara District, Karnataka, some 200 kilometers away from the Kyasanur Forest. In the village of Koyyur, 248 people were stricken by the mysterious disease, 60 of whom died. Three months after its onset, the illness was identified as KFD. In the six-month period between December 1982 and May 1983, over 20 villages were affected by KFD, over 1,000 cases were treated at hospitals, and over 100 deaths were directly attributed to the disease. In 1984 the epidemic escalated. With 31 villages in the taluk affected, 605 people were admitted to hospitals, 136 of whom died (*Karnataka Sunday Herald*, 30 December 1984). During the period 1982–1984, mortality rates in hospitals for the disease ranged from 12 percent to 18 percent.[2]

In this ethnographic account of KFD, I shall consider the way in which this unfamiliar, debilitating disease was perceived and treated by South Kanarese villagers during the epidemic. First, I will focus on the social and historical conditions that provide the basis for the explanatory models of KFD which South Kanarese villagers fashioned out of the wide range of explanations for misfortune available to them as cultural resources. Highlighted will be the way in which certain aspects of the disease were incorporated into social construction of its etiology. The analysis will also show that Indian villagers accept multiple frames of reference for explaining the causes of a single misfortune. Villagers viewed different ideas of causality as though they were "pieces of a puzzle" (Beals 1976) which were assumed to fit together in some unified way that ordinary humans could not fathom. The question I shall consider, following Babb (1983, 171), is why villagers adopted one idea of causality rather than another. As he noted:

> The same misfortune may be viewed in more than one frame of reference, even by the same individual. If this is so, then the most important question becomes that of why one frame of reference might be adopted rather than another. It seems reasonable that at least part of the answer lies in the different ways in which theories of misfortune deal with the problem of human responsibility. (Babb 1983, 171)

Looking beyond changing and coextensive ideas of etiology, I shall also examine the manner in which these ideas affected health-care decision making. What I shall describe is a community experiencing rapid social and ecological change while desperately trying to develop plans for action during an epidemic crisis. What I ultimately seek to do is to place KFD in the context of a distinctively Tuluva sense of history and natural order, a sense of history reproduced and embodied during ritual performance. Data upon which this account of KFD is rendered were collected during the epidemic of 1984. Contextual information on South Kanarese health culture is drawn from three and a half years of intermittent anthropological fieldwork begun in 1974.

Characteristics of the Disease

Kyasanur forest disease is closely related to tick-borne encephalitis. The KFD virus has been isolated in the blood of various species of small forest animals, and the tick *Haemaphysalis spinigera*, feeding on the blood of these animals, serves as the vector for the virus. The KFD virus is a pathogen that has long existed as part of an established ecosystem in South Kanara. Human modification of that ecosystem through deforestation has produced the epidemic occurrence of the disease (Banerjee and Bhat 1984; Boshell 1969). The first outbreaks of KFD in Shimoga and the later outbreaks in Beltangady were both preceded by deforestation and the creation of an interface of scrub between villages and forest. In the case of Beltangady, two months prior to the KFD epidemic virgin forest began being cleared to make way for a cashew plantation financed by an international development agency.

The widespread death of black-faced and rhesus monkeys signaled the advent of the epidemic in both Shimoga and Beltangady. As a consequence of deforestation, these monkeys were compelled to spend more time on the ground and became increasingly exposed to the vector. The virus proved highly virulent among monkeys, and ultimately humans, who also proved to be suitable hosts. Cattle-rearing contributed to the transmission of KFD to human settlements. Since cattle have a low susceptibility to the disease, they provide an excellent reservoir for concentrating, propagating, and maintaining the vector. Cows provide a rich source of nourishment for ticks by grazing in the scrub at forest margins. During the monsoon season, the mature ticks lay their eggs under leaves on well-trodden cattle paths, and the emergence of nymphs, after the rains have subsided, coincides with the epizootic and epidemic aspects of the disease. Thus, the first appearance of the disease usually occurs in December, with a peak incidence in January/February, when the tick vectors are in their nymphal stage. By May the epidemic subsides.

Another feature of KFD outbreaks is their localized nature. In any one season the disease strikes only a few villages and then moves on to others the following year. This pattern, which is attributed to heightened levels of immunity in afflicted villages, is presented in table 10.1, which provides figures on incidence and gross mortality for thirteen villages in Belthangady Taluk during the 1983 and 1984 seasons. Besides being localized, KFD may also appear in epidemic form for a few years and then seemingly die out until a force of infected ticks builds up.

A final point about KFD in South Kanara is that it is a disease of development (Hughes and Hunter 1970) which especially affects the poor. At greatest risk are agricultural workers, especially Harijans, who were most exposed to the forest interface and tick-bearing cattle. Members of a local KFD relief committee estimated that 50 percent of those infected by KFD regularly tended cattle.

TULUVA COSMOLOGY AND SOCIAL CHANGE

An understanding of the community's response to KFD requires familiarity with both South Kanarese cosmology and land reform in the area. South Kanara or Tulunad (Land of the Tulu speakers) was until recently a conglomerate of feudal kingdoms ruled by petty kings. Feudal relationships comprise an important dimension of Tuluva cosmology and are expressed in legends and ritual performances. During the decade preceding the KFD epidemic, land reform legislation disrupted long-established feudal relationships and the rituals associated with them. To understand these changes

TABLE 10.1.   Villages in Belthangady Taluk Where at Least One Death Was
Reported to Health Authorities

	Dec. 1982–June 1983 (7 months)		Dec. 1983–March 1984 (4 months)	
	Attacks	Deaths	Attacks	Deaths
Bandar	2	1	16	4
Belal	306	35	28	7
Belthangady			31	7
Dharmasthala	293	24	10	3
Kaliya			20	4
Kokkada			4	2
Koyyur	25	1	200	54
Laila			12	2
Melanthabettu			1	1
Nidle	65	5		
Patrame	170	24		
Puduvettu	8	1		
Ujire	167	7	59	18
TOTAL	**936**	**98**	**381**	**102**
Other cases reported not leading to morality	127		14	

and their relationship to the KFD epidemic, we must review several specific features of Tuluva cosmology.

The Tuluva universe consists of three realms: the domain of humans which exists in opposition to both the wild and the supernatural (Claus 1978a). In this tripartite division, the supernatural mediates between the forest, as the realm of the wild, and the cultivated and ordered realm of humans. The landlord as petty king is a temporal sovereign whose warrant to exploit nature in the name of his subjects requires periodic renewal through tribute to patron deities.[3]

Whenever and wherever the realm of spirits and the realm of humans meet, there is danger. This danger, associated with the forest, is not due to its innate malevolence or to the malevolence of supernatural beings, but rather to the constant danger of the encroachment of both into the realm of ordered society. When forest and supernatural beings are controlled and their influence regulated, they are sources of vitality and benefit to humans. When uncontrolled, chaos results as manifested in crop failure, epidemics, and the violent death of humans and domestic animals.

For each social sphere in which humans interact (household, village, kingdom), there are local patron deities, *bhuta*. Rituals are periodically performed to propitiate these deities. At the broadest local level, the feudal king has traditionally borne a responsibility to his subjects to maintain the boundaries of the kingdom and to conduct transactions with guardian deities of the domain. In return, subjects have traditionally sworn allegiance and paid tribute in kind, *geni*, to the king. They also participate by caste in elaborate *bhuta* possession cult rituals (*kola* and *nema*), which express the ideals of kingdom and village unity, as well as caste interdependence.

Traditionally, *bhuta* cult rituals served judicial and law enforcement functions, as well as being occasions of worship. With the implementation of land reform in the mid-1970s, former tenants became small landowners. A loss of *geni* and lands meant that many royal families became unable to conduct large-scale *bhuta* rituals for their domains. A temporary decline in village-level *bhuta* rituals occurred in Belthangady Taluk following land reform five to eight years prior to the KFD outbreak.[4]

It is believed that if one neglects routine obligations and vows to patron *bhuta*, they will be quick to reveal their displeasure by imposing illness and misfortune. If neglect persists, they may even seek vengeance through violent or sudden death. Thus, sudden illnesses, particularly those involving the passing of blood, are commonly attributed to *bhuta*. Although the stakes of transgression and nonfulfillment of vows to *bhuta* are high, these breaches occur frequently because of life exigencies, escalating costs of performing rituals, disputes between social factions, and so on.

Periodic rituals are also performed at home for household deities, totemic spirits, and departed ancestors, who together constitute a family cult. These cults are fluid, evolving, and subject to manipulation by individual family members. New spirits may enter the cults by causing misfortune to individual family members. After they are appeased, they are enjoined to remain as protectors. Occasions of misfortune may be attributed to any one of a number of known spirits or to a new spirit making its identity known for the first time. Consulting oracles and astrologers is thus commonplace in order to identify interfering spirits.

Coexisting with, and in some cases encompassing, the local *bhuta* cult in South Kanara District is the pan-Indian Hindu tradition. Tuluva people perceive no clear division of function between local *bhuta* and pan-Indian deities (*deva*), who are commonly given local identities and characteristics and are at times even conjoined with *bhuta* (Claus 1973; Nichter 1977). Both types of deities are turned to in times of need, but, as in mundane life, villagers first approach more familiar sources of influence for problems requiring immediate attention.

CAUSAL INTERPRETATION OF KFD

It would be misleading to describe South Kanarese health culture as being predominantly personalistic or naturalistic (Foster 1976). In the Tuluva universe, spirits can cause physiological imbalances that take on a course of their own, and both physiological and social imbalances may attract spirits that prey on the most vulnerable as well as those most disruptive of the sociomoral order. When spirits strike they may do so through curses, touch, or the wind as well as worms, germs, or insects. Some illnesses are thought to initiate from contact with spirits due to either anger, affection, or chance. Once in existence, however, they may constitute contagious sicknesses capable of being transmitted to others by way of natural substances.

South Kanarese popular health culture has been significantly influenced by Tuluva spirit cults, Āyurveda, and astrology, as well as by a growing knowledge of cosmopolitan (allopathic) medicines made available by medical doctors and commercial vendors. Use of curative resources is thus eclectic with few people resorting to only one form of diagnosis or treatment. In the case of most serious illnesses, several kinds of knowledge are considered by the family in the course of consulting practitioners and weighing treatment options.

While in some instances symptom sets are clearly recognized as distinct illnesses or diseases, in many instances symptoms do not fit neat, mutually exclusive illness categories. Identification and labeling of an illness is a process that occurs over time, as signs and symptoms unfold (Nichter 1979), and diagnoses are always provisional. If the symptoms do not subside or they flair up again, people reconsider the sickness in light of several possibilities: (a) that all the causes were not addressed; (b) that new causal factors have compounded the nature of the problem; (c) that the illness transformed into another illness; or (d) that either the medicine or practitioner was ineffective. Causal thinking about illness is thus complex and is influenced by perceived and expected therapeutic results.

Given this complexity, it is important to assess social, cultural, psychological, and historical factors that also influence the production of illness knowledge. In the case of KFD, notions of causality involved statements about power and relations of dependency in the Tuluva cosmos, socioeconomic and ecological change, curative resources, and the psychological needs of the population. In order to appreciate fully the range of ideas that emerged about the causes of KFD, one must therefore maintain the kind of multilevel perspective advocated by Glick (1967) as a heuristic.

The Wrath of Bhuta in the Context of Land Reform

Several natural characteristics of KFD readily lent themselves to interpretations involving *bhuta* spirits. First, the symptoms of KFD matched the signs of *bhuta upadra* (trouble)—sudden high fever, body pain, and the passing of blood. Second, the epidemic outbreak of KFD was initially limited to isolated villages, which suggested some moral transgressions in these communities. Finally, the failure of doctors to control the disease gave credence to ideas about supernatural causation. Thus, villagers began to interpret the disease in terms of transgressions against *bhuta* spirits. Two explanatory stories sprang up at about the same time in the areas most severely affected by the epidemic. One story focused on the transgressions of outsiders and the other on the sociomoral transgressions of a royal family.

> I. At the end of December, just prior to the outbreak of the epidemic, a large *benga* tree (*Pterocarpus marsupium*), which was the abode of a *bhuta* called Rakteshavari, was marked to be cut by a Muslim timber contractor from outside the district. The people of the area pleaded that the tree not be cut, because of its sacred character. When, despite their protestations, the tree was cut, people described the red sap that seeped out of the severed trunk as blood. Within a few days, a large monkey that had lived in the tree died, as did the contractor. Several of the tree cutters became ill and sought protection at the local Dharmasthala temple. The head of the temple blessed them and told them to seek medical advice. Some of the cutters died, and soon afterwards many villagers also became ill and died.

> II. Many years ago there was a quarrel between the *bhuta* of Koyyur kingdom and the patron *bhuta* spirits of Dharmasthala temple, a famous and prosperous pilgrimage center for the god Manjunatha. Following the defeat of the Dharmasthala *bhuta*, members of the royal family of Koyyur were barred by their patron *bhuta* from visiting the temple. This taboo was respected until just before the epidemic, when the eldest son of the Koyyur royal family, who had become a good friend of the head of Dharmasthala temple, borrowed some money from him. Subsequently, the prince's wife and child went to the temple to give offerings. On returning to Koyyur, the child fell seriously ill. When it was suggested that the illness might be related to problems with the Dharmasthala *bhuta*, the head of the temple intervened and decided to settle the long dispute between the *bhuta* of the two kingdoms. Soon after he approached a Jain priest for this purpose, the head of the Koyyur family died suddenly at the age of forty-seven. This untimely death was taken as a sign that the dispute was still unresolved.

In accord with the second story and the interpretation of a popular local astrologer, the epidemic resulted from the wrath of the guardian *bhuta* of Koyyur kingdom. The Koyyur king lost his control of the kingdom through poor management of his lands, unpaid debts, and failure to respect the words of his patron *bhuta*. As a result, the kingdom was no longer protected against the encroachment of malevolent forces from the forest. The astrologer thus saw KFD as coming from the forest in the context of an unbalanced ecology, a corrupt administration, and a weak king unable to secure the boundaries of his kingdom.

As the epidemic spread, rituals to both village and family deities proliferated, not only in afflicted villages but also in neighboring ones. Scarce resources were increasingly diverted to these performances. In many cases, offerings were prompted by anxieties associated with land reform. These

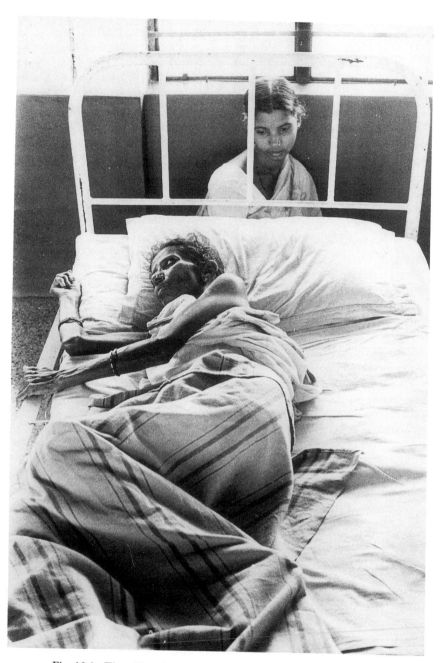

Fig. 10.1. The afflicted and kin attendant. (Photo by Mimi Nichter)

anxieties concerned the ongoing duties of royal families to former subjects, the duties of former tenants to royal families, and the respective duties of each to guardian deities. In addition, village rituals to patron *bhuta* had not been performed for some time, because these rituals, formerly paid out of *geni*, were now beyond the means of local royalty with reduced land holdings.

An appreciation of the anxiety experienced by former tenants is rendered by a consideration of the way many landlords in the region had used the *bhuta* cult to intimidate tenants during land reform implementation. This was done in two ways. First, by holding large impressive rituals, landlords reminded villagers of both the power of the *bhuta* and the feudal obligations structuring social relations. Second, rumors were spread about the ill fate of those who had filed for land and/or had disrupted the routine flow of tribute. Astrologers and exorcists indirectly contributed to the impression that *bhuta* caused misfortune in keeping with prevalent patterns of social discord. From 1974 to 1976, I encountered several landlords who had effectively used the *bhuta* cult to delay tenants from filing for land rights, convince tenants to file for land rights but continue to pay a part of *geni*, or at least to continue performing traditional agricultural labor obligations in their paddy fields.

Cultural practice is complex and not merely an epiphenomena of political economy. Praxis is influenced by multiple ideologies, values, and imperatives articulated in everyday life as well as ritual contexts. A political economic analysis of the *bhuta* cult as a means of social control and the domination of the tenant proletariat by the landholding bourgeoisie is insightful, but insufficient for a complete understanding of how *bhuta* cults were linked to KFD. Required is an indigenous sense of history based upon a broader appreciation of relationships of exchange that structure the Tuluva moral universe. The following case facilitates discussion of this issue.

In April 1984, during the peak of the *bhuta* cult ritual season, as well as the KFD epidemic cycle, I attended a *bhuta kola* in a household ten miles from a village afflicted with KFD. Once a yearly event, this ritual had not been performed since land reform. The *kola* was sponsored at considerable expense by members of a local royal family who had lost much of their lands to land reform. When interviewed, members of the royal family stated that they had personal reasons for sponsoring a *kola*. Women and cattle had experienced acute illnesses the year before. These troubles had been divined by an astrologer to be a sign of warning from a dissatisfied patron *bhuta*. The family continued to feel vulnerable despite the protective talismans they had received from an exorcist.

The ritual was well attended, and former tenant families voluntarily contributed whatever resources they could as offerings without any coercion from the royal family. One reason for the large attendance was clearly concern about KFD, which was viewed in two different ways by the royal family and former tenants. It was seen as a trouble that their patron *bhuta* could either help keep out of the kingdom through protection, or a form of wrath

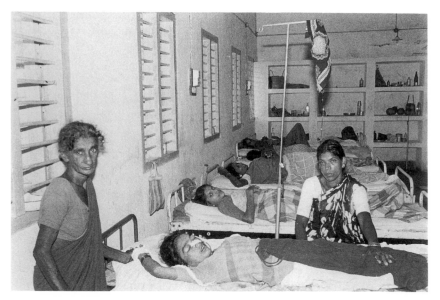

Fig. 10.2. The KFD ward. (Photo by Mimi Nichter)

that the *bhuta* could bring upon the kingdom through the vehicle of infected ticks—beings of malevolence from within the forest. Members of the royal family spoke of a sense of responsibility to the community that prompted the performance of a *kola*. A sense of responsibility was also articulated by former tenants. Ten former tenants who had successfully filed for land over the last eight years were interviewed. All believed that it was their duty to support the royal family in their performance of *bhuta* rituals through contributions and ritual services. Their voluntary contributions were given with a sense of pride and responsibility as well as a sense of fear and dread of KFD.

KFD, an unknown disease associated with the forest, served to reinforce a precapitalist form of social organization at a time of economic change. Respect for the royal family and the reproduction of feudal relationships were evident despite the fact that relationships of servitude expressed by rights to land and labor had all but disappeared. Despite economic change, former tenants continued to play the role of subjects during ritual occasions when a sense of a lived history was articulated. Reasons for respecting royalty extended beyond status and pageantry to an imperative. Agriculturalists remained dependents of the royal family because their right to cultivate land was not simply a question of secular land ownership. Displays of danger and power, like KFD, reminded all that human prosperity was dependent upon a renewable warrant obtained from patron *bhuta* by the local "king." Obtaining this warrant required offerings of the fruit of the land, ritual service, and displays of devotion. Claus (1978*a*, 1978*b*) has noted that during *kola* performances, tenants are referred to as fictive kin of the landlord. As dependent kin, the well-being of tenants is as closely tied to their service to the cult of the "landlord" as their own family cult. Consequently, a sign of vulnerability in the royal family signals vulnerability in the community at large. In the case described above, vulnerability was clearly manifest at a time of the encroaching malevolence of KFD.

Seeking the Advice of Astrologers

Despite *bhuta kola* rituals, the KFD epidemic continued to escalate. Villagers were perplexed about why some of the afflicted died, while others lived. Although *bhuta* stories, like the two noted above, served as explanations for the generalized presence of the disease, they proved insufficient for the families of the afflicted. In increasing numbers, villagers began to consult diviners and astrologers for more information about pending debts to *bhuta* that had been made by family members in the form of vows (*harike*). *Harike* are thought to be transferred within a household from one generation to the next on the death of the member who made the vow. During the second epidemic season of KFD, a popular astrologer reported a growing concern among families that their own deities might be responsible for the affliction. Clients wanted to know if family deities were involved in causing the illness, in failing to protect the family from it, in increasing the severity or duration of the illness, or in causing medicines to fail to take effect. Observation of astrologer-client interactions revealed that such concerns were usually elicited by the astrologer who assisted clients in articulating doubts in the course of divination.

The process of "speculation" is an important aspect of the astrologer's vocation and a key to his ability to engage clients in the hermeneutic process of arriving at a negotiated diagnosis of the problem (Nichter 1981; Young 1981). This diagnosis draws upon circumstantial evidence, the astrologer's background knowledge of the community, his reading of nonverbal cues, and his interpretation of signs (Pugh 1983, 1984). Often an astrologer engages in what Margaret Trawick (personal communication) has described as "skillfully ambiguous communication." I cite below an example bearing relevance to KFD.

A popular astrologer consulted during the epidemic hailed from neighboring Kerala state and a caste renowned for astrology. When he came to South Kanara, he worked to become conversant in the two regional languages, Tulu and Kannada. He also studied the folkways of both patrilineal and matrilineal castes residing in the region. He candidly described to me how he had carefully observed caste customs and learned about the patron *bhuta* of villages as well as castes. A Tuluva exorcist had spoken to him at great length about local sources of social conflict and he maintained a referral relationship with him.

During the KFD epidemic, the astrologer was confronted by many clients who would simply ask, "What is the trouble befalling my family?" The astrologer's most common divination was *bhumi dosha*, land-related problems. This replay was "specifically ambiguous" in the sense that land trouble could refer to a wide range of problems. Land-related problems could refer to *bhuta* problems associated with either one's family or village, to problems related to jealous kin or malevolent neighbors, or to problems relating to the construction of one's house. After the astrologer's retort of *bhumi dosa* a client commonly inquired about ill or newly deceased family members. The astrologer would then link *bhumi dosa* to the illness through an intermediary such as family or village *bhuta*, ancestor spirits, and so forth. Through a series of rhetorical comments made by the astrologer, the hidden anxieties of clients would become increasingly apparent. While the specificity of the astrologer's comments would seemingly increase, they would never be framed in a close-ended fashion. His statements always remained open-ended, to allow for interpretation and reinterpretation. In any case, clients did not expect all the astrologers' initial statements to be on target, only a large enough percentage to foster confidence and establish credibility. A divination session produced negotiated knowledge (Young 1981, Nichter 1981).

Of particular relevance to the KFD epidemic was the way in which the astrologer approached afflicted families. The astrologer recognized that death in public hospitals was deemed inauspicious, because the spirit of the deceased would not receive satisfaction. Surviving family members would be troubled until costly rituals were performed to appease their kin's spirit. An appreciation of this complex influenced the astrologer when clients approached him for advice on where to seek treatment for ill family members. The astrologer would not refer patients to two special hospitals set up for treatment of KFD patients and suggested instead that the best medicine could be secured in a particular direction, one not associated with either of the two hospitals. In other words, the astrologer sanctioned use of medical services, but from private practitioners who would provide home treatment.

Mariamman

In early 1984 Mariamman, a pan-Indian female deity associated with pox diseases, began being linked to KFD. Three reasons for this linkage may be noted. First, the Koyyur king had maintained a shrine to the deity Wandadurga, a local female *bhuta* who was conjoined with Mariamman by some devotees. Second, Mariamman is associated with devastating epidemic illnesses that are marked by symptoms of "heat." More specifically, she is linked to diseases that spread beyond one village and the jurisdiction of one set of guardian deities. At the time Mariamman was being implicated, KFD had spread to new villages, where attempts to appease local patron *bhuta* appeared to have failed. Third, with the eradication of smallpox, Mariamman had become dispossessed of an awesome sign of her destructive power, a deity bereft of divine force.[5] The symptoms of KFD (high fever, thirst, and hemorrhaging) happened to accord with Mariamman's qualities of heat and anger (Beck 1969; Nicholas 1981; Wadley 1980). In addition, the epidemiology of KFD matches that of other diseases associated with the deity like poxes and measles, which also flare up in December, and die down in May with the onset of the monsoons.[6]

The link between KFD and Mariamman was also fostered by castes, such as the Gowda, who have a special devotional relationship with the deity.[7] For the first time in two decades in Belthangady Taluk, elder members of the carpenter caste were called upon during the epidemic to prepare wooden Mari dolls for use in transvillage Mari rituals. These rituals involve transporting symbols of ritual impurity from one village boundary to another. Eventually the collective impurities of the region are deposited into the sea or a deep forest. Such rituals require large-scale community participation, as well as the ritual expertise of high-caste Brahmans. The involvement of Mari signaled regional, not just local, concern about KFD and a general awareness that the problem was spreading. It also assigned responsibility for the illness beyond patron *bhuta* to more generalized ideas of causality.

References to Karma and Fate

By April 1984, Mari rituals had become commonplace throughout the region, yet the illness still persisted. An increasing number of people started speaking of the illness in terms that reflected a general sense of both powerlessness and meaninglessness. Direct and indirect reference to karma and fate became more common. Local usage of the term *karma*, as distinct from the more ethicized Brahmanic notion, generally took on an undifferentiated quality, aptly described by Daniel (1983, 299) in his discussion of the meaning of karma in Tamil Nad:

> When they use the term karma to describe or characterize a particular misfortune for which no plausible explanation is possible, what comes to their mind is not a whole series of ethicized causal reasonings but a sense of the meaninglessness of it all.

Karmic explanations for KFD were usually offered in the same context as more specific explanations relating to deities. For example, nonafflicted community members would assign the ultimate cause of an afflicted neighbor's death to karma. They referred not to particular sins, *pappa*, that a person had accumulated but to an unknowable karmic debt (Obeyesekere 1968, 21). A general statement about another's karma to some degree distanced the destiny of the afflicted from oneself.

In discussions with those directly afflicted with KFD, I recorded no reference to karma at all. Occasionally, however, reference was made by sufferers themselves to *hanne baraha*, the writing on one's forehead, a general expression of unqualified fate determined at birth. As noted by Sheryl Daniel (1983) and Babb (1983), headwriting establishes a frame of ultimate reference in which individuals have no control over their actions and are thus not responsible for their destiny. Following up on cases when headwriting was referred to by the nonafflicted, I found no instance when this notion precluded the person from acting to cure the disease. On this note, Babb (1983, 176–178) has observed:

> When malice of deities or spirits are cited as causal agents, what is stressed is the immediacy and urgency of human problems. . . . To attribute misfortune to the anger of a deity is to connect it with a cause with which the afflicted persons can deal directly. It seems probable that this is one of the reasons Hindu villagers so infrequently allude to the karma doctrine in relation to specific misfortunes. Nonkarmic explanations seem to convey a Malinowskian confidence in the immediate efficacy of human actions. . . . Karmic theory implicates the entire world-career of the self not lending itself easily to the isolation of specific causes of particular misfortunes.

While Babb is correct in calling attention to the active result of identifying instrumental causality, he does not fully appreciate the importance of references to karma or headwriting that occur in conjunction with more specific supernatural explanations of causality. The Tuluva conception of karma extends beyond the world career of an individual self to a corporate self and a family's cumulative debts to *bhuta* through unspecified time. These more remote causal explanations for KFD, like headwriting, served to distance survivors from immediate responsibility for the ailments of their kin and thus helped them cope with the crisis. Another karma-related reference was *Devaru shikse*. This term was commonly used by villagers with reference to the death of a child from KFD.

By mid-1984, villagers knew from health workers and the media that ticks from the forest carried KFD. What remained puzzling was that children continued to contract the disease, even though they were prohibited from going to the forest. While health workers propagated important general information about KFD, they failed to emphasize that ticks could easily be transferred to children by other means such as through tick-laden clothing. Given this puzzling situation of children dying apparently without contact with known instrumental causes of the disease, some villagers interpreted the deaths as a curse by the gods, related to the "karma of the land." Generally, this phrase was simply an expression of helplessness. In other instances it took on a more specific meaning related to the qualities of space and time within the region. Here the phrase may be contrasted with references to the Kali Yuga, a Brahmanic notion of time periods having distinct qualitative characteristics. The second more marked reference to "karma of the land" evokes Daniel's (1984) discussion of the relationship between an individual and his native place or territory. Daniel argues that this relationship entails embodiment in the sense that the substance of place mixes with bodily substance. The karma of a place and a person are enmeshed. Since a child is the most vulnerable fruit of the body and the native place, *uru*, a child is the most sensitive barometer of the quality of a population's relationship with the land.

To what extent did references to karma constitute a statement of fatalism? More relevant to our concerns, did karmic explanations for KFD reduce villagers' inclination to engage in curative or preventive health actions? What we find is that reference to unmarked karma served as a coping resource while curative and preventive health-related actions were engaged in by the community. Talk about karma or headwriting neither impeded interest in nor curtailed the seeking of information about instrumental causes of KFD. I would emphasize, along with Babb (1983) and Nicholas (1981), that there is little evidence that Hindus are any more inclined than other people to ignore proximate causes of human misfortune.

DISCUSSION OF KFD CAUSALITY

Writing on India, Ursala Sharma (1973) has noted that explanations for misfortune can be arranged on a scale of varying degrees of responsibility imputed to the sufferer or to others. In the present case, we see a two-way movement in the production of ideas involving responsibility for KFD causality. In two early KFD narratives, concern was focused on transgressions against *bhuta* spirits by individuals—outsiders and members of a royal family. Next, attention was paid to feudal relations of tribute and warrant that linked the vulnerability of specific locales to failed obligations to deities following the aftermath of land reform. This gave way to notions of deity dissatisfaction linking illness to debts, vows, and unperformed family cult rituals. In some instances astrologers and oracles directed responsibility toward identifiable discord in the family while in other cases it was diffused in time and place either by reference to debts of the dead or spirits who followed the unsuspecting home. When the appeasement of village and family patron spirits did not abate the illness, villagers began to turn their attention toward the pan-Indian deity Māriamman. Māriamman is associated with dramatic illness bridging larger intervillage domains of social space. This signaled a projection of responsibility away from more immediate social domains. Finally, interpretations incorporating more general and less marked notions of causality became more prevalent when people's inability to control the spread of the epidemic through ritual or medicine became apparent. A rise in references to unmarked fate corresponded to the increased performance of such all purpose Pan-Indian rituals as Sathya Narayana Puja and rituals to the nine planets, Nava Graha puja.

In order to outline multilevel ideas of KFD causality it is necessary to modify the concepts of etiology introduced by Glick (1967). The following four levels of causality may initially be identified:

predisposing cause: transgressions, failure to uphold feudal relations with deities involving tribute and warrant, unfulfilled vows
efficient cause: bhuta, Māriamman
instrumental cause: a spirit wind, curses, ticks
ultimate cause: unmarked karma, headwriting as fate

Our outline is not yet complete. Missing are "at risk" factors that lend themselves to states of vulnerability. In the case of KFD these include impurities (removed during Māriamman rituals), heat (reduced by the drinking of tender coconuts during KFD season), and the negative effect of planets (mitigated by Nava Graha rituals) which might place one at risk for illness in general or confound the effectiveness of treatment.

UTILIZATION OF MEDICAL RESOURCES

Thus far we have explored beliefs about KFD and its causes. We now turn to the effects both of these beliefs and of economic factors on the use of local health-care resources. To appreciate these relationships more fully, however, we must first outline the clinical background of KFD.

The initial symptoms of the disease are not unlike various forms of malaise common in Karnataka: respiratory illnesses with fever are widespread during winter season, and diarrhea is common during summer. The fact that KFD affects people differently further compounds the difficulties of differential diagnosis, especially under conditions where rapid laboratory diagnosis was impossible. In addition, the major symptoms that resulted in death from KFD changed between 1983 and 1984 with lung complications and encephalopathy prevalent in the first year, and hemorrhage in the second. In short, diagnosis of KFD either by laypersons or professionals is difficult. Treatment of the disease is symptomatic. The prior nutritional state of victims is an important factor in their recovery, especially since anorexia is common during the height of the disease. As might be expected, the disease is debilitating and survivors are often incapacitated or weak for one to two months afterward. Relapse is also common and may constitute a second phase of the illness. Faced with rather enigmatic and generalized symptoms, sufferers turned to a variety of sources for health care.

Hospitals

As soon as KFD was identified in Belthangady Taluk, the head of Dharmasthala temple offered to set up a special hospital to treat the afflicted. This gesture was no doubt prompted by a sense of compassion and duty; Dhar-

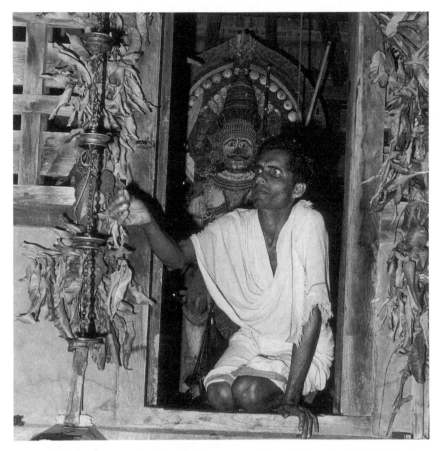

Fig. 10.3. Priest possessed with the village patron *bhuta*. (Photo by Mark Nichter)

masthala temple has long been active in charitable works. In addition, head-lines in statewide newspapers, such as "KFD Kills One Person a Day in Belthangady Taluk," significantly reduced the number of pilgrims visiting the temple and consequently the revenues received through offerings.

A tuberculosis hospital managed by Dharmasthala temple was converted into a KFD facility, with basic services provided free to patients. The only stipulation made of the relatives of the afflicted was that a healthy family member remain with the patient as an attendant. Not all KFD sufferers took advantage of the hospital, however, because of the aforementioned etiological ideas that associated KFD with the wrath of the Koyyur *bhuta* against Dhar-masthala. As a result, a second hospital was established less than three kilo-meters away under the auspices of the government.

While the staff of both hospitals worked with great dedication and were praised by the community at large, many of the afflicted refused to seek assistance from either hospital for both cultural and economic reasons. Early on in the epidemic both KFD hospitals became stigmatized as a place to die, because most of the afflicted who first went for treatment to them were in the acute stage of the disease, some five to eight days after onset. Since the fever and body pain that characterize the onset of KFD resemble the malaise that marks the onset of other, less serious diseases, families did not perceive the need for hospital care until fever persisted or bleeding occurred. Often nurses reprimanded the families of these patients for not bringing the sick in sooner, with the result that family members simply began lying about patients' histories. Not uncommonly, patients arrived at the hospital in a state of dehydration, in part brought on by cultural restrictions prohibiting the intake of large quantities of liquid during bouts of fever or diarrhea. Consequently, the death rate at the two hospitals was high, and their reputations for death became established.

Reasons why villagers were reluctant to enter hospitals to receive medical aid involved both their belief system and the economics of a bad death. In a context where the death rate inside the hospital appeared to be no lower than that outside the hospital, villagers debated the merits of sending the afflicted to the hospital against the demerits of having a family member die at the hospital. An unsatisfied spirit, *preyta*, caused by a bad death in hospital, is believed to trouble kinsmen. The need to appease such a spirit through expensive rituals would have to be weighed against the family's subsistence needs. Some families, after considering risk, decided against hospitalization. They looked beyond death to the well-being of the spirit and the family. The cultural concept of a good death is little appreciated by biomedical practitioners.

Another concern in the health-seeking behavior of families was the loss of a healthy wage earner who would be required to attend to the patient at the hospital. Between 1983 and 1984 food relief was unavailable to the families of the afflicted, although it had been promised by state and local government authorities.[8] The only aid came from sporadic donations of rice by the Lions and Rotary clubs.

The popularity of the hospital was further reduced by the set-up of the wards, where no attempts were made to separate patients by age or by the severity of illness. A feverish patient was commonly forced to listen to the moans of a neighbor who was receiving a glucose drip or, even worse, to observe the deteriorating condition of a neighbor who was hemorrhaging to death.

Private Practitioners

Private practitioners played a notable role during the epidemic. Government hospital staff estimated that some 60 percent or more of their patients had

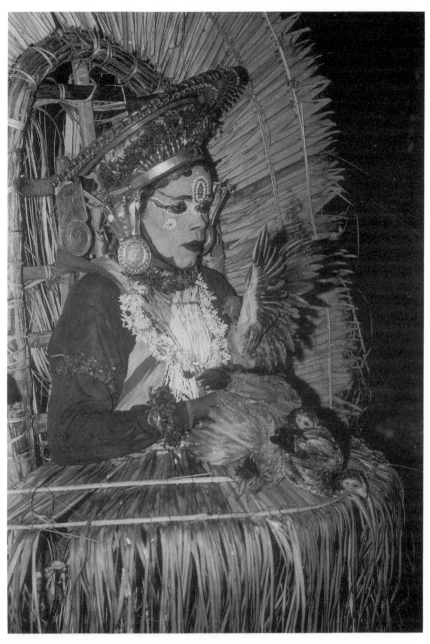

Fig. 10.4. Spirit dancer accepts blood offerings and promises protection to the village. (Photo by Mark Nichter)

undertaken treatment first from a private practitioner. In general, these practitioners referred patients to the hospital only when the disease became acute, since they did not want their reputations to be tainted by the death of a patient. These delayed referrals added to the image of the hospital as a place of death. The number of persons with KFD who never attended a hospital, relying only on the services of practitioners—allopathic, Āyurvedic, or eclectic—remains undetermined, but it is no doubt considerable. In one newspaper article, for example, a local reporter estimated that in 1984, 1,068 cases of KFD were admitted to hospitals, while the number of people afflicted with the disease was more than 3,000.

The popularity of private practitioners and the confidence placed in them by the public is worth exploring through a case study. The practitioner, a middle-aged native of the region, had a licentiate diploma from a school of Āyurvedic medicine, where limited training had also been provided in "emergency" allopathic medicine. He was moderately popular before the KFD epidemic but became renowned for his treatment of the illness. His popularity was based in part on his practice of identifying a wide range of his patients' ailments as KFD, especially after their cure, giving villagers the impression that his success rate was much higher than that of the hospital. In addition, he only treated the acutely ill if they began therapy early on in the disease. Those who consulted him for the first time in the acute stage of the illness were sent to the hospital. For this reason, far more people consulted him during the epidemic soon after they developed even minor symptoms. This practitioner's popularity was also based on the fact that his charges for the home treatment of KFD were deemed fair and reasonable by layperson's standards (Nichter 1983). Since his fee (Rs. 5–8) was about equivalent to the daily wages for an adult laborer, it did not much exceed the cost of receiving free treatment from the hospital, when one figured in the lost wages of a family member who was required to stay with the ill, to say nothing of the cost of family visits. If the patient died at home, the family would also save money by not having to deal with spirit problems and expensive rituals.

A major source of the practitioner's popularity in treating KFD was his sensitivity to popular health beliefs, both about the disease and about allopathic and Āyurvedic medications. Although villagers associated KFD with deities as an efficient cause and ticks as an instrumental cause, they linked individual susceptibility to KFD with overheat. A similar idea exists for pox diseases. In addition to linking the deity Māriamman to chicken pox, villagers associate pox epidemics, occurring in summer months, with overheat. A convergence of etiological and physiological ideas about illness causality and risk (Young 1976) is apparent. Among the poor, those most affected by KFD, it was common to link increased susceptibility to the illness to heat resulting from greater exposure to the sun and higher consumption of "heaty foods."

To reduce heat as a risk factor for the illness, lay preventive health behavior focused on cooling the body, by the drinking of cooling tender coconut water.

Beliefs about hot and cold also affected consumption of medicines, particularly among the elderly. Because the local population generally considered allopathic medicines as heating to the body and the cause of general debility after acute symptoms subsided (Nichter 1980), they tended to curtail the quantity of allopathic medicine they consumed. When told to take more than three different allopathic medicines per day, the elderly suspected that this dosage would weaken their bodies and prove harmful. Some patients, therefore, reduced the quantity of medicine they consumed, while others discontinued medication after acute symptoms subsided. Hospital staff attributed relapse and secondary infection to such noncompliance behavior.

In contrast, the private practitioner prescribed a mix of medicines that patients saw as more balanced and health-promoting than those offered at the hospital. For example, his prescriptions commonly included both antiviral (Septilin) and antibacterial (ampicillin) medications as well as an Āyurvedic antihemorrhagenic agent and a popular herbal liver tonic (Liv 52). Inclusion of the latter accorded with popular ideas that such KFD symptoms as vomiting, giddiness, and internal bleeding arose from *pitta*, a humor linked with the liver. The practitioner's advice to eat only vegetables accorded with religious ideology emphasizing purity during illnesses associated with deities. Likewise, his advice against consuming foods considered *nanju*, toxic, within the local folk dietetic system accorded with common sense. While the practitioner's advice to patients to avoid drinking excessive tender coconut water (because of his concern about its high potassium content) did surprise patients, he reassured them by advising the substitution of lemon water and the juice of the local fruit *punar puli* (*Garcinia indica*), both folk remedies for *pitta*, as well as for excessive heat.

Two other aspects of the practitioner's treatment are noteworthy. First, he never administered glucose or saline drips—much feared symbols of approaching death in the hospital. Instead, he managed minor states of dehydration with an oral rehydration solution and referred cases of severe dehydration to the hospital. Second, he was quite liberal in his administration of diazepam to patients having a wide variety of illnesses. He was attentive (perhaps overattentive) to anxiety about KFD in the wake of the epidemic. In sum, the practitioner's popularity was related to: (1) "after-the-cure" identification of illness with KFD; (2) a negotiation of care within the folk health culture; (3) dissociation with symbols of "approaching death"; and (4) treatment of anxiety as routine practice. Hospital clinicians offered good technical treatment, but made little effort to accommodate their treatment to folk health culture, or to explain the reasons for their suggestions about diet. Although attentive, nurses tended to be condescending to families of the afflicted. Fear of being scolded impeded villagers from asking questions or airing health concerns. It must be kept in mind, however, that staff were terribly overworked and in need of personal distance during this time of massive death. Although all forms of medical assistance were praised by the community, the reputation of private practitioners, like the one described, increased most during the epidemic. Astrologers and diviners tended to refer patients either directly or indirectly, to this type of practitioner.

Convalescence

If one survives KFD until the fourteenth day, chances of recovery are high. However, it is common for a relapse to occur four or five weeks after onset and for a person to be weak for some months after fever has abated. In cases of relapse, villagers tended to attribute their vulnerability to bad stars and planets rather than to spirits or karma. Medical doctors implicated nutrition in speed of recovery. However, following illness, a great many villagers found themselves and their families in dire economic circumstances, which forced them to eat less, with the result that they experienced relapse and renewed inability to work. In addition, once villagers became convinced that the forest and the ticks were instrumentally responsible for the illness, they became wary of going to the forest interface for wage labor, and so grew poorer.

GOVERNMENT INTERVENTION

Local politicians tried to downplay the link between KFD and deforestation. They argued that woodcutters from Shimoga must have brought infected ticks into the area. Consequently, for the first two years the district and state governments responded to KFD with strictly curative, or (more aptly put) palliative assistance. A hospital was set up, doctors assigned, and a mobile medical unit dispatched.

A group of educated, community-minded members of Belthangady Taluk independently prepared literature on KFD and appealed to the government to take preventive measures and provide nutritional relief to afflicted villagers, not just medical care. The KFD Relief Committee was set up by community members who lobbied for government assistance through increased press coverage. Instead of immediately establishing a nutritional intervention program and undertaking preventive measures, such as cattle spraying which would no doubt have prevented many deaths, the government promised a technical medical fix—the development of a vaccine.[9] They emphasized spraying of cut timber being shipped out of the taluk.

Ironically, district officials warned community members against taking preventive environmental measures within the area, like spraying cattle or underbrush, on the grounds that this might threaten the local ecological balance. Community members were outraged that officials who had condoned cutting the forest now voiced a concern for ecology. In the monsoon season of

1985, after considerable publicity organized by the KFD Relief Committee, cattle spraying was undertaken. Few cases of KFD were reported in 1986, and district health officials were quick to take credit for the eradication of KFD, much to the chagrin of the KFD Relief Committee.

In all these activities, the government failed to tap community self-help as a resource in the management of the disease. Could the community participation that evolved in ritual propitiation of deities have been directed toward public health action if guidance had been provided? Interviews with organizers of Mari rituals revealed that their effort to appease this spiritual cause of KFD did not preclude an interest in controlling ticks as an instrumental cause of the disease.

Though the KFD Relief Committee received praise in the press throughout the epidemic, their efforts were forestalled by the government. The group called for an investigation into why forests were cut down when suitable lands for plantations could have been found elsewhere. They questioned why government officials and the international banking organization that financed the plantation scheme did not act more responsibly to investigate the social and ecological ramifications of this "development program." In sum, they saw KFD as a "disease of development" (Hughes and Hunter 1970) while the government saw it as a disease involving viruses and ticks.

CONCLUSION

> Nature is not only a biological entity, but is also something whose distinctions are used by the mythic imagination to think with—so that this nature is also an enchanting landscape in which the history of the conquest itself acquires the role of the sorcerer. (Taussig 1984, 94)

Culture entails the production, reproduction, transformation, and embodiment of ideology through praxis. In Tulunad, the performance of *bhuta* rituals articulate power relations that underlie both kin-oriented and tributary modes of production (Wolf 1981).[10] The social relations upon which a feudal political economy was structured are sanctioned by Tuluva cosmology and embodied within Tuluva religious life. In the past, the ideology of dominant Tuluva culture was supported by repressive, in some instances, violent social institutions, as well as more subtle aspects of feudal hegemony (Gramsci 1971). These include paternalistic landlord-tenant relations expressed during *bhuta* cult rituals through the idiom of kinship, duty, and justice. As a result of land reform legislation, the political conditions for external repression have now largely been mitigated. What remains are subtle statements of feudal hegemony in Tuluva cosmology, myth, and ritual performance that are used by different kinds of actors to reproduce a familiar history or to transform history in accord with changing social relations.

It is within this larger historical context that interpretations of KFD need be understood. The symptom attributes and tragic outcome of KFD resonate with Tuluva beliefs in which justice and the wrath of *bhuta* are associated with the themes of tribute and warrant, moral obligations to the group, and the destructive consequences of selfishness, pride, and transgression. The tragedy of KFD at a time of social change appealed to the particularities of a distinctly Tuluva sense of history and natural order. This sense is typified in Tuluva legend and ritual by the need to control and contain the forest and is represented symbolically by a yearly ritual hunt into the forest, led by the king of each *sime* (Claus 1978*a*). Prior to the hunt, the patron *bhuta* of the *sime* are propitiated by the people of the land for the success of the hunt, a metaphor for the containment of nature ensuring domestic prosperity. In the past, it was the forest's encroachment into the world of humans that led to the destruction of order, for example, the destruction of fields by wild boar and elephants. In the case of KFD, it was the encroachment of humans into the forest, coupled with a patent disregard for ecology, that led to the catastrophic epidemic. The forest's contact with humans through virus-infected ticks in a disrupted ecosphere was perceived as complementary to the *bhuta*'s contact with humans in a disrupted social universe. Within an ordered ecology, the activity of ticks are kept within bounds by a balance of nature. In a similar way, within an ordered social universe, the activity of spirits are controlled for the benefit of man by ritual transactions involving the rights and obligations of tribute and warrant. Thus conceived, the case of KFD is truly a *bhumi dosha*, a trouble of the land, merging the ancient and modern relations of people, the state, and the environment.

EPILOGUE

Briefly revisiting the village of Koyyur in 1988, I found that in the absence of a KFD outbreak during the past three years, many households had stopped spraying cattle for ticks. Farmers were largely aware that the disease was spread by ticks that accumulate on cattle, but many of them associated the KFD problem with more general troubles and sources of malevolence. Several informants spoke of the curse of KFD as having passed, yet rituals to local deities continued to be performed routinely and with vigilance. Ritual activity in the region as a whole had also increased.[11] While a dispute between Dharmasthala and Koyyur *bhuta* was still recognized, a rural development project funded by Dharmasthala temple was being initiated in Koyyur providing aid for agriculture and reforestation. Few households declined assistance on the grounds that local deities might be angered.

I visited the region again in 1990. No outbreak of KFD had been reported for six years in South Kanara, although local newspapers carried stories of outbreaks in the adjoining districts of North Kanara and Shimoga. Local activist groups took credit for having pressured the district and state governments into a sustained cattle spraying program that broke the chain of KFD infection. Activists primarily spoke of community education and the power of the press, and a few had contacted groups in other districts to whom they sent educational materials about KFD.

Of particular interest to me was the current activity of community activists mobilized by KFD in 1984. Several had taken up environmental issues, including social forestry (Save the Ghats campaign), as well as an adult literacy program. These causes kept them in the public view. An important role they had come to serve was to foster a dialogue about the "development of underdevelopment," although not using this term. Apparently, a mistrust of development agencies was an important outcome of KFD. This encouraged a general questioning of expert agricultural advice. For example, one KFD activist challenged advice given to farmers regarding the cultivation of one species of cocoa in lieu of another one that yielded a greater fat content. Another questioned the government's motives in popularizing cashew instead of rubber in Karnataka, but not in neighboring Kerala state. A third became active in questioning the political economic motivations underlying eucalyptus reforestation schemes. My impression was that former members of KFD community action groups had established a public voice that extended beyond the epidemic that first inspired dialogue.

ACKNOWLEDGMENTS

I would like to thank Mimi Nichter for her assistance in collecting field data during the KFD epidemic and Sham Pa Daithota and members of the KFD Relief Committee for their encouragement, provision of data on mortality and morbidity, and many hours of discussion. Thanks also go to Alan Harwood, Peter Claus, and Val Daniel for constructive criticism on a previous draft of this paper. A shorter form of this paper has been published under the title, Kyasanur forest disease: an ethnography of a disease of development, *Medical Anthropology Quarterly* 1 (1987): 406–423.

NOTES

1. KFD has been known to cause disease in both monkeys and people in the Shimoga, North Kanara, Chickmagalur, and South Kanara districts of Karnataka, India. Serological evidence of the activity of a similar virus has been found in Gujarat, Rajasthan, Maharasthra, West Bengal, and Tamil Nadu (Bhat 1984). In Karnataka the disease has spread in five different directions from its original outbreak area. The heaviest incidence of the disease has been in South Kanara.

2. According to the KFD hospital run by Dharmasthala temple, the morbidity and mortality rates for females exceeded that of males in both 1983 and 1984. Doctors attributed higher mortality rates to a lower general nutritional status among women.

In 1983, 158 women, 147 men, and 44 children were treated at the Dharmasthala hospital. Of these, 42 had died, thus yielding a mortality rate of 12 percent. The sex ratio of children treated was nearly equal. In the government hospital almost 480 cases were treated between December 1983 and May 1984, with a mortality rate of approximately 18 percent.

3. There are interregional variations in the Tuluva feudal structure, which are beyond the scope of this paper. The term *kingdom* is also used loosely. Historically, Tulunad's social structure has been composed of feudal relationships between administrative and political estates established around ecological tracts of paddy land. Differences between high-status palaces (*aramane*) and smaller manor houses (*beedu* and *guttu*) are of little relevance to us here. Use of the term *royalty* applies to landlord families around whom an integrated system of agriculture and religious activity revolved.

4. Although there was a decline in village level *bhuta* rituals in the mid-1970s following intensive land reform, there has been a marked rise in ritual performance in the 1980s. Growing prosperity in the region has increased individual contributions for this purpose as a means of increasing individual, caste, and village prestige. In many villages, members of landed families working outside the district have used the sponsorship of *kola* as a means of reestablishing their presence and prestige in their native place. In the Belthangady area, KFD was clearly a factor strengthening village-level *bhuta* worship.

5. Egnor (1982), in a study of Mariamman in Tamilnad, noted that the characteristics of the deity accord with the epidemiological features of smallpox. The deity's affinity for women, particularly pregnant women, corresponds to higher rates of mortality within this group. She also notes that smallpox is a convenient symbol for problems associated with poverty, a fact underscoring the special devotion of the poor to the deity. In response to the question of what has become of Mariamman's power now that smallpox has disappeared, Egnor cites a case in which tuberculosis was associated with the deity.

6. A few Gowda informants tied the fact that KFD ceased during monsoon season to *bhuta* worship. *Bhuta* are not worshiped during the month of *Ati* (July-August), a month considered inauspicious throughout South India, as it marks the sun's movement into the southern hemisphere. While bhuta are worshiped prior to agricultural operations, large *bhuta* rituals such as *kola* and *nema*, are held only after the rains have stopped, in January to late April. The idea expressed by one key informant was that at the time of customary *kola* and *nema*, *bhuta* spirits became most angered if they were not remembered. It was when people were supposed to be most active toward *bhuta* that *bhuta* became most active toward people.

7. Mariamman's chief devotees in Belthangady hail from castes that have migrated to South Kanara from the Deccan Plateau, an area where Mariamman is a more important deity. Among one of these castes, the Gowda, a yearly ritual hunt of wild boar associated with the symbolic control of nature, is performed after worship to Mari.

8. In 1984, the state and central government promised to pay the families of KFD mortality victims Rs 2500 ($250). As of May 1984, no one I interviewed had received any form of relief aid. Aid did not, therefore, provide an incentive to seek hospital care.

9. A trial vaccine was developed for KFD in 1971 by the National Institute of Virology, Pune, and the Haffkine Institute, Bombay. Two doses of this vaccine were found to establish immunity in 59 percent of persons inoculated. Experts believed that three doses would protect 70 percent of the population, if supplies were available (*Blitz* 1984). According to newspaper reports, money was allocated by the Karnataka State Government to produce the vaccine at a Shimoga laboratory. Reports indicate, however, that equipping and staffing the unit were so badly mismanaged that production will be impeded for some time (*Current Magazine* 1985, *Times of Deccan* 1984).

10. Bhuta cult performance and oral tradition articulate the values of both kin-oriented and tributory modes of production. A tributary mode of production is distinguished by the appropriation of goods from non-kin through the overt or subtle exercise of power as well as legitimacy of rule through religious charter. It is beyond the scope of this paper to discuss how kin-based and tributory ideologies have interrelated in Tulunad. Suffice it to say that they are complementary in the sense that both are based upon relations of recripocal exchange which structure an encompassing Tuluva moral universe. These ideologies are challenged by the social relations of a market economy. Capitalist expansion in Tulunad has not necessarily meant the abandon of previous ideologies. Capital is often invested in ritual as a means of obtaining prestige as well as insuring future bounty as per the dictates of the Tuluva moral universe. On the mediation of "regimes of value" (Appadurai 1986) through ritual activities, see Parry and Bloch (1989).

11. Of course, catastrophic illness in the form of KFD has not alone fostered *bhuta* ritual activity. Other factors have played a role. Chief among these is increased wealth flowing into the district from the gulf and rises in wages which supersede rises in commodity prices. This translates into increased disposable income. A means of turning gulf money into social status is the sponsoring of *bhuta* rituals that elsewhere in the district are becoming more "glitzy" and embellished with political speeches. Increased disposable income on the part of small landholders and coolie laborers has contributed to ritual activity in the household as well as attendance at larger possession rituals. The point that I wish to make is that in Belthangady Taluk, KFD has emerged as a visible demonstration of the powers that govern the land. It remains to be seen the manner in which the rich oral tradition will integrate this dramatic episode of Tuluva history.

REFERENCES

Agárwal, A.
    1985   Beyond pretty trees and tigers. *South Asian Anthropologist* 6 (1): 25–40.
Appadurai, Arjun.
    1986   Commodities and the politics of value. In *The Social Life of Things*, ed. Arjun Appadurai. Cambridge: Cambridge University Press.
Babb, Lawrence
    1983   Destiny and responsibility: Karma in popular Hinduism. In *Karma: An Anthropological Inquiry*, ed. Charles Keyes and E. V. Daniel, 163–184. Berkeley, Los Angeles, London: University of California Press.

Banerjee, K., and H. R. Bhat
   1984   Kysanur forest disease. In *Virus Ecology*, ed. K. Banerjee and H. R. Bhat, 123–138. New Delhi: South Asian Publishers.
Beals, Allan
   1976   Strategies of resort to curers in South India. In *Asian Medical Systems*, ed. Charles Leslie, 184–200. Berkeley, Los Angeles, London: University of California Press.
Beck, Brenda
   1969   Color and heat in South Indian ritual. *Man* 4: 553–572.
Bhat, H. R.
   1984   *Public Health and Environment. Karnataka State of Environment Report 1983–84.* Bangalore, India.
Blitz
   1984   Editorial: monkey fever kills one a day. 31 March 1984. Bangalore, Karnataka, India.
Boshell, M. J.
   1969   Kysanur forest disease: ecological considerations. *American Journal of Tropical Medicine and Hygiene* 18 (1): 67–80.
Claus, Peter
   1973   Possession, protection, and punishment as attributes of deities in a South Indian village. *Man in India* 53 (3): 231–242.
   1978*a*   Oral tradition, royal cults and materials for a reconsideration of the caste system in South India. *Journal of Indian Folkloristics* 1 (1): 1–25.
   1978*b*   Heroes and heroines in the conceptual framework of Tulu culture. *Journal of Indian Folkloristics* 1 (2): 28–42.
Current Magazine
   1985   KFD vaccine still a dream. 12 January 1985. Bangalore, Karnataka, India.
Daniel, E. V.
   1983   Karma: the uses of an idea. In *Karma: An Anthropological Inquiry*, ed. Charles Keyes and E. V. Daniel, 287–300. Berkeley, Los Angeles, London: University of California Press.
   1984   *Fluid Signs.* Berkeley, Los Angeles, London: University of California Press.
Daniel, Sheryl
   1983   The tool box approach of the Tamil to the issues of moral responsibility and human destiny. In *Karma: An Anthropological Inquiry*, ed. Charles Keyes and E. V. Daniels, 27–62. Berkeley, Los Angeles, London: University of California Press.
Egnor, Margaret
   1982   The changed mother or what the smallpox goddess did when there was no more smallpox. *Contributions to Asian Studies* 18: 26–45.
Foster, G.
   1976   Disease etiologies in nonwestern medical systems. *American Anthropologist* 78: 773–782.

Glick, M.
  1967   Medicine as an ethnographic category: the Gimi of the New Guinea
          Highlands. *Ethnology* 6: 31–56.
Gramsci, A.
  1971   The intellectuals. In *Selections from the Prison Notebooks*, ed. Q. Hoare and
          G. Smith. London: Lawrence and Wishart Press.
Hughes, Charles, and John Hunter
  1970   Disease and development in Africa. *Social Science and Medicine* 3: 443–493.
Nicholas, Ralph
  1981   The goddess Sitala and epidemic smallpox in Bengal. *Journal of Asian
          Studies* 41 (1): 21–44.
Nichter, Mark
  1977   The Joga and Maya of the Tuluva Buta. *Eastern Anthropologist* 30 (2):
          139–155.
  1979   The language of illness. *Anthropos* 74: 181–201.
  1980   The layperson's perception of medicine as perspective into the utilization
          of multiple therapy systems in the Indian context. *Social Science and Medi-
          cine* 156: 225–233.
  1981   Negotiation of the illness experience: the influence of Ayurvedic therapy
          on the psychosocial dimension of illness. *Culture, Medicine and Psychiatry* 5:
          5–24.
  1983   Paying for what ails you: sociocultural issues influencing the ways and
          means of therapy payment in South India. *Social Science and Medicine* 17
          (14): 957–965.
Obeyesekere, Gananath
  1968   Theodicy, sin and salvation in a sociology of Buddhism. In *Dialectic in
          Practical Religion*, ed. Edmund Leach, 7–40. Cambridge: Cambridge Uni-
          versity Press.
Parry, Jonathan, and Maurice Bloch (eds).
  1989   *Money and the Morality of Exchange*. Cambridge: Cambridge University
          Press.
Pugh, Judy
  1983   Astrological counseling in contemporary India. *Culture, Medicine and
          Psychiatry* 7: 1–21.
  1984   Concepts of person and situation in North Indian counseling: the case of
          astrology. *Contributions to Asian Studies* 18: 85–105.
Sharma, Ursula
  1973   Theodicy and the doctrine of Karma. *Man* 8: 347–364.
Sunday Herald
  1984   Article: death from the forest. 30 December 1984. Bangalore, Karnataka,
          India.
Taussig, M.
  1984   History as sorcery. *Representations* 7: 87–109.
Times of Deccan
  1984   Editorial: monkeying with health. 16 March 1984. Bangalore, Karnata-
          ka, India.

Wadley, Susan
   1980   Sitala: the cool one. *Asian Folklore Studies* 39 (1): 33–62.
Wolf, Eric.
   1981   *Europe and the People Without a History.* Berkeley: University of California Press.
Young, Allan
   1976   Internalizing and externalizing illness. *Social Science and Medicine* 10: 147–156.
   1981   The creation of medical knowledge: some problems in interpretation. *Social Science and Medicine* 15b: 379–386.

.

PART THREE

Islamic Humoral Traditions

In comparison to the emerging bodies of new historically informed research on East and South Asian medical anthropology, studies of Islamic health care appear to be scattered and unrelated. Perhaps this is because the civilization encompasses regional cultures from the Atlantic Coast of Africa to the South Pacific, and is so diverse that only a powerful writer could initiate a dialogue on the medical anthropology of Muslim communities. Nevertheless, a few Indonesian, Indian, and Egyptian social scientists work in this field, along with a larger number of Western ethnologists. Bernard Greenwood, a physician anthropologist, Ann Sweetser, Judy Pugh, and other scholars completed Ph.D. dissertations on health care in Muslim communities at Cambridge University, Harvard, the University of Chicago, and other universities. Outstanding work has been published by Unni Wikan, Soheir Morsy, Beatrix Pfleiderer, and others, including the authors of the two essays in this concluding section of our book.

Perhaps the following essay by Byron and Mary Jo DelVecchio Good will begin the dialogue on Islamic medical ethnology, for they address a central issue: How can a medical cosmology "given classic formulation in ancient Greece seem uniquely suited to map the life world of extraordinarily diverse Muslim societies?" In part, they say, Foucault points the way in analyzing the mode of thought grounded in systems of correspondences, where "to search for meaning is to bring to light a resemblance." But this is only one of five kinds of cultural analysis that they propose, including the analysis of "deep semantic codes that cut across diverse explanatory forms, symbolic oppositions, and illness idioms" that Byron Good (1977) used in his Iranian research. Finally, they suggest that the universality of Islamic humoral thought resides in an episteme that links male-female correspondences to the

monogenetic theory of biological reproduction, and to the honor-shame complex of Mediterranean civilization which also affects other Islamic cultures.

Carol Laderman's essay complements the argument set forth by the
Goods, and elaborates the indigenous Malay humoral thinking that provided
a "welcoming soil" for the Greco-Arabic tradition. While the Goods review a
substantial part of current ethnological research, Laderman's work in
Malaya sets standards for the great amount of ethnography that remains
to be carried out in South Asian Muslim communities, as well as in other
regions of Islamic culture.

REFERENCES

Good, Byron
    1977   The heart of what's the matter: the semantics of illness in Iran. *Culture,
    Medicine and Psychiatry* 1 (1): 25–58.

ELEVEN

The Comparative Study of Greco-Islamic Medicine: The Integration of Medical Knowledge into Local Symbolic Contexts

Byron Good
Mary-Jo DelVecchio Good

INTRODUCTION

Some twenty years ago, Hildred Geertz (1968) wrote of a paradox in the study of *latah*, the Malay term for a behavioral syndrome provoked by startling vulnerable individuals. Despite the appearance of similar phenomena in a variety of Asian societies—from Siberia to the Malayo-Indonesian archipelago—this so-called culture-bound behavioral disorder appears, she argued, to be "tailor-made for Javanese," that is, uniquely suited to express basic Javanese values concerning the person and social life. Despite advances in our understanding of *latah* and claims that the problem has been resolved (Simons 1985), the paradox identified by Geertz remains: a distinctive behavioral syndrome appearing in widely diverse cultures takes on local meanings so compellingly that it appears uniquely suited to articulate important dimensions of each local culture, as though it had sprung naturally from that environment.

Students of Greco-Islamic medicine[1] face a similar but even more complex form of this paradox. Despite the origins of the Islamic medical traditions in classical Greece and in ancient Middle Eastern hermetic and religious traditions, local forms of this tradition often seem particularly apt for expressing distress and managing illness in ways that reveal paradigmatic aspects of reality in societies from urban North Africa to small tribal societies, in Muslim India and Pakistan, and in many other Asian societies. Diseases and symptom complexes, interpreted in language almost identical to that used by the Greeks, become "master illnesses," to use a term from Susan Sontag, and the sources for speculation on central value concerns of these diverse societies. Unique constellations of social stresses, arising from local power arrangements, are "embodied," experienced and communicated as distinctive forms of bodily distress, although the language of experience reflects its Greek origins. Symbolic oppositions such as hot/cold and wet/dry express the character of men and women or human emotions in contemporary Muslim societies, and govern dietary practice and popular thinking about health. Illness narratives, using idioms recognizably Greek in origin, link personal meanings and biography to social values, as they rationalize treatment or negotiate symptoms. Thus, medical traditions given classic formulation in ancient Greece seem uniquely suited to map the life world of extraordinarily diverse Muslim societies.

This paper outlines an approach to the analysis of medical systems which casts light on this paradox. Ecological models that focus on the adaptive aspects of medical systems, and political economy models essential for understanding the organization and distribution of health services, are not much help in studying the integration of learned medical traditions into the life world of specific communities. For this purpose, cultural analysis is required. This perspective considers medical systems to be systems of meanings, symbolic forms used to construct and interpret personal experience and social reality, forms of discourse and medical knowledge used to express, negotiate, and reconstruct illness realities, and thus essential aspects of the systems of practice which constitute social and power relations.

In an important set of papers, Morsy (1978a, 1978b, 1980, 1981) argued that cultural analyses of Middle Eastern medicine treat sickness simply as "psychosocial and physical maladaptation" (1981, 160), concentrating exclusively on the cognitive dimension of medical culture, rather than exploring the links between local power relations and the expression and management of sickness. We agree with this critique of much of the literature; yet Morsy herself fails to attend systematically to the cultural forms that allow such links to be formed. How do Greek medical texts—or even Islamic texts—provide the language for expressing power relations in an Egyptian village or for articulating resistance to structured inequality? How do popular forms of Greco-Islamic medicine achieve authority, the links to power and efficacy that allow practitioners to treat sickness and at the same time to reproduce local power relations? While answers to such questions are implicit in Morsy's work, they are seldom central to her analysis.

In this paper, we will be concerned with symbolic dimensions of Greco-Islamic medicine, the counterpart to Āyurveda and classical Chinese medicine, rather than with sacred medicine, concentrating on ethnographic rather than historical aspects of its integration into local Muslim cultures. We conclude with a discussion of the "cultural authority" (Starr 1982) of Islamic medicine and biology, using this perspective as a vantage to explore their relation to codes of power, sexuality, and the sacred and to consider medical revivalism.

THE SYMBOLIC INTEGRATION OF GRECO-ISLAMIC MEDICINE INTO LOCAL CULTURES

In the following pages, we discuss five aspects of the symbolic organization of Islamic medicine which seem particularly important for analyzing how Greco-Islamic medicine is integrated into local cultures and for comparing forms of medicine in diverse Islamic societies. Examples will be drawn from our work in Iran.

Medical Cosmology and Epistemology

Greek medicine, and later Greco-Islamic medicine, are only comprehensible in relation to classical cosmology and its underlying *episteme*, those assumptions that determine what constitutes knowledge and sources of power and efficacy (compare with Foucault 1970). Although many details of the cosmology of the classic texts are not part of contemporary world view, the classical *episteme* is still important for understanding popular medicine in Islamic societies today. Its presence as an organizing *episteme* is one way that Greco-Islamic medicine is integrated with local cultures.

Islamic cosmology was built up from the Ptolemaic conception of concentric spheres, the Aristotelian understanding of the elements fire, water, earth, and air, and the Plotinian view of the emanations of pure intelligences and souls (B. Good 1977*a*; Nasr 1964, 1968). These ideas were joined in a view of nature as a hierarchy of being that could be analyzed as a series of oppositions and correspondences. Analogical reasoning treated the universe as macrocosm perfectly reflected in the human microcosm. These Greek elements were combined with intense Islamic monotheism, elements of Qur'anic cosmology, mystical practices, pilgrimage and shrine traditions, and with the Middle Eastern Hermetic or wisdom (*hikmat*) tradition. Islamic/Galenic medicine was one of the speculative sciences, along with astrology, numerology, and "the science of the secrets of letters," all of which were grounded in common assumptions about the structure of the universe, the relationship between orders of reality, and an underlying *episteme* based on analogy and sympathy (Foucault 1970). The traditional classics of Islamic medicine, as well as the popularizations of these classics in the textual genre of Medicine of the Prophet, in the practice of folk specialists, and in popular medicine, conceptualized physiology, pathology, and medical care within this framework.

In the classic formulation, the world is divided between the spheres of the planets and intelligences or angels, which have perfect form and movement but neither generation nor decay, and the sublunary world of generation and corruption, in which form and matter are codependent and in continuous transformation. The sublunary world consists of the earth, with its mineral, plant, and animal kingdoms, representing distinctive ontological levels. Qur'anic formulations were integrated with these Greek concepts, so that the seven earths and seven heavens, the Divine Pedestal and Throne, the cosmic mountain *Qaf* and the cosmic tree were elements of sacred history and sacred geography that provided the matrix for "natural history" (Nasr 1968, 108–125).

Humans are unique among sublunary beings. Unlike other beings who represent a single level of the ontological hierarchy, humans are microcosms of the entire universe. They are material beings, constituted, as are other sublunary beings, of a unique compounding of the four simple elements arranged in a form characteristic of the species. But they are also constituted of a soul (*nafs*), or rational faculty, that transcends corporeality and is open to the realm of pure form or intellect. This hierarchy within the person is represented, following Plato and Galen, as three souls or faculties: the vegetative or natural faculty associated with the liver, the animal or vital faculty associated with the heart, and the rational faculty associated with the brain.

Islamic cosmologists and scientists did not divide the universe between the natural and the supernatural realms. It was a unified hierarchy ordered along a gradient "from corporeality to incorporeality, from body to intellect," in the words Tambiah has used to describe the Thai cosmology (1970, 36). The claims to knowledge that now appear to lie on opposite sides of the natural/supernatural divide, the natural sciences and the occult, and which have been grounded in opposing systems of verification, were joined in a single *episteme*. Medicine, astrology, and numerology were grounded in common assumptions about the relationship between orders of reality, the relation of language to nature, and what is required if one is to have certain knowledge of anything. Each level of the cosmic hierarchy was an analogue, so that analogy provided the reasoning that revealed the whole.

In a lucid chapter in *The Order of Things*, Foucault outlined an analysis of the *episteme* of Renaissance learning, a cosmology based in Greek texts and their Islamic interpretations. The relationships among elements in the hierarchical orders were understood in classical epistemology to be of four types: "*Convenientia, aemulatio, analogy*, and *sympathy* tell us how the world must fold in upon itself, duplicate itself, reflect itself, or form a chain with itself so that things can resemble one another" (1970, 25–26). These relationships are grounded in a ternary semiology:

> It is ternary, since it requires the formal domain of marks, the content indicated by them, and the similitudes that link the marks to the things designated by them; but since resemblance is the form of the signs as well as their content, the three distinct elements of this articulation are resolved into a single form. (Foucault 1970, 42)

This view of symbolization determined assumptions about meaning, knowledge, and causal influences. "To search for a meaning is to bring to light a resemblance. To search for the law governing signs is to discover the things that are alike. The grammar of beings is an exegesis of these things" (Foucault 1970, 29).

A similar *episteme* was the basis for the medieval Islamic sciences, including medicine, and remains apparent in contemporary discourse. Ordered sets of correspondences were produced in long lists of structural homologies and elements that resemble or have sympathy for one another. Such correspondences were said to determine an individual's physiological temperament (*tabi'i*) in relation to gender, life cycle, and geography. They revealed the relationships among symptoms or diseases, the sufferer's temperament, and the characteristics of the seasons, and they were used to predict the influences particular foods or medications would have on any particular individual. This *episteme* made comprehensible the conjunction of Greco-Islamic physiology and medicine with astrology and numerology.

In parts of the Islamic world, the classical cosmology and epistemology continue to frame popular physiology and home-based medical care, including interpretations of individual psychological and physiological temperament, seasonal and life cycle changes, and treatments by herbal medicine sellers and sacred healers who use astrology and numerology. Specific elements of Greco-Islamic physiology may be found, for example, in popular understandings of procreation, birth rituals, attempts at birth control, and symptoms associated with contraception (M. Good 1980; Delaney 1986, 1987). They are evident in popular notions of physiological "fluidity" and of "restorative balance" in *baladi* medical culture in Cairo (Early 1988), in elaborate theories of physiology and the pathophysiology of digestion, circulation, and illness in Iran (B. Good 1977*a*), as well as in the somatopsychic discourses on heart and nerves in Iranian culture (B. Good 1977*b*; Good and Good 1982; Pliskin 1987). And they are evident in those Muslim societies, including Iran and Malaysia, in which humoral theories still govern popular dietary rules and prohibitions (see Laderman 1981 and her chapter in this book). However, our argument is not that bits and pieces of traditional Greco-Islamic medicine persist in discrete popular beliefs about sexuality or physiology or popular cures, but that for important segments of the Islamic world, the classical epistemology still provides the conditions for meaningful adherence to seemingly diverse practices and beliefs, and that a reading of medical practices from the perspective of the classical cosmology and *episteme* makes them comprehensible.

Although important for parts of the Islamic world, the classical cosmology and epistemology are far from universally accepted or integrated into local cultures. Tambiah has described how a similar classical cosmology produced a "fantastically ornate" popular cosmology in Thailand (Tambiah 1970, 33). In much of the Middle East the opposite seems to have occurred. The dual universe of God and man, the latter including jinns or spirits, was never replaced by, or fully integrated into, the hierarchy of being of neo-platonic speculation. Therapies derived from the power of sacred words (Coville 1985), the healing power residing in exceptional individuals (for example, Bilu 1988), and the centrality of sacred places, especially the tombs of saints or the Imams (Pfleiderer 1988), maintained a distinctive ontology and episte-mology. It should be noted, because there have often been misconceptions of this matter (for example, Burgel 1976; Gallagher 1983, 8–10), that sacred medicine as a distinctive and competing system was not maintained through the literature on the Medicine of the Prophet (*Tibb ul-Nabbi*). This literature seems to be primarily a set of popular treatises and pamphlets, written throughout Islamic history (into the present) and in many societies, which synthesizes classical Greco-Islamic medicine, popular health culture, and Islamic culture and religion. This popular culture literature presents sim-plified accounts of the classical texts, interspersed with sayings of the Prophet providing advice on such diverse matters as diet, childrearing, dress, and good citizenship. Sections on medical ethics closely linked to the Greek litera-ture on this topic are often included (see, for example, Elgood 1962; Levey 1967; Early 1985a). Sacred medicine, maintained in diverse forms at shrines and by religious folk healers, popular ritual practices, and organized posses-sion cults (see Safa 1988 for a recent account), is not explicated in this litera-ture and was never fully integrated with the Greco-Islamic cosmology, epis-temology, and medical practices.

Symbolic Oppositions and Correspondences
A second form of cultural analysis important for understanding such integra-tion is to examine symbolic oppositions and correspondences and both the breadth and the depth of their elaboration in social practice, cultural forms, and ritual life. Classical Greek and Islamic cultures provided a veritable "generative grammar" of hierarchically ordered sets of oppositions and cor-respondences, linked by a common semiology. The hot/cold moist/dry dis-tinctions provided organizing principles for classifying organs, humors, dis-eases and remedies, personality types, the life cycle, gender differences, the seasons of the year, foods and herbal remedies, and other dimensions of life. Al-Ruhawi provided a classic statement of the relations among these:

> Some people have divided age into four divisions and have said that the com-plexion of each one is similar to the complexion of the mixtures of the body and its parts, and related to the seasons of the year. They have declared that in childhood there is heat and moisture similar to the complexion of blood, air, and the season of spring; in the young there is heat and dryness like the com-plexion of yellow bile, fire and the season of summer; in the mature man's

age, there is coldness and moisture like the nature of phlegm, water, and the season of winter; in the aged, there is coldness and dryness like the nature of black bile, soil and autumn. (Levey 1967, 48)

Physiological processes were viewed within the logic of this system. Metabolism was understood as step-wise transformations of aliments into humors through a process analogous to cooking, utilizing the body's innate heat; substances are increasingly refined, providing vital humors, while the baser sediments are eliminated from the body. A counter process of putrification or rotting, deriving from foreign heat, produces morbid humors (B. Good 1977a).

These oppositions and correspondences have differing levels of elaboration and significance as basic symbolic operators in different communities where the Greco-Islamic tradition exists. In Iran, they seem to be quite extensive but to lack cultural intensity. Males are considered relatively hotter than females, the young relatively hotter than the old. As individuals age, their bodies become increasingly cool; a woman's womb becomes increasingly cool and dry, rendering her infertile. Rituals are said to heat or cool the passions (Good and Good 1988). These oppositions from the Greek tradition are linked to religious distinctions between pure (*pak*) and impure (*najes*). In contemporary popular medicine, foods, herbal remedies, and illnesses are organized in these terms, and this is one means by which the classical humoral tradition is integrated into popular Iranian culture. On the other hand, in contrast with the historically conceptualized Moharram rituals and the symbols associated with them, the symbolic operators from Islamic medicine are lacking in cultural or emotional intensity in Iran.

The literature on medicine in Muslim societies indicates great variation in the extent to which the classical oppositions and correspondences are known and integrated into social practice, and differences in both their extent and the depth of their cultural intensity. For example, popular medicine in Cairo is organized around a fundamental opposition between *baladi* and *afrangi*, literally "neighborhood" and "foreign" (Early 1988). This distinction symbolizes many dimensions of traditional Egyptian lifestyle in the poor neighborhoods in contrast with that among modern residents of cosmopolitan quarters. *Baladi* is authentic and good, essential and natural, while *afrangi* is inauthentic and bad, superficial and unnatural. This opposition corresponds with distinctions in popular medicine: *hilal* (permitted by Islam) causes and cures, grounded in restoration of natural humoral balance, is contrasted with *halal* (forbidden) or foreign causes of illness, such as microbes, and with unnatural and invasive medical therapeutics. Even supernatural causes of illness are divided between *baladi asyad*, or good spirits, including an individual's spiritual double (*qarina*), and *afrangi afarit*, or foreign, evil spirits. Thus, in Cairo, oppositions and correspondences from classical medicine are linked to a set of symbolic markers that represent both extensive and intensive dimensions of social and affective life. Evidence is less clear for most Muslim societies. Laderman's work (for example, 1981) indicates that symbolic oppositions from Greco-Islamic medicine are widely ramified in Malay social life. Delaney's work from Turkey (1987) suggests that even in a society in which humoral reasoning is largely absent from popular medicine, Greco-Islamic physiology rationalizes gender differences as it does in Iran (M. Good 1980), and thus expresses a fundamental structural principle in the society.

Semantic Networks

We have argued elsewhere that a primary means by which Islamic medicine has been integrated symbolically into Iranian culture is through its links to semantic networks, deep semantic codes that cut across diverse explanatory forms, symbolic oppositions, and illness idioms. The heart, conceived in classical Greek and Islamic terms, is a highly polysemous symbol, linked to domains of personal meanings as well as socially organized and value-laden domains of public experience (B. Good 1977b). The heart thus takes on specific constellations of meanings that change as the social and political context changes. As individuals negotiate troubling experiences, Islamic medicine is not only symbolically integrated into Iranian culture; it is also literally "embodied" in somatic experience. Similarly, depression is not only associated with typical physiological symptoms associated with neuroendocrine dysfunction, but it is also clearly associated with highly specific semantic domains grounded in popular Islamic medicine and ethnopsychology (Good, Good, and Moradi 1985). We believe analysis of semantic illness networks provides a primary means of understanding the integration of Islamic medicine into radically diverse cultural contexts.

Clinical Knowledge and Practice

Integration of Islamic medicine into local life worlds was achieved in clinical practice by specialists—hakims, herbal medicine sellers, midwives, traditional orthopedic specialists, astrologers, and others. Unfortunately, the literature on clinical knowledge and specialized forms of clinical practice is unusually weak. This is in part because hakims no longer practice in most Islamic societies, unlike the professionalized specialists of Āyurveda or classical Chinese medicine. However, few studies of the practice of hakims in Pakistan and India have been undertaken. We have much less historical or ethnographic information about the symbolic organization of traditional Islamic medical practice or the structure of clinical knowledge than we have for most of the other great medical traditions, and surprisingly little of the ethnographic research focuses specifically on the clinical knowledge and practice of folk practitioners.

The study of clinical practice and forms of clinical knowledge are especially important since the learned tradition is essentially speculative and theoretical, systematically refined to record universal and comprehensive truths free of internal contradiction. High systems of medicine are developed with an aim to understanding disease and its cure, but it is primarily in clinical practice that knowledge and techniques are developed for applying the system to real phenomena, constructing illness realities, and activating curative powers in particular cases. Traditional Greco-Islamic medical science was based in part on clinical observation and practice, but so great were the rational constraints of the scientific perspective that common sense knowledge—the effectiveness of particular herbs known to the old women or the structure of an organ as observed by butchers—did not make its way into the theoretical system. In addition, it is precisely in clinical practice that negotiations between scientific knowledge and the culturally embedded experience of the client or patient occurs. The clinician is necessarily the hermeneutic specialist, interpreting fragmentary discourse (symptoms and complaints) and seeking contexts for explanation and understanding that provide leverage for treatment. This is a critical area for research on the forms of knowledge and practice that mediate between Greco-Islamic medicine and local social life.

Illness Narratives

Since Islamic medicine is culturally embedded as practical reason and reproduced in illness narratives, analysis of these narratives provides a further key to understanding the integration of Islamic medicine into specific cultural and communicative contexts. Recent research has focused new attention on performative dimensions of medical discourses (Brodie 1988; Kleinman 1988). Studies of the self and of emotion, illness, and healing in the Middle East have begun to attend to discourse and narrative (Good, Good, and Fischer 1988; Anderson and Eickelman 1985). However, the only research to focus specific attention on naturally occurring illness narratives in Islamic societies has been Early's work in *baladi* Cairo (1982, 1985a, 1988). Recording everyday narratives of women concerning illness and care-seeking, Early wrote that such narratives serve two important functions: "They provide a biographical context and experiential reference for perception and diagnosis of illness; second, they facilitate transformation of diagnosis and prognosis" (1982, 1492). In such illness narratives, medical discourse links personal biography to local cultural values, as sufferers and care providers struggle to make illness meaningful, to determine appropriate therapeutic responses, and to justify past actions. Islamic medicine is thus embedded in stories, and such stories provide a medium for interpreting symbolic forms originating in Greece many centuries ago in relation to current forms of suffering and social life.

THE CULTURAL AUTHORITY OF GRECO-ISLAMIC MEDICINE

Paul Starr (1982) has argued that cultural authority for biomedicine was gained through its links to science. Capitalizing on the growing publicity, commercial value, and popular esteem of scientific discoveries in the nineteenth century, physicians achieved a level of autonomy and professional dominance unique among the professions. We have argued that Greco-Islamic medicine was variously integrated into local cultures through several identifiable processes, but we have still to ask how it achieved cultural authority, how it came to be seen as a source of therapeutic efficacy and healing power, and how its practitioners achieved social legitimacy. We will address two aspects of this problem by briefly examining the issues of medical revivalism over the past century and the role of Islamic medicine in reproducing core values and social relations associated with gender in Muslim societies. (We purposely leave aside questions of the physiological efficacy of Greco-Islamic therapeutics and the role of such efficacy in cultural authority.)

When Āyurveda and classical Chinese medicine were disparaged by colonial administrators and allopathic physicians in the nineteenth and early twentieth centuries, sophisticated advocates of these medical systems responded with efforts to reform them and improve their status (Croizier 1968, 1976; Leslie 1973). This medical revivalism is hardly surprising, given the extent to which their cultural authority was diminished by the increasing authority of cosmopolitan medicine. What seems remarkable is that with the exception of colonial India, hakims or other advocates of Greco-Islamic medicine made no sustained efforts to organize professionally to maintain the legitimacy of their practice. For example, Gallagher (1983, 83–101) found that the decree of 1888 that legally curtailed the practice of Islamic medicine in Tunisia was met with little response. Using as justification the need to control epidemics and improve the public health, European medicine was legitimized, and colonial propagandists interpreted the medical transition in the light of imperialist ideology: "Tunisians, like other Muslims, because of religion and culture, were said to be passive or fatalistic in the face of epidemic disease and so stood to gain from guidance by a more enlightened civilization" (Gallagher 1983, 100–101). Similarly, in Iran, although hakims to the Qajar court resisted the growing influence of European physicians and the political and commercial uses of the Quarantine Services to regulate trade through Iran, the passage and gradual enforcement of the licensing law that gave sole right to practice to physicians trained in Western medicine were met with little resistance (B. Good 1981). What does this indicate about the cultural authority of Greco-Islamic medicine in this period? While practitioners of biomedicine sought to enhance their authority through linking medicine to science, and while Āyurvedic and Chinese medical practitioners and advocates sought to counter biomedical authority by joining medicine to powerful nationalist sentiments and political movements, practitioners of Islamic medicine seldom claimed legitimacy from either science or nationalism. Greco-Islamic medicine is literally Tibb Unani, Greek Medicine, not Iranian or Tunisian or even Islamic medicine. For example, in 1943 Ayatollah Khomeini (in *Kashef Asrar*, "Revealing the Secrets") argued that *Tibb Unani* was still superior to European medicine, except for surgery, and blamed Europeans for the lack of trained hakims and for hospitals not treating the poor. However, after he came to power his main attack was on aspects of psychiatry that he believed compete with religion, and he did not call for a revival of Islamic medicine as part of his fundamentalism. Yet, Greco-Islamic medicine, often called *tibb-e qadim* or "old medicine" in the town in which we conducted research, continued to be widely practiced and integrated into popular medical culture.

In addition to a history of governmental legitimation and association with intellectual and political centers, what are the sources of cultural authority of Greco-Islamic medicine in Muslim communities? Although it has some associations with religious conceptions of power, its cultural authority—unlike that of sacred medicine—is not grounded in these concepts. Though rooted in a sacred cosmology, Tibb Unani nevertheless has a distinctively secular cast. Delaney's work from Turkey offers one suggestion about the cultural authorization of Greco-Islamic medicine. She argues that fundamental conceptions of male-female relations and honor and shame refer ultimately to theories of procreation. Men provide the generative seed, women the field within which the seed grows. Men's honor resides in shielding their wives from access to other men, thus ensuring the legitimacy of their children. This cultural model is grounded in Islamic cosmology, biology, and medicine.

> In this cosmological system the material, unregenerate, and eventually perishable aspects of life and women associated with it are devalued in relation to and encompassed by the creativity and spiritual essence of men and God. It is not a relation of opposition and duality, for that would imply separate but potentially equal status; instead, it is a relation of hierarchy, dominance, and encompassment. As the world is dependent on and encompassed by God, so too are women dependent on and encompassed by men (Delaney 1987, 44).

Thus, she argues, the honor/shame complex "is a distinctive system in which power, sex, and the sacred are interrelated and seen to be rooted in the verities of biology. The 'truth' of biology is, in this case, the particular (and peculiar) theory of monogenesis" (Delaney, 45). The biology of monogenesis, which holds that men's seed alone provides the creative source for fathering children, differs from that of Galen, who held that embryos are the joint product of fluid from testis and ovary (see M. Good 1980 for a fuller description). However, the monogenetic theory is widespread in the Islamic world, and is accepted as a part of Greco-Islamic physiology. It seems likely that not only are power, sex, and the sacred rooted in the "verities of biology," but that this biology came to have cultural authority in part because it provided a model that linked power, sex, and the sacred. This sketch of the authorization of Greco-Islamic biology and therefore medicine through its role in reproducing a cultural ideology of gender and power suggests an important direction for future cultural analysis.

ACKNOWLEDGMENTS

Our thanks to Charles Leslie for his careful editing and useful commentary on this paper.

NOTE

1. The term "Greco-Islamic medicine" will be used throughout this paper, alternating at times with "Islamic medicine" or "Tibb Unani." Although any label is problematic, we use this phrase to refer to that cosmopolitan medical tradition that grew out of translation of Greek texts and was elaborated in diverse communities of Islamic civilization. We prefer the term to "Arabic medicine," even though the texts were predominantly written in Arabic, because both literary and popular forms of this tradition flourished in non-Arabic languages (for example, many of the texts were translated originally from Greek into Persian, only secondarily from Persian into Arabic) and in local cultures that were Muslim but not Arabic. "Tibb Unani" or simply "Tibb" were often used by practitioners and intellectuals, and at times were popular designations for this tradition. We have elsewhere used "Galenic-Islamic medicine," but the tradition drew from the wider Greek corpus. "Islamic" in Greco-Islamic refers to Islamic civilization rather than religion. Many of the leading physicians and scholars were Jewish or Christian rather than Muslim, and Greco-Islamic medicine has served Hindus and many other non-Muslim peoples. Nonetheless, the medical tradition is essentially rooted in Islamic civilization.

REFERENCES

Anderson, Jon W., and Dale F. Eickelman, eds.
    1985   Self and society in the Middle East. *Special Issue of Anthropological Quarterly* 58 (4).
Bilu, Yoram
    1988   Rabbi Yaacov Wazana: a Jewish healer in the Atlas Mountains. *Culture, Medicine and Psychiatry* 12: 113–135.
Brodie, Howard
    1988   *Illness Stories*. New Haven: Yale University Press.
Burgel, J. Christoph
    1976   Secular and religious features of medieval Arabic medicine. In *Asian Medical Systems*, ed. Charles Leslie, 44–62. Berkeley, Los Angeles, London: University of California Press.

Coville, Elizabeth
    1985   Healing words in the Malayo-Indonesian Archipelago. Manuscript pre-
            sented at the AAA Annual Meetings, Dec. 4–8, 1985.
Croizier, Ralph C.
    1968   *Traditional Medicine in Modern China: Science, Nationalism, and the Tensions of
            Cultural Change.* Cambridge: Harvard University Press.
    1976   The ideology of medical revivalism in modern China. In *Asian Medical
            Systems,* ed. Charles Leslie, 341–355. Berkeley, Los Angeles, London:
            University of California Press.
Delaney, Carol
    1986   Mortal flow: menstruation in Turkish village society. In *Blood Magic:
            Explorations in the Anthropology of Menstruation,* ed. Thomas Buckley and
            Alma Gottlieb, 83–106. Berkeley, Los Angeles, London: University of
            California Press.
    1987   Seeds of honor, fields of shame. In *Honor and Shame and the Unity of the
            Mediterranean,* ed. David Gilmore. American Anthropological Associa-
            tion, Special Publication 22. Washington: AAA.
Early, Evelyn
    1982   The logic of well-being: therapeutic narratives in Cairo, Egypt. *Social
            Science and Medicine* 16: 1491–1497.
    1985a   Catharsis and creation: the everyday narratives of Baladi women of
            Cairo. *Anthropological Quarterly* 58: 172–181.
    1985b   From prophetic to Islamic literature: the canonized and the kiosk.
            Manuscript presented at AAA Annual Meetings, Dec. 4–8, 1985.
    1988   The Baladi curative system of Cairo, Egypt. *Culture, Medicine and Psychia-
            try* 12: 65–83.
Elgood, Cyril
    1962   Tibb-ul-Nabbi or Medicine of the Prophet: Being a translation of two
            works of the same name. *Osiris* 13: 33–192.
Foucault, Michel
    1970   *The Order of Things.* New York: Vintage Books.
Gallagher, Nancy Elizabeth
    1983   *Medicine and Power in Tunisia 1780–1900.* Cambridge: Cambridge Univer-
            sity Press.
Geertz, Hildred
    1968   Latah in Java: a theoretical paradox. *Indonesia* 5: 93–104.
Good, Byron
    1977a   The heart of what's the matter: the structure of medical discourse in a
            provincial Iranian town. Ph.D. diss., Dept. of Anthropology, University
            of Chicago.
    1977b   The heart of what's the matter: the semantics of illness in Iran. *Culture,
            Medicine and Psychiatry* 1: 25–58.
    1981   The transformation of health care in modern Iranian history. In *Modern
            Iran: The Dialectics of Continuity and Change,* ed. M. Bonine and N. Keddie.
            Albany: SUNY Press.
Good, Byron, and Mary-Jo DelVecchio Good
    1982   Toward a meaning-centered analysis of popular illness categories:
            "Fright Illness" and "Heart Distress" in Iran. In *Cultural Conceptions of*

Mental Health and Therapy, ed. A. J. Marsella and G. M. White, 141–166. Dordrecht, Holland: D. Reidel Publishing Co.

Good, Mary-Jo DelVecchio
1980   Of blood and babies: the relationship of popular Islamic physiology to fertility. *Social Science and Medicine* 14B: 147–156.

Good, Mary-Jo DelVecchio, and Byron J. Good
1988   Ritual, the state, and the transformation of emotional discourse in Iranian society. *Culture, Medicine and Psychiatry* 12: 43–63.

Good, Mary-Jo DelVecchio, Byron J. Good, and Michael M. J. Fischer
1988   Introduction: Discourse and the study of emotion, illness and healing. *Culture, Medicine and Psychiatry* 12: 1–8.

Good, Byron, Mary-Jo DelVecchio Good, and Robert Moradi
1985   The interpretation of Iranian depressive illness and dysphoric affect. In *Culture and Depression*, ed. Arthur Kleinman and Byron Good, 311–368. Berkeley, Los Angeles, London: University of California Press.

Kleinman, Arthur
1988   *The Illness Narratives: Suffering, Healing and the Human Condition*. New York: Basic Books.

Laderman, Carol
1981   Symbolic and empirical reality: a new approach to the analysis of food avoidances. *American Ethnologist* 8: 468–493.

Leslie, Charles
1973   The professionalizing ideology of medical revivalism. In *Entrepreneurship and Modernization of Occupational Cultures in South Asia*, ed. Milton Singer, 216–242. Durham, N.C.: Duke University Press.

Levey, Martin
1967   Medical ethics of medieval Islam, with special reference to Al-Ruhawi's "Practical Ethics of the Physician." *Transactions of the American Philosophical Society*, New Series, vol. 57, pt. 3.

Morsy, Soheir A.
1978a   Sex roles, power and illness in an Egyptian village. *American Ethnologist* 5: 130.
1978b   Sex differences and folk illness in an Egyptian village. In *Women in the Muslim World*, ed. Lois Beck and Nikki Keddie, 599–616. Cambridge: Harvard University Press.
1980   Body concepts and health care: illustrations from an Egyptian village. *Human Organization* 39: 92–96.
1981   Towards a political economy of health: a critical note on the medical anthropology of the Middle East. *Social Science and Medicine* 15B: 159–163.

Nasr, Seyyed Hossein
1964   *An Introduction to Islamic Cosmological Doctrines*. Cambridge: Harvard University Press.
1968   *Science and Civilization in Islam*. New York: New American Library.

Pfleiderer, Beatrix
1988   The semiotics of ritual healing in a North Indian Muslim shrine. *Social Science and Medicine* 27 (5): 417–424.

Pliskin, Karen
  1987   *Silent Boundaries*. New Haven: Yale University Press.
Safa, Kaveh
  1988   Reading Saedi's *Ahl-e Hava*: pattern and significance in spirit possession
           beliefs on the southern coasts of Iran. *Culture, Medicine and Psychiatry* 12:
           85–111.
Simons, Ronald
  1985   Resolution of the Latah paradox. In *The Culture-Bound Syndromes: Folk
           Illnesses of Psychiatric and Anthropological Interest*, ed. R. C. Simons and C. C.
           Hughes. Dordrecht, Holland: D. Reidel Pub. Co.
Starr, Paul
  1982   *The Social Transformation of American Medicine*. New York: Basic Books.
Tambiah, S. J.
  1970   *Buddhism and the Spirit Cults in Northeast Thailand*. Cambridge: Cambridge
           University Press.

TWELVE

A Welcoming Soil: Islamic Humoralism on the Malay Peninsula

Carol Laderman

The bases of medical thought in three of the world's great civilizations, ancient Greece, India, and China, are remarkably similar. All define health as the balance of universal and opposing elements, though each plays its own variation on the broad theme of humoral pathology. The similarities can be explained, in part, by early, continuing, and deliberate cross-fertilization. In the ancient world, Greek and Indian humoral traditions traveled from east to west and back again through Persia (Filliozat 1964). In the centuries following Chinese conversion to Buddhism, Chinese pilgrim-monks traveled to India and returned bearing Indian medical texts in Chinese translation (Huard and Wong 1968).

Malaya, located on the periphery of both the Indian and the Chinese spheres of influence and trade, has exchanged medical and philosophical ideas as well as goods with representatives of both cultures for close to two thousand years. Although we cannot date the first Indian voyages to Malaya with any precision, there is evidence dating from the third century A.D. of a growing ocean-borne trade. Success of this trade depended on the establishment of restapling ports in the Malay archipelago, where Indian merchants could remain during the monsoon season before returning home. Third-century Chinese sources mention a terminus port for Indian shipping, apparently located near the Melaka Straits (Andaya and Andaya 1982). Indian traders were drawn to Malaya in search of gold and silver, aromatic woods, and spices. Their religious concepts, notions of kingship, and the vocabulary of Sanskrit pervaded Malay life and thought, although nothing in legend or history points to a dramatic conversion such as occurred with the adoption of Islam. There appears to have been little in the way of actual colonization, although there is evidence of small coastal and riverine settlements and remains of Buddhist temples dating from A.D. 300–550 in Kedah (Ryan 1965).

Hindu, as well as Buddhist, inscriptions, attributed to the fourth century, have been found in Prai (Province Wellesley) as well as in Kedah.

Few Chinese sources prior to the fifth century mention Southeast Asia, but there is suggestive evidence of earlier contact, such as the fragments of Han Dynasty (206 B.C.–A.D. 221) pottery found in Malaya. From the fifth century on, Chinese trade in luxury items from western Asia, which had previously been carried overland, made increasing use of the sea. Harbors in the Melaka Straits provided shelters for the sailing ships that had to wait for the winds to change before continuing on their voyages or returning home. Although the influence of Chinese thought and culture in Malaya was not as pervasive as that of India, the association of China and Malaya has been long and continuous.

By the fourteenth century, when Greek-Arabic medical theories reached Malaya along with Islam, its inhabitants had had more than a thousand years of exposure to similar Āyurvedic theories, tempered by contact with Chinese medicine. Over the centuries, Islamic humoral theory has been shaped by and integrated into Malay thought. Elaborated humoral ideas of contemporary Malays extend from such mundane matters as food and illness to the workings of the universe and the nature of its inhabitants, both seen and unseen.

Historians have theorized that the establishment of peaceful relationships between traders and natives was aided by an exchange of medical treatments, amulets, herbs, and other curative and preventive ingredients (for example, Ferrand 1919; Coèdes 1968; Winstedt 1935; Golomb 1985). The sharing of *materia medica* and *materia magica* and their practical application is a common feature of culture contact. The transfer of the underlying theories behind treatments is considerably rarer.

It has become increasingly evident in societies throughout the world that people will often accept the treatments a foreign medical system provides while rejecting their theoretical basis. The prestige of a donor culture whose technology is not only more sophisticated than the recipients' own, but whose religion has been accepted as the true faith, is a powerful stimulus to the acceptance of other aspects of the exogenous culture. It is doubtful, however, that foreign ideas will take root and flourish as thoroughly as humoral theories have done among Malays in the absence of a preexisting worldview that could incorporate them without dissonance.

Just as the humoral system brought to the New World by Spaniards found acceptance among Native Americans who believed the universe to be ordered by a balance of opposites, so may such theories have found points of resemblance in pre-Hindu Malayan beliefs about sickness and health, humanity, and the cosmos. Since we lack written records of Malay life and thought in ancient times, we must turn for clues to ethnographic accounts of the Negritos, Senoi, and Proto-Malays, the aboriginal peoples (*Orang Asli*) of the interior of Malaya, who were converted neither to Hinduism nor to Islam.

Concepts of Heat and Cold among Orang Asli

Although they do not employ a humoral classificatory system, a hot-cold opposition is dominant in the cosmological, medical, and social theories of all Orang Asli groups. Whether on the physical or the spiritual plane, the distinction refers to actual temperatures and is not related to either the Chinese or Malay concepts of humoral "heating" or "cooling" properties (Endicott 1979). The heat of the sun and all its earthly reflections are associated with excrement, blood, misfortune, disease, and death (Endicott 1979; Howell 1981; Wazir-Jahan Karim 1981; Roseman 1991). Heat, in fact, is the primary cause of human mortality. The Chewong believe that our world has become hot and unhealthy owing to its burning sun, the heat emanating from the slaughter of animals, and the accumulation of urine and feces. The Original People, who live on another world with a cool sun, have cool white blood and cool eyes. They, unlike us, never sicken or die. The Batek Negrito place their benevolent supernaturals on the moon, but they, too, attribute their immortality to their cool breath, colorless blood, and cool bodies.

The hot blood of humanity makes us mortal, and the need to eat hot bloody animal flesh accelerates the process. Those who take animal life may expose themselves, as well, to *badi*, a hot spiritual force found in all living things, but concentrated especially in human corpses and jungle animals, and released upon death (Mohammad Hood Salleh 1978).

Although humans must eat meat and other foods that have been rendered less wholesome through their exposure to heat by cooking, it is possible to avoid the harmful effects of the sun's heat by depending upon the jungle for one's sustenance rather than venturing out into the open for the long hours necessary to cultivate one's garden. This is the argument most often advanced by Batek Negritos for resisting agriculture, an activity that removes one from the coolness and comfort of the forest and exposes one to the harmful rays of the sun (Endicott 1979).

Coolness is considered to be so vital to health that, should a Negrito or Senoi take ill in a jungle clearing, the entire group will immediately withdraw to the forest. The jungle is not only cool in itself, it is the source of cooling herbs and leaves, used internally and externally to counteract the heat of disease (P. Laird and S. Nagata, personal communication). It is, as well, the only environment in which spells become truly effective.

Disease is most often associated with heat, whether carried by malevolent spirits or resulting from *badi*. Treatments of aboriginal healers are designed to remove the heat and substitute coolness. Skeat and Blagden (1906) cite spells used by Senoi and Aboriginal Malay healers to plead with supernatural forces to "Cool the heat, be cool, be cold," "Let the hot grow cold and frigid," "Give coolness within the body." Like the immortal gods they resemble, healers' bodies are superhumanly cool, and they take steps to retain their coolness by bathing in cold water and sleeping far from the fire. Their eyes are especially cool, enabling them to see the true nature of things, hidden to ordinary people. After removing their patients from the hot clearing to the cool jungle, they blow their cooling breath upon their patients' backs, treat them with cooling medications, call upon beneficent spirits to assist them in magically infusing the sick body with refreshing (sometimes invisible) liquid, which they draw from a bowl placed under hanging leaf ornaments, or from their own breasts, and carry the patient's ailing soul to the sky, where supernaturals bathe it in cooling dew.

Heat and dryness are associated with psychic as well as physical discomfort. The Temiar describe longing for the absent beloved, longing of the living for the dead, and longing of the male healer for his female spirit-guide, as a hot, dry wind. "One hears it in one's ear like wind: 'Yaaw-waaw-waaw.' If we sit, dream, we hear this in our ear; it's uncomfortable. We must have a singing ceremony, it orders us to have a trance-dancing ceremony. Only then are we relieved. Otherwise, after a while, we would go mad. [It] is like a hot, dry wind rustling the leaves when there is no rain; we must hold a ceremony" (Roseman 1984).

Coolness and moisture are associated with everything positive in aboriginal society: self-control, harmony, fertility, health, and life. Heat epitomizes disease, death, destruction, and disorder, not only within the individual person but, metaphorically, within aboriginal society. Not only are the spirits of disease hot, but so is one who causes monthly bleeding in women and punishes incest by hurling a hot lightning bolt at the perpetrators. Proscribed sexual relations themselves are referred to as "hot," as are other threats to society, such as the incompatibility between mother and child attributed to the mother's "hot body," which may destroy the child unless it is removed to another household. Violent emotions, aggressive behavior, and drunkenness, all potentially disruptive to the harmony of aboriginal society, are manifestations of heat and call for cooling remedies (P. Laird, personal communication).

While coolness is much preferred to heat, extreme cold can harm the body. The problem is rare in normal life, except for a woman who has recently given birth. During pregnancy, a Senoi mother-to-be and her midwife should be ceremonially bathed "to make them supernaturally 'cool,' that is, healthy" (Dentan 1965). While in labor, women are aspersed with cold water to keep them cool and healthy and protect them from destructive heat. After a woman has delivered, however, her body is no longer normally cool, but has become very cold and vulnerable. She must avoid decreasing her heat further by refraining from drinking or bathing in cold water. She adds to her heat by tying sashes containing warmed leaves or ashes around her waist, bathing herself and her newborn child in warm water, and lying near a fire source (a practice known as "mother roasting," widespread throughout Southeast Asia, as is the theory of the healer's cooling breath) (for example, Hart, Rajadhon, and Coughlin 1965; Laderman 1981, 1984, 1991; Errington 1983).

These beliefs, which make general statements about heat and cold, set the stage for the acceptance of an exogenous humoral theory that systematically categorized particular diseases, treatments, and foods according to the hot, cold, wet, and dry properties of their components. Indianized Malays had undoubtedly been influenced by Āyurvedic theory before the arrival of the Greek-Arabic medical system, based upon Galen's humoral concepts, which reached the Malay peninsula in the fourteenth century along with Islam and was incorporated into the medicine and cosmology of Islamicized Malays. Islamic humoralism differed from indigenous theories in two important respects: (1) it attempted to deal with illness according to a rational, scientific approach, which located the problem in the natural world and measured degrees of humoral qualities precisely; and (2) the aboriginal emphasis on the danger of heat and value of coolness was reversed.

Medieval Islamic Humoral Theory

According to medieval humoral theory, foods, diseases, medicines, and many other aspects of nature could be scientifically classified according to their inherent qualities of heat, cold, dryness, and moisture. Heat and cold did not refer, necessarily, to thermal qualities; that is, squash hot off the stove was still considered to be extremely cold. Classifications used by Islamic theoreticians were far from the generalized hot and cold notions of the aboriginal Malays. Not only were foods, and so forth, rated as to humoral degrees, but their precise positions were often calculated as well, for example, in terms of "the beginning of the third degree" or "the end of the second." Health handbooks, such as the *Regimen Sanitatis Salernitanum* (Harington 1920) and the *Tacuinum Sanitatis* (Cogliati 1976) (translated into Latin from the work of Ibn Botlan), advised readers as to the effects of foods, their usefulness and dangers, and the means of neutralizing them. For example, cucumbers, which are cold and humid in the third degree, are useful in cooling fevers, but may cause pain in the loins and stomach. They can be neutralized by the addition of honey and oil (both "hot"). Spinach, cold and humid in the second degree, should be fried with "hot" salt and spices to balance its humoral qualities.

Although medieval Islamic humoral theory emphasized the importance of balance for the maintenance of health, the ideal human body was not located on the humoral scale midway between the cold and hot, wet and dry polarities, but was hot and moist in the second degree (McVaugh 1975). (Temperance should lie between the first degree hot and first degree cold.) Heat that is not natural to the body could imperil it by causing putrefaction. Internal heat, however, was not only believed to increase the virility and courage of its possessor, it was considered "the great instrument with which the system . . . destroys hot things which are inimical to life . . . and protects also against injurious cold." Cold "produces only weakness and damage. It is for this reason that heat is called the innate heat while cold is not termed the innate cold" (Shah 1966).

Medieval physicians, such as Avicenna (Krueger 1963), Averroes (Blumberg 1961), Ibn Ridwan (Dols 1984), Ibn Botlan (Cogliati 1976), and Maimonides (1981), advised their patients to live prudent lives, since moderation in all things produced innate heat. Moderate amounts of sleep, a moderate degree of wakefulness, moderate exercise, moderate mental exertion, moderate quantities of food, moderate use of hot baths, moderate indulgence in pleasurable activities, moderation in the expression of emotions—all of these are beneficial to human well-being. Excess of any kind is destructive to health since it disturbs the innate heat. Thus, extremes of atmospheric temperature or topical applications, both hot or cold, are destructive to innate heat, excessive activity disperses it, excessive repose suppresses it, excessive food and drink smothers it, insufficient food depletes it, strong emotions and too much pleasure destroy it—all are productive of cold, the absence of health. (Anger, in fact, was considered to deplete the innate heat by causing it to boil within the heart.) The predominance of heat and moisture ensures long life, since death is nothing more than cold and dryness.

When one considers the negative connotations of cold in medieval Islamic medical theory, it is not surprising to learn that women, the imperfect half of humanity, are naturally colder than men, and moister, since "their greater cold leads to the excessive formation of excrements" (Krueger 1963). Females are deficient in heat from the time of their conception. They are produced from the imperfect semen of their fathers' left testicles and deposited in the left side of their mothers' wombs, both of which are naturally colder than those on the right (Maclean 1980; Maimonides 1970). Women's slower metabolism burns food less efficiently. The residue changes to fat, which is stored to nourish their unborn babies and, later, used in milk production. The female form, broader in the hips and narrower in the shoulders than the male, is due to deficiency of heat, the driving force that sends matter up toward the head. Women's brains, therefore, lack the mental characteristics of heat: courage, liberality, moral strength, and honesty. Their lesser amounts of innate heat make women weaker and more vulnerable to sickness, particularly in their womanly parts and functions. They were advised to avoid sitting on cold stones, staying too long in a cold bath, and drinking cold water, since this would further deplete their innate heat and cause the uterus to ache, or even to slip its moorings (Rowland 1981). A cold, wet womb is a sterile womb, since "just as a wet soil and too much rain [it] will destroy seeds" (Elgood 1970).

The production of male seed was encouraged by the external application of heat, and by a diet which emphasized foods that increase heat and excluded foods that increase cold. Although medieval and Renaissance theoreticians were careful to measure humoral qualities in precise degrees, a layman could arrive at a rough estimation by using this rule of thumb: those foods which taste sweet, salty, bitter, or sharp were heating, as are oils, fats, alcohol, and the flesh of animals, while those foods which are sour, astringent, or tasteless were cooling.

Once the seed was planted, it could still be imperiled by the mother's coldness. Miscarriage and premature labor were usually attributed to a disproportionate measure of cold and damp within the womb. Childbirth further depleted a woman's innate heat, putting her into a colder-than-normal condition for the duration of the postpartum period.

The intensely pleasurable sex act was considered to be fraught with danger for the male. Intercourse depleted his body of hot, moist semen, decreasing his body's strength, and rendering his brain dry (Gorlin 1961). Averroes counseled moderation in sexual activity, explaining that those whose lust is excessive often die young, while Maimonides (1981) warned that only "one in a thousand dies of other diseases, the rest of the thousand of sexual overindulgence." Men were advised to avoid cold water and fruits after intercourse, and to shun old women and women who had recently delivered, since both were extremely cold and would rob the man of his innate heat. The young mother would regain her heat in time, but the old, of both sexes, were permanently cold, a cold that increased with age, ending with death, the total absence of heat. A man who aspired to a long and healthy life, therefore, should locate himself in a warm climate, conduct himself with moderation in all things, avoid cold foods except in hot weather (unless they were balanced by heating ingredients), and marry a young wife.

Many of the precepts of medieval Islamic theory were incorporated into the Malay medical system, and continue to be salient today, but acceptance was selective. Some beliefs have remained essentially unchanged, others have been modified, and still others were never accepted, since they reversed the hot and cold polarities of pre-Islamic, aboriginal cosmology.

Malay Humoralism

Malaya was introduced to Islam and its elaborate post-Galenic humoral traditions during the fourteenth and fifteenth centuries by Indian merchants (and an occasional Persian or Arab trader), who combined proselytization with commerce. Sparsely settled and provincial to all major centers of humoral theory, Malaya received a less than perfect transfer of knowledge through the agency of nonprofessionals and low-level practitioners. This may help to explain why humoral classifications became less precise, why moisture and dryness virtually disappeared as independent qualities (in common with contemporary humoral systems found in similarly provincial areas), and why a neutral category, neither hot nor cold, took on importance.

The universe of contemporary Malays is composed of the four elements of Greek-Arabic doctrine, earth, air, fire, and water (rather than the universal building blocks of China or India). Their humoral concerns are very salient: Within days after arriving at my village in Trengganu, I was warned that eating *durian* fruit in conjunction with hospital-type medicines was dangerous, since their combined heat might prove fatal, and that papaya should be limited to the noon meal, when the body is at its hottest and can withstand the coldness of the fruit.

Although Malays do not attempt to categorize foods according to precise humoral degrees, their rationales concerning their heating or cooling qualities are essentially those of medieval Islamic theory. Both agree that hot foods include alcohol, fats, oils, the flesh of animals, and foods which are salty, bitter, or spicy; while cold foods are sour or astringent. Malays add other criteria to these basic humoral distinctions: juicy fruits and vegetables, plants that exude viscous matter reminiscent of phlegm (the cold humor), or those that need a great deal of moisture to grow, are cold, as are vines and creepers (which cling or are dependent upon larger plants and therefore partake of feminine, and therefore cooler, qualities). Islamic humoral theory differentiated between the active qualities of heat and coolness, and the passive qualities of moisture and dryness, and assigned both active and passive qualities in independent assortment. Thus, sugar was hot and moist, spinach cold and moist, and garlic hot and dry. Contemporary Malays speak only of hot and cold foods, but it is clear from their discussions of humoral characteristics that "passive humors," rather than acting independently, are tied to the "active humors." Moisture is associated with coolness and dryness with heat, whether in terms of the innate qualities of foods and medicines, in connection with physiological processes, such as the cooling properties of sweat, or in relation to the seasons. In Malaysia, the dry season is the hottest time of the year, while the monsoon season is justifiably known as the cold season. According to the Malay view of nature, rain should be associated with cold, and dryness with heat. That is why sunshowers (called *hujan panas*, or literally "hot rain"), because of their anomalous position in nature's scheme, are believed to carry risks to the health of vulnerable people.

Although the daily diet of contemporary Malays differs from that of medieval Arabs or Europeans in the species of foods available, where foods overlap there is a surprising amount of agreement as to their humoral qualities. For example, all would agree that cucumbers, squash, and spinach are very cold, that meats and egg yolks are quite hot, and that, while sugar and honey both are heating, honey is hotter. Like the medieval theoreticians, Malays believe that humoral qualities of foods can be neutralized by eating them in conjunction with ingredients of opposite qualities, but that intensely cold foods, such as squash, should be eaten only during the hottest months.

Humoral concerns become most pressing during illnesses and other times of physical vulnerability. Most diseases are attributed to natural causes, and their treatments, in the main, follow rationally along an Islamic humoral model. These include dietary changes, ingestion and topical application of medicines (most of which are classified humorally), massage (believed to break up the lumps of cold phlegm that cause muscular pain, and allow the hot blood to flow properly), and thermal treatments, such as steam inhalation and cold compresses.

Diseases are classified by the following criteria, which interpret empirical evidence in the light of humoral reasoning:

1. External heat: those illnesses, such as fever or boils, that are hot to the touch.
2. Internal heat: illnesses that make the patient experience hot or burning sensations, such as sore throat or heartburn.
3. Visible signs: hemorrhages are evidence that the hot element has boiled over; clotted phlegm indicates that the cold element has become still colder.
4. Deficiency or excess of a humor deduced from internal evidence: Anemia is cold since its sufferers lack blood; vertigo and hypertension are hot since an excess of blood is presumed to have gone to the head (considered by Malays to be normally hotter than the rest of the body), thereby overheating it.
5. Pulse reading: A fast pulse denotes heat, since its speed is owing to the rate at which blood travels through the veins; a slow pulse is a sign that inner cold has thickened the blood and made it sluggish.
6. Behavioral considerations: Some forms of madness are thought to occur as a result of the brain overheating, causing violent and angry behavior. Such behavior is called *panas* (literally, hot). Madness can result from too much thought (such as excessive amounts of studying), or violent emotions. Prescribing hot medicines for hot conditions can also lead to madness when their combined heat reaches the brain.
7. Response to treatments: If illnesses respond to treatments already classified as hot or cold, this indicates that these illnesses have the opposite humoral quality, that is, asthma is cold since it responds to steam inhalation; heatstroke is hot since it responds to cold water.
8. In reference to age: Malays follow medieval Islamic medical theory in attributing a greater degree of cold to the aged. Since rheumatism is most often found in old people, it is classified as cold.

Malays are so convinced of the empirical reality of humoral qualities that, when I sent off food samples to the Institute for Medical Research for nutrient testing, my neighbors were sure that the Institute would also test for inherent heat and cold.

The great majority of illnesses are attributed by Malays to natural causes, and treatments follow along a humoral model. Illnesses that do not respond to these treatments, or which otherwise deviate from the normal course, are often blamed on incursions from the unseen world and must be treated by means other than dietary changes and pharmaceuticals. Etiology and treatment, although they do not locate the problem in the natural world and would not qualify as either scientific or rational by Galenic standards, are congruent with a humoral model employing the Greek-Arabic concept of a four-fold universe. The spirits, lacking the earthy and watery components of fleshly bodies, consist only of superheated air. By blowing on their victim's back, they upset his humoral balance. Treatment involves increasing the cool and moist elements and ridding the body of excess heat and air. Healers employ "neutralizing rice paste," recite spells, blowing their magically cooled breath on their patients, and bathe them in cooling water.

Divinations employed to discover the cause of these illnesses also follow a humoral model. One method uses rice popped by dry heat. The shaman places handfuls of this rice on a pillow and counts out the grains in pairs, two each for earth, air, fire, and water. If the count ends on earth, it might point to a cold illness, or one caused by the earth spirits. If it falls on fire, it might signify that the patient has incurred someone's hot wrath, whether human or spirit, or it might simply mean that the condition was hot. Another method consists of reading the flame of a beeswax candle. No other type of candle can be substituted. The bee partakes of the spirits' unholy heat. Found in the jungle, beyond human control (at least on the east coast of Malaysia), and commanding a remarkably hot sting, bees are called friends of the spirits (Laderman 1991).

Malay incantations invariably include Koranic sentences and other appeals to Allah, his Prophet, and his saints. Although Malays have reinterpreted their beliefs about the spirits, using stories about the angel Gabriel, the Light of Mohammad, and other Islamic references (Laderman 1984, 1991), their treatments for extranormal problems are fundamentally the same as those of non-Islamic Orang Asli.

The Malay belief in the dangers of *badi*, that hot, impersonal, destructive spiritual force that emanates from the corpses of jungle animals and human beings, which also parallels beliefs of the Orang Asli, makes no appeal to Islam for the authentication of its power. Badi holds particular danger for the unborn, working indirectly through their parents. To avoid its risks, prospective fathers are advised to forgo hunting for the duration of their wives' pregnancies, and mothers-to-be are warned against visits of condolence to homes of yet-unburied dead (Laderman 1984).

Malays locate the normal, healthy male body in the very center of the hot-cold continuum, rather than toward the hot polarity preferred by Islamic humoral doctrine. Some believe that women are slightly colder than men, owing to their monthly loss of blood, the hot body humor, however this is not considered an important distinction, nor is it elaborated upon as it was in medieval Islamic theory. It is important to stay near the humoral center, and nature assists one by encouraging the outpouring of cooling sweat during the hot dry season. Freely flowing sweat in the presence of heat is considered essential to the maintenance of health. This concept disagrees with medieval Islamic theory: Maimonides (1970) maintained that "sweat is an abnormal occurrence because the body is such that if a man conducts himself properly and eats natural foods and digests them properly, [a healthy man] will not sweat excessively."

In common with all adherents to humoral theory, and in common as well with Orang Asli, Malays believe that childbirth precipitates a woman into an abnormally cold state, which they attempt to redress by means of dietary changes that follow a humoral pattern, and by treatments, such as "mother-roasting," bathing with warm water, and tying protective sashes about their waists, that can be interpreted humorally but are also the counterparts of Orang Asli postpartum procedures.

Conclusions

Although Islam was successfully implanted in Malaya, and Islamic concepts are used by Malays to interpret and reinterpret empirical realities, the pre-Islamic aboriginal view of the workings of the cosmos, and the positive valence of coolness in the universe and its human microcosm, still fundamental to Malay thought, have radically altered the received theories of Islamic humoralism.

Moderation in all aspects of life is seen as a positive good by contemporary Malays and Orang Asli, as it was by medieval theoreticians. Overeating to the point of obesity is derided by Malays, and drunkenness or drug use puts one beyond the pale. Malays rarely exhibit strong emotions in public; neither great joy at a wedding or birth, nor grief at a funeral. Most Malays, in fact, deny that they have ever experienced such feelings. Although they would agree with Avicenna et al. (see Blumberg 1961; Dols 1984; Elgood 1970; Gorlin 1961; Krueger 1963; Shah 1966) about the benefits to one's health accrued by following the middle road, the humoral associations of Malays with such behavior are the polar opposites of those of medieval Islam.

While Greek-Arabic medical theory stresses the importance of the "innate heat," Malays associate coolness with self-control and health, and heat with vulnerability to illness. Violent emotions, like anger and passionate love, are hot and dangerous and can lead to an overheated brain and madness. A person quick to anger is known as *"panas hati"* (literally, "hot-livered"); the heat rises from the liver, the center of emotions which is ordinarily cool, to the head, which is ordinarily warm. Malays believe that the head is normally hotter than the rest of the body, and try to avoid heating it further. That is why newborn babies, who are in other respects cold compared to adults, are washed in warm water, except for their heads, which are subjected to cold water. This is in direct contradiction to the advice of medieval Islamic physicians who recommended that "the whole body should be washed, but water used on the head may be very hot" and never cold or lukewarm, since the head was considered to be the source of phlegm, the cold humor (Maimonides 1981).

All other humoral systems associate sterility with cold wombs, conception with coital heat, and pregnancy with either an intensely heated condition for the mother, or one which begins with a hot mother who is gradually polarized toward the cold direction due to loss of her own blood, used in her baby's development (Fabrega 1974; Thakkur 1965; Pillsbury 1982). Malays, on the contrary, believe conception cannot take place unless both parents' bodies are in a cool state, an event that occurs once a month on "the day the seeds fall." The mother's body must continue to be cool throughout her pregnancy to safeguard the developing child, at first a lump of blood which may be liquefied by heat, and later, a creature in danger of being driven from the womb prematurely by heat. Prospective mothers must guard their unborn children against fevers and "hot" medicines, while women who find themselves inconveniently pregnant do their utmost to destroy the fetus by making their wombs uncomfortably hot, using "hot" medicines and heating massage (Laderman 1984).

The Malay identification of heat with destruction and coolness with life and health is reflected in their daily language. *Sejuk* (literally, coolness) can be used as a synonym for "healthful, energetic, and pleasant." *Menyejukkan* (to make cool) can mean "to calm, to revive, to repair, to amuse." A person whose liver is cool (*hati sejuk*) is tranquil and carefree. In contrast, *panas* (heat) can be used as a synonym for unlucky, ominous, disastrous. Those with *panas rezeki* (hot livelihood) are poor unfortunates. A generally ill-tempered person is described as a "glowing ember" (*panas bara*); a person quick to anger has a "hot liver" or "hot blood" (*panas hati, panas darah*). *Memanaskan hati* (to cause the liver to become hot) means to instill hatred in one's breast. That is why black magic is called *ilmu panas* (the hot science), predicated as it is on carrying out its mission of hatred (Awang and Khan 1977; Iskandar 1970; Wilkinson 1959).

Malay preference for coolness and anxiety about heat extends beyond individual health concerns to concern for the health of the body politic. A successful sultan embodies the coolness that balances the destructive heat of nature, men's emotions, and the spirit world. The highest praise a ruler can receive is that his reign was cold (*perentah-nya sejuk*). An ordinary Malay, while limited in his powers, can still help to keep universal balance toward the cold polarity by reciting "the blessed cooling prayers" of Islamic obligation (Zainal-Abidin 1947).

Aboriginal peoples of Malaya have many ideas concerning the effects of foods in health and disease. Some of these are related to heat, although not in its humoral sense. There was nothing to prevent the acceptance of a system that accorded humoral qualities to foods and much to encourage it in specific aboriginal food beliefs as well as in the basic hot/cold opposition dominant in aboriginal cosmology. Many of the criteria for assigning foods to the hot category employed by adherents of humoral systems may have already existed as characteristics of hot foods in Negrito and Senoi nonhumoral belief systems before contact. Both Negritos and Senoi agree that animal flesh is hot, owing to its blood, and some Senoi also add salt, chilies, and sugar to their "hot" category, all of which are also humorally hot according to medieval Islamic and contemporary Malay theory. The Semelai, a group of aboriginal Malays, also believe that some foods may become hot as a result of the inherence of the hot destructive force of badi.

Malaya proved a remarkably receptive soil for Islamic religion and medical theories. Their humoral theory provided Islamicized Malays with a new grammar with which to organize ideas about humanity and the universe. Medieval Greek-Arabic humoral theories concerning foods, medicines, and diseases whose etiology stems from the natural world appear in simplified but otherwise virtually unchanged form in contemporary rural Malaysia. Malay attributions of heat or cold to particular foods, and the reasons behind these attributions, would be very familiar and acceptable to their medieval Arab and European counterparts. Their conceptions of the values and dangers of heat and cold in the universe and within the human body, however, would not.

The aboriginal peoples of Malaya found nothing discordant in Islamic humoral dietary beliefs. Their ideas concerning the workings of the human body and the relations between the unseen world and the earthly life of mortals, however, were in direct opposition to the tenets of Greek-Arabic medical theory, both in their reversal of the hot and cold polarities, and in their inclusion of "nonrational" etiologies.

Although contemporary Malays are wary of the jungle, fearing its wild inhabitants, both visible and invisible, the positive value that Orang Asli have always given to coolness and moisture, strongly associated with the rain forest, has remained an integral part of Malay cosmology. This positive evaluation of the cool polarity, although contrary to Islamic humoral doctrine, has its counterpart in aspects of Islamic religious doctrine, which, curiously, reinforced aboriginal Malay ideas about heat and cold in the universal macrocosm and within the human body's microcosm.

The Islamic conception of the afterlife stresses the pleasure of coolness and moisture and the destructiveness of heat. Paradise is a garden watered by running streams in a cool shade where the righteous drink from a refreshing spring. "In paradise there are a great river of water, a great river of honey, a great river of milk, and a great river of wine" (Koran 1956). There the righteous will feel "the north wind blow and scatter fragrance on their faces and their clothing" (Mishkat Al-Masabih 1965). The home of the unrighteous will be a scorching fire, a Destroying Flame, a place where garments of fire are prepared for unbelievers. Further reinforcement of the dangers of spiritual heat come from the Islamic belief that the jinn were created from fire.

Orang Asli who have considered the possibility of an afterlife conceive of it as a cool place of fruit trees, where the dead remain (Schebesta 1957), or where only the worthiest stay, the rest being reborn. Most, however, are extremely skeptical about the likelihood of any life after death (Dentan 1964). Their beliefs are strongly centered on life, and on the daily interactions between mortals and spirits. Neither they nor contemporary rural Malays recognize a clear division between the "natural" world and the "supernatural." Malays do not speak of naturally caused illnesses, in contrast to those caused by supernatural means. The terms employed are *biasa* (usual) and *luar biasa* (unusual), referring to the greater frequency of illnesses having no spiritual etiology.

Operating alongside the Malay model of disease causation based on the Greek-Arabic system that locates medical problems in the sensory world is a theory that certain illnesses are caused by disembodied hot spirits. Treatments for these illnesses and beliefs concerning their etiology closely parallel those of Orang Asli, although Malays have reinterpreted these ideas and practices using an Islamic and/or humoral idiom. Their ideals of coolness as attributes of beneficent spiritual powers and important components of treatments for illnesses caused by maleficent spiritual powers are echoed in their belief that coolness is necessary for the creation and development of the spirit made flesh in conception and pregnancy. In accepting the doctrine of humors, Malays have kept its "rational" superstructure, as well as individual categories, but have retained a vision of the universe (mankind writ large), and of humanity (the cosmos in miniature), that is its mirror image. Because they were able to identify the aboriginal belief in the coolness of the Immortals and their world with the coolness of the Islamic Paradise, and because they continued to believe in a participatory relationship between the human microcosm and celestial ideal, the Malays succeeded in detaching the grammar of the Islamic humoral system from its emphasis on the ideal of innate heat.

The seeds of Islamic thought, transplanted on the peninsula, have proliferated to every corner of Malay life. Seeds sown in a foreign soil, however nourishing, often throw up sports, hybrids, and new combinations of familiar characteristics, and such was the case with humoralism among the Malays.

ACKNOWLEDGMENTS

Research for this article was supported by the Social Science Research Council, the Danforth Foundation, National Institute of Mental Health Training Grant 5 F31 MH05 352-03, and by the University of California International Center for Medical Research through research grant AI 100541 to the Department of Epidemiology and International Health, University of California, San Francisco, from the National Institute of Allergy and Infectious Diseases, National Institutes of Health, U.S. Public Health Services. It was done under the auspices of the Institute for Medical Research of the Malaysian Ministry of Health.

I would particularly like to thank my husband, Gabriel Laderman, for his invaluable suggestions.

REFERENCES

Andaya, B. W., and L. Andaya
    1982   *A History of Malaysia.* London: The MacMillan Press Ltd.
Awang Sudjai Hairul, and Yusoff Khan
    1977   *Kamus Lengkap.* Petaling Jaya: Pustaka Zaman.
Blumberg, H.
    1961   *Averroes' Epitome of Parva Naturalis.* Cambridge, Mass.: The Mediaeval Academy of America.
Coèdes, G.
    1968   *The Indianized States of Southeast Asia.* Honolulu: East-West Center.
Cogliati, Arano L.
    1976   *The Medieval Health Handbook (Tacuinum Sanitatis).* New York: George Braziller.
Dentan, R. K.
    1964   Senoi. In *Ethnic Groups of Mainland Southeast Asia*, ed. F. K. Lebar, G. C. Hickey, and J. K. Musgrove. New Haven: HRAF Press.
    1965   Some senoi semai dietary restrictions: a study of food behavior in a Malayan Hill Tribe, Ph.D. diss. Dept. of Anthropology, Yale University, 1965.
Dols, M. W.
    1984   *Medieval Islamic Medicine.* Berkeley, Los Angeles, London: University of California Press.
Elgood, C.
    1970   *Safavid Medical Practice.* London: Luzac and Co., Ltd.
Endicott, K.
    1979   *Batek Negrito Religion.* Oxford: Clarendon Press.

Errington, S.
  1983   Embodied Sumange' in Luwu. *Journal Asian Studies* 42: 545.
Fabrega, H., Jr.
  1974   *Disease and Social Behavior: An Interdisciplinary Perspective.* Cambridge: MIT Press.
Ferrand, G.
  1919   Le K'Ouen-Louen et les anciennes navigations interoceaniques dans le Mers du Sud. *Journal Asiatique* Eleventh Series, July–August.
Filliozat, J.
  1964   *The Classical Doctrine of Indian Medicine: Its Origins and Its Greek Parallels.* Delhi: Munshiram Manoharlal.
Golomb, Louis
  1985   *An Anthropology of Curing in Multiethnic Thailand.* Illinois Studies in Anthropology no. 15. Urbana and Chicago: University of Illinois Press.
Gorlin, E., ed.
  1961   *Maimonides "On Sexual Intercourse."* Brooklyn: Rambash Publishing Co.
Harington, Sir J.
  1920   *The School of Salernum: Regimen Sanitatis Salernitanum.* New York: P. B. Hoeber.
Hart, D. V., P. A. Rajadhon, and R. Coughlin
  1965   *Southeast Asian Birth Customs: Three Studies in Human Reproduction.* New Haven: HRAF Press.
Howell, S.
  1981   *Society and Cosmos: Chewong of Peninsular Malaysia.* Singapore: Oxford University Press.
Huard, P., and M. Wong
  1968   *Chinese Medicine.* London: World University Library.
Iskandar, T.
  1970   *Kamus Dewan.* Kuala Lumpur: Dewan Pustaka dan Bahasa.
Koran
  1956   Trans. N. J. Dawood. Harmondsworth: Penguin Books.
Krueger, H. C.
  1963   *Avicenna's Poem on Medicine.* Springfield, IL: Charles C. Thomas.
Laderman, C.
  1981   Symbolic and empirical reality: a new approach to the analysis of food avoidances. *American Ethnologist* 8: 468.
  1984   *Wives and Midwives: Childbirth and Nutrition in Rural Malaysia.* Berkeley, Los Angeles, London: University of California Press.
  1991   *Taming the Wind of Desire: Psychology, Medicine, and Aesthetics in Malay Shamanistic Performance.* Berkeley, Los Angeles, Oxford: University of California Press.
Maclean, I.
  1980   *The Renaissance Notion of Woman.* London: Cambridge University Press.
Maimonides
  1970   *Medical Aphorisms,* ed. and trans. F. Rosner and S. Munter. New York: Yeshiva University Press.

1981   *The Book of Knowledge*, trans. H. M. Russell and Rabbi J. Weinberg. Edinburgh: Royal College of Physicians.

McVaugh, M.
1975   Discussion of medicinal degrees at Montpellier by Henry of Winchester. *Bulletin of the History of Medicine* 9: 57.

Mishkat Al-Masabih.
1965   Trans. J. Robson. Lahore: Sh. Muhammad Ashraf.

Mohammad Hood Salleh
1978   Semelai rituals of curing, Ph.D. diss. St. Catherine's College, Oxford University.

Pillsbury, B. L. K.
1982   Doing the month: confinement and convalesence of Chinese women after childbirth. In *Anthropology of Human Birth*, ed. M. A. Kay. Philadelphia: F. A. Davis Co.

Roseman, M.
1984   The social structuring of sound: The Temiar example. *Ethnomusicology* 28: 411.
1991   *Healing Sounds from the Malaysian Rainforest: Temiar Music and Medicine*. Berkeley, Los Angeles, Oxford: University of California Press.

Rowland, B.
1981   *The Medieval Woman's Guide to Health*. Kent, Ohio: Kent State University Press.

Ryan, N. J.
1965   *The Making of Modern Malaya: A History from Earliest Times to Independence*, 2d ed. Kuala Lumpur: Oxford University Press.

Schebesta, P.
1957   Die Negrito Asiens. *Studia Instituti Anthropos* 13: 11.

Shah, M. H.
1966   *The General Principles of Avicenna's Canon of Medicine*. Karachi: Naveed Clinic.

Skeat, W. W., and C. O. Blagden
1906   *Pagan Races of the Malay Peninsula*. 2 vols. London: Macmillan and Co., Ltd.

Thakkur, C. G.
1965   *Introduction to Ayurveda*. Bombay: The Times of India Press.

Wazir-Jahan Karim
1981   *Ma'Betisek Concepts of Living Things*. New Jersey: The Athlone Press.

Wilkinson, R. J.
1959   *A Malay-English Dictionary*. London: Macmillan.

Winstedt, R. O.
1935   *A History of Malaya*, vol. 13, pt. 1. *Journal of the Royal Asiatic Society, Malay Branch*.

Zainal-Abidin bin Ahmad
1947   The various significations of the Malay word *sejok*. *Journal of the Royal Asiatic Society, Malay Branch* 20 (2): 41.

CONTRIBUTORS

Judith B. Farquhar is Associate Professor of Anthropology at the University of North Carolina, Chapel Hill.

Byron J. Good is Associate Professor of Medical Anthropology in the Department of Social Medicine and Health Policy, Harvard Medical School, and Editor-in-Chief of *Culture, Medicine and Psychiatry*.

Mary-Jo DelVecchio Good is Associate Professor of Medical Sociology in the Department of Social Medicine and Health Policy, Harvard Medical School, and Associate Editor of *Culture, Medicine and Psychiatry*.

Shigehisa Kuriyama is Assistant Professor of the History of Science in the Institute of the Liberal Arts at Emory University, Atlanta.

Carol Laderman is Professor and Chair of the Department of Anthropology at City College of the City University of New York.

Charles Leslie is Emeritus Professor of Anthropology in the Center for Science and Culture at the University of Delaware, Newark.

Margaret Lock is Professor of Anthropology in the Department of the Humanities and Social Studies in Medicine and the Department of Anthropology, McGill University, Montreal.

Mark A. Nichter is Associate Professor in the Department of Anthropology and the Department of Family and Community Medicine, University of Arizona, Tucson.

Gananath Obeyesekere is Professor of Anthropology at Princeton University, Princeton, New Jersey.

Gary Seaman is Associate Professor of Anthropology at the University of Southern California, Los Angeles.

Margaret Trawick is Professor and Chair, Department of Social Anthropology, Massey University, New Zealand.

Paul U. Unschuld is Professor and Director of the Institute for the History of Medicine, Munich University, Munich.

Allan Young is Professor of Anthropology in the Department of the Humanities and Social Studies in Medicine and the Department of Anthropology, McGill University, Montreal.

Francis Zimmermann is a Director of Studies in South Asian Anthropology and the History of Science, School of Advanced Studies in the Social Sciences, Paris.

INDEX

Designer: U.C. Press Staff
Compositor: Asco Trade Typesetting Ltd.
Text: 10/12 Baskerville
Display: Baskerville
Printer: Maple-Vail Book Manufacturing Group
Binder: Maple-Vail Book Manufacturing Group